617.413
EAR

WG 630
EAP

MFT Library Services

D1486138

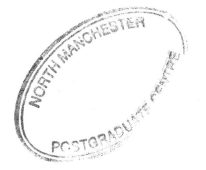

JACK TAYLOR LIBRARY
ROCHDALE EDUCATION CENTRE
ROCHDALE INFIRMARY
ROCHDALE OL12 0NB

ary **Services**

WITHDRAWN FROM STOCK

The Evidence for Vascular Surgery

Edited by Jonothan J Earnshaw & John A Murie

A Joint Vascular Research Group book

Second Edition

tfm Publishing Limited
Castle Hill Barns
Harley
Shrewsbury
SY5 6LX
UK

Tel: +44 (0)1952 510061
Fax: +44 (0)1952 510192
E-mail: nikki@tfmpublishing.com
Web site: www.tfmpublishing.com

Design & Typesetting: Nikki Bramhill BSc (Hons) Dip Law Solicitor

Cover photographs courtesy of:
Top right: Mr Mike Gough, The General Infirmary at Leeds
Top left: Mr John Wolfe, St. Mary's Vascular Unit and Mohamad Hamady, Consultant Interventional Radiologist, St. Mary's Hospital.
Bottom left and right: Mr Jonothan Earnshaw, Gloucestershire Royal Hospital

First Edition   © 2007

ISBN 10: 1 903378 45 1
ISBN 13: 978 1 903378 45 8

The entire contents of *The Evidence for Vascular Surgery* is copyright tfm Publishing Ltd. Apart from any fair dealing for the purposes of research or private study, or criticism or review, as permitted under the Copyright, Designs and Patents Act 1988, this publication may not be reproduced, stored in a retrieval system or transmitted in any form or by any means, electronic, digital, mechanical, photocopying, recording or otherwise, without the prior written permission of the publisher.

Neither the authors, the editors nor the publisher can accept responsibility for any injury or damage to persons or property occasioned through the implementation of any ideas or use of any product described herein. Neither can they accept any responsibility for errors, omissions or misrepresentations, howsoever caused.

Whilst every care is taken by the authors, the editors and the publisher to ensure that all information and data in this book are as accurate as possible at the time of going to press, it is recommended that readers seek independent verification of advice on drug or other product usage, surgical techniques and clinical processes prior to their use.

The authors, editors and publisher gratefully acknowledge the permission granted to reproduce the copyright material where applicable in this book. Every effort has been made to trace copyright holders and to obtain their permission for the use of copyright material. The publisher apologizes for any errors or omissions and would be grateful if notified of any corrections that should be incorporated in future reprints or editions of this book.

Printed by Gutenberg Press Ltd., Gudja Road, Tarxien, PLA 19, Malta.

Tel: +356 21897037; Fax: +356 21800069.

Contents

Contributors

Jonathan D Beard FRCS ChM Consultant Vascular Surgeon, Sheffield Vascular Institute, Northern General Hospital, Sheffield, UK

Andrew W Bradbury BSc MB ChB MD MBA FRCSEd Professor of Vascular Surgery, Birmingham University Department of Vascular Surgery, Heart of England NHS Trust, Birmingham, UK

Marcus J Brooks FRCS MA MD Specialist Registrar, Regional Vascular Unit, St. Mary's Hospital, London, UK

Bruce Campbell MS FRCP FRCS Consultant Surgeon and Professor, Royal Devon and Exeter Hospital and Peninsula Medical School, Exeter, UK

Tom Carrell MA MChir FRCS Consultant Vascular Surgeon, Department of General and Vascular Surgery, Guy's and St. Thomas' Hospitals NHS Foundation Trust, London, UK

Gillian Cockerill PhD Senior Lecturer in Vascular Biology, St. George's Vascular Institute, London, UK

Andrew R Cowan FRCS Consultant Surgeon, Exeter Vascular Service, Royal Devon and Exeter Hospitals, Exeter, UK and Peninsula Medical School, Exeter, UK

Simon G Darke MS FRCS Consultant Surgeon, Royal Bournemouth Hospital, Bournemouth, UK

Katy AL Darvall MB ChB MRCS Research Fellow, Birmingham University Department of Vascular Surgery, Heart of England NHS Trust, Birmingham, UK

Neil Davies MB BS FRCS FRCR Consultant Radiologist, Department of Radiology, Royal Free Hospital, London, UK

Jonathan J Earnshaw DM FRCS Consultant Vascular Surgeon, Gloucestershire Royal Hospital, Gloucester, UK

Robert K Fisher MD FRCS Vascular Specialist Registrar, Regional Vascular Unit, Royal Liverpool University Hospital, Liverpool, UK

Robert B Galland MD FRCS Consultant Surgeon, Department of Vascular Surgery, Royal Berkshire Hospital, Reading, UK

Christopher P Gibbons MA DPhil MCh FRCS Consultant Vascular Surgeon, Morriston Hospital, Swansea, UK

Geoffrey Gilling-Smith MS FRCS Consultant Vascular Surgeon, Royal Liverpool University Hospital, Liverpool, UK

Antony Goode MB BS BSc MRCP FRCR Consultant Radiologist, Department of Radiology, Royal Free Hospital, London, UK

Michael J Gough MB ChB ChM FRCS Consultant Vascular Surgeon, Leeds Vascular Institute, The General Infirmary at Leeds, Leeds, UK

George Hamilton FRCS Professor of Vascular Surgery, Vascular Unit, University Department of Surgery, Royal Free Hampstead NHS Trust, Royal Free & University College School of Medicine, London, UK

Denis W Harkin MD FRCS EBSQ-VASC Senior Lecturer & Consultant Vascular Surgeon, Regional Vascular Surgery Unit, Royal Victoria Hospital, Belfast, Northern Ireland

Peter L Harris MD FRCS Professor of Vascular Surgery, Regional Vascular Unit, Royal Liverpool University Hospital, Liverpool, UK

Brian P Heather MS FRCS Consultant Vascular Surgeon, Gloucestershire Royal Hospital, Gloucester, UK

Shazia M Khan MRCS MSc Specialist Registrar in Vascular Surgery, Sheffield Vascular Institute, Northern General Hospital, Sheffield, UK

Peter Lamont MD FRCS Consultant Vascular Surgeon, Bristol Royal Infirmary, Bristol, UK

Timothy A Lees MD FRCS Consultant Vascular Surgeon, Freeman Hospital, Newcastle upon Tyne, UK

Ian Loftus MD FRCS Consultant Vascular Surgeon, St. George's Vascular Institute, London, UK

Felicity J Meyer MA BM BCh FRCS Consultant Vascular Surgeon, Department of General and Vascular Surgery, Norfolk and Norwich University Hospital, Norwich, UK

John A Murie MA BSc MD FRCS Consultant Vascular Surgeon and Honorary Senior Lecturer, The Royal Infirmary of Edinburgh, Edinburgh, UK

Sanjay Nalachandran FRCS Clinical Fellow, Freeman Hospital, Newcastle upon Tyne, UK

A Ross Naylor MD FRCS Professor of Vascular Surgery, Leicester Royal Infirmary, Leicester, UK

Crispian Oates MSc MIPEM AVS Consultant Physicist, Newcastle General Hospital, Newcastle upon Tyne, UK

Tim J Parkinson MB BS MRCS(Glasg) Vascular Research Fellow, Northern Vascular Centre, Freeman Hospital, Newcastle upon Tyne, UK

Jeremy MT Perkins MD FRCS Consultant Surgeon, Department of Vascular Surgery, John Radcliffe Hospital, Oxford, UK

David A Ratliff MD FRCP FRCS (Eng & Ed) Consultant Vascular Surgeon, Northampton General Hospital, Northampton, UK

John D Rose FRCP FRCR Consultant Radiologist, Northern Vascular Centre, Freeman Hospital, Newcastle upon Tyne, UK

Cliff Shearman BSc MB BS FRCS MS Professor of Vascular Surgery, University of Southampton, Southampton General Hospital, Southampton, UK

Frank CT Smith BSc MD FRCS FRCSEd Consultant Senior Lecturer in Vascular Surgery, Bristol Royal Infirmary, Bristol, UK

Peter R Taylor MA MChir FRCS Consultant Vascular Surgeon, Department of General and Vascular Surgery, Guy's and St. Thomas' Hospitals NHS Foundation Trust, London, UK

John F Thompson MS FRCSEd FRCS Consultant Surgeon, Exeter Vascular Service, Royal Devon and Exeter Hospitals, Exeter, UK and Peninsula Medical School, Exeter, UK

Matt Thompson MD FRCS Professor of Vascular Surgery, St. George's Vascular Institute, London, UK

John HN Wolfe FRCS MS Consultant Vascular Surgeon, Regional Vascular Unit, St. Mary's Hospital, London, UK

Kenneth R Woodburn MD FRCSG (Gen) Consultant Vascular Surgeon, Honorary Clinical Lecturer, Peninsula Medical School, and the Vascular Unit, Royal Cornwall Hospitals Trust, Truro, Cornwall, UK

Mike G Wyatt MSc MD FRCS Consultant Vascular Surgeon, Northern Vascular Centre, Freeman Hospital, Newcastle upon Tyne, UK

Dominic Yu MB BS MRCPI FRCR Consultant Radiologist, Department of Radiology, Royal Free Hospital, London, UK

Foreword

In the eight years since the first edition of *The Evidence for Vascular Surgery*, there have been many changes in our specialty. In particular, an increasing number of endovascular treatment options are available to challenge conventional open procedures, as we predicted in the Foreword to the first edition. An expanding volume of scientific evidence is accumulating to aid clinicians make choices when various interventions are possible. There have been one or two large trials, such as EVAR I and II, which will undoubtedly inform the management of aneurysms, and a host of smaller ones that give useful advice for everyday clinical decisions. The aim of this book is to summarise the best available evidence for the treatment of common vascular diseases.

The first edition of *The Evidence for Vascular Surgery* was described as a "longed for addition to the literature", and as a text that "cannot be compared with any other book on vascular surgery" (*Lancet* 2000; 355: 1918). At the time it was different; a book to help clinicians sift through surgical research and use it to make sensible decisions for clinical practice. The challenge for the second edition is to produce something better still; a text that will be valuable to everyone who manages patients with vascular diseases. We have therefore consolidated some of the chapters from the first edition, and introduced new ones following advice from colleagues and readers. We have used authors that mostly belong to the Joint Vascular Research Group (JVRG), a collection of vascular specialists who conduct collaborative research projects. More information about the Group can be found on its website www.jvrg.org.uk.

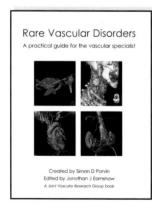

The JVRG has produced a number of other textbooks, including most recently *Rare Vascular Disorders - A practical guide for the vascular specialist*, which looks at unusual conditions for which there is little evidence to guide intervention. It should be seen as an ideal companion text to *The Evidence for Vascular Surgery* which focuses on common problems met every day by the vascular specialist.

The Editors are enormously grateful to everyone who has contributed to this book, and in particular to Nikki Bramhill at tfm, our publisher, who has pulled everything together so expertly.

Jonothan J Earnshaw
John A Murie

Chapter 1

The nature of surgical evidence and evidence-based practice

John A Murie MA BSc MD FRCS, Consultant Vascular Surgeon and Honorary Senior Lecturer
The Royal Infirmary of Edinburgh, Edinburgh, UK

Introduction

Evidence is grounds for belief in something. Medicine in general, and surgery in particular, have not always followed an evidential path, but in recent times - the scientific era - evidence has been one of the great driving forces. Over the last few years it has become obvious that not all evidence is of equal value, and an evidential hierarchy has been suggested as a useful tool when considering the strengths and weaknesses of propositions. The following levels are the most well known:

- Ia - evidence obtained from systematic review of meta-analysis of randomised controlled trials;
- Ib - evidence obtained from at least one randomised controlled trial;
- IIa - evidence obtained from at least one well-designed controlled study without randomisation;
- IIb - evidence obtained from at least one other type of well-designed quasi-experimental study;
- III - evidence obtained from well-designed non-experimental descriptive studies, such as comparative studies, correlation studies and case studies;
- IV - evidence obtained from expert committee reports or opinions and/or clinical experience of respected authorities.

From the above hierarchy, recommendations for clinical practice can be grouped into the following grades:

- A - at least one randomised controlled trial as part of a body of literature of overall good quality and consistency addressing the specific recommendation (evidence levels Ia and Ib);
- B - well-conducted clinical studies but no randomised clinical trials on the topic of recommendation (evidence levels IIa, IIb, III);
- C - expert committee reports or opinions and/or clinical experience of respected authorities. This grading indicates that directly applicable clinical studies of good quality are absent (evidence level IV).

The above schemes are used throughout the chapters in this book and they are a real advance in evaluating the results of clinical science.

Another advance in assessing scientific work that has achieved prominence in recent years has been the introduction of the formal search strategy into the surgical literature. Not so long ago it was commonplace to come across a review article that contained a commentary based solely on those original papers that favoured the personal bias of the review author. Today, reputable journals will publish review work only if an assurance is given that all the appropriate literature has been competently searched and a clear explanation given of what has been included, what has been excluded, and the reasons why. This has isolated the old art form of the prediced review to the realms of the medicolegal report.

The problem with researchers and authors

In an ideal world the literature would contain a full and proper description of all the studies ever carried out, but the scientific world is far from ideal. It is surprising how most readers accept the written word as reflecting ultimate truth, when a moment's reflection must surely convince even the most credulous that this cannot be so. Researchers and authors are human, and just as prone to insanity, perverse incentive and ignorance as everyone else. Gross fabrication of data might be uncommon, but it happens even at the highest level and outright lies appear in even the most prestigious journals. To support such a claim one need look only at the Woo Suk Hwang affair earlier this year [1]. This South Korean professor had achieved worldwide fame and near pop star adulation in stem cell research, choosing to publish his work in journals such as the *Lancet* and *Science*, but it all came to a sad end on the front pages of newspapers internationally when his claims to have used cloning techniques to create stem cell lines of 11 people were proved fraudulent.

It is probable that data mismanagement is far commoner than outright fabrication; in one study of scientific behaviour only 0.3% of researchers admitted to falsifying data while no less than 15.3% admitted to excluding observations or data points from analyses based on a gut feeling that they were inaccurate [2]. To this must be added failing to present data that contradict one's own previous research (6.0%), overlooking others' use of flawed data or questionable interpretation of data (12.5%), changing the design, methodology or results of a study in response to pressure from a funding source (15.5%), republishing the same data (4.7%) and so on. Very occasionally some of this behaviour can be attributed to the ignorance of a young researcher on how to

conduct a scientific project, but far more often it is a matter of dishonesty for personal gain, be it money or prestige.

In addition to misconduct in data handling there is the problem of vested interest. Surgical instrumentation, implantable devices and drugs now play a greater part than ever before in healthcare, and their costs are high. With these increased costs has come an ever greater industry presence in medicine. Sometimes industry is an active partner in a research project, with full access to data and its interpretation, and with an axe to grind. More often industry is the silent partner, contributing in a general sense to departmental 'research' funds, and offering international travel and high quality accommodation to facilitate doctors' attendance at professional conferences. Is this likely to affect a surgeon's attitude to an instrument or prosthesis? Industry also specifically targets so-called 'opinion formers', easing their way around the world in business class seats to spread the word on how good the product is. Vested interest occurs in other forms too, but industrial connections, with their need for a return on an ever-enlarging investment, are the greatest cause for concern.

The problem with journals and editors

Surgical evidence appears mostly in journals. Journals, to remain healthy, have two concerns. First, they must attract papers; second, they must attract a readership. Why do authors choose to send work to one journal rather than another in the same field? The single biggest influence is perceived 'high quality', after which comes high impact factor. The impact factor of a journal is simply a measure of how often that journal's articles are cited. For a given (index) year, it is the number of citations made to articles appearing in the journal during the index year, divided by the number of articles published in the journal in the two previous years. Most editors feel, in general, that articles expressing a 'positive' result are more likely to appeal to readers (who are potential authors) and are more frequently cited than 'negative' articles (articles coming to no firm conclusion or expressing doubt about some approach). Such an attitude, of course, is recognised by researchers who, over time,

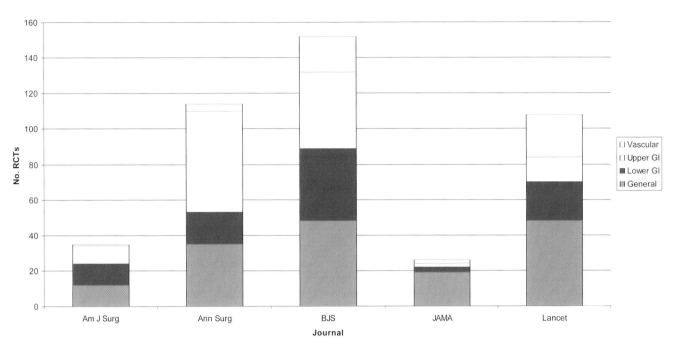

Figure 1. The number and type of randomised clinical trials published in major surgical journals 1998-2005.

are effectively discouraged from submitting 'negative' work for publication, resulting in a positive feedback or vicious cycle. The result of this dysfunctional situation is that the literature is loaded with positive bias - inadvisable operations appear to produce wonderful results, prostheses perform with a brilliance that is stunning and drugs have perfect actions with few or no side effects.

Over the last couple of years the importance of the 'missing literature' has been recognised by editors and a plan is now afoot to redress the balance. Many of the most reputable journals now require all comparative prospective studies to be registered on a freely available website before they commence, if they are to be considered for publication at some future point [3]. This should ensure that there is a detailed record, free to all, of all such prospective work, including trials that produce a 'negative' result. The plan is not perfect, of course, as it is still likely to leave a positive spin within the pages of the journals, but at least reviewers will have access to unpublished 'negative' results and those conducting meta-analyses

will be able to revert to authors for complete 'negative' or other unpublished data.

Evidence-based practice

Evidence-based medicine is usually defined as 'the conscientious, explicit, and judicious use of current best evidence in making decisions about the care of individual patients' [4]. But is the evidence available adequate to make this notion a practical proposition? In broad terms only about 24% of surgical activity is based on level Ia/Ib evidence [5] and only 3.4% of all publications in the leading surgical journals are randomised controlled trials [6] (Figure 1). This represents a base of work that seems adequate to provide some guidance in the clinical sphere, but it is not a big base and, regretfully, many published guidelines reflect little more than level III/IV evidence. Clearly, there is room for improvement.

Even when high quality evidence is available, it rarely penetrates into clinical activity with ease. Many surgeons are resistant to change, others besotted with the latest gadgetry; personal opinion and hubris go largely unchallenged. Even in enlightened departments, dissemination of evidence-based guidelines has often done little to improve clinical practice, and some have concluded that the dream of expecting busy clinicians to follow this process is impractical [7, 8]. This has led to the synthesis of evidence into systematic reviews, development of computer-based clinical decision support systems, and improving access to useful information via the internet [9].

Such attempts to improve implementation of evidence-based practice are worthy, but they are unlikely to succeed without a change of departmental culture. Any success of evidence-based surgery will depend on the support of staff members, education of surgical trainees and regular practice within a patient-centred approach. Some hospitals hold an annual course for new staff and have weekly time set aside for discussion of evidence-based activity, using a standard format. 'Number needed to treat' and 'number needed to harm' are used rather than p-values, as the former are more informative measures of effect size. It is advisable to have one or two senior members of staff trained in evidence-based techniques who can take responsibility for the programme [10].

Conclusions

Surgical evidence and its effect on clinical practice depend on many factors. Some of these are sound, positive and encouraging, others are a cause of concern. The level of evidence hierarchy and the grading of recommendations are useful tools that focus the mind on the power of the available data. The recognition of evidence-based practice as a real entity is also important, as are attempts at its formal introduction into the clinical setting. Encouraging, too, is the fact that the 'missing evidence', which stems from failure to publish negative or equivocal results, has been recognised and is currently being addressed by the major journals. It would be laudable if the knowledge of how poor the surgical database actually is stimulates good research in the future [11].

References

1. Murphy TJ. On being downstream from faked scientific reports. *Br Med J* 2006; 332: 674.
2. Martinson BC, Anderson MS, de Vries R. Scientists behaving badly. *Nature* 2005; 435: 737-8.
3. De Angelis CD, Drazen JM, Frizelle FA, *et al.* Is this clinical trial fully registered? - A statement from the International Committee of Medical Journal Editors. *N Engl J Med* 2005; 352: 2436-8.
4. Sackett DL, Rosenberg WMC, Muir Gray JA, *et al.* Evidence-based medicine: what is and what isn't. *Br Med J* 1996; 312: 71-2.
5. Howes N, Chagla L, Thorpe M, McCulloch P. Surgical practice is evidence-based. *Br J Surg* 1997; 84: 1220-3.
6. Wente MN, Seiler CM, Uhl W, Buchler M. Perspectives of evidence-based surgery. *Dig Surg* 2003; 20: 263-9.
7. Guyatt GH, Meade MO, Jaeschke RZ, *et al.* Practitioners of evidence-based care: not all clinicians need to appraise evidence from scratch but all need some skills. *Br Med J* 2000; 320: 954-5.
8. McColl A, Smith H, White P, Field J. General practitioners' perceptions of the route of evidence-based medicine: a questionnaire survey. *Br Med J* 1998; 316: 361-5.
9. Applying evidence to health care delivery. In: *Crossing the Quality Chasm*. National Institute of Medicine. Washington, DC: National Academy Press, 2001; 145-63.
10. Ubbink DT, Legemate DA. Evidence-based surgery. *Br J Surg* 2004; 91: 1091-2.
11. Lara PN Jr, Higdon R, Lim N, *et al.* Prospective evaluation of cancer clinical trial accrual patterns: identifying potential barriers to enrolment. *J Clin Oncol* 2001; 19: 1728-33.

Chapter 2

Indications for carotid endarterectomy

Jeremy MT Perkins MD FRCS, Consultant Surgeon
Department of Vascular Surgery, John Radcliffe Hospital, Oxford, UK
Robert B Galland MD FRCS, Consultant Surgeon
Department of Vascular Surgery, Royal Berkshire Hospital, Reading, UK

Introduction

Carotid surgery started in the 1950s when a number of different operations were described for treating atheromatous stenosis of the carotid artery. All have been largely abandoned except for carotid endarterectomy, which is now the operation of choice. The indications for carotid endarterectomy and the technical aspects of the operation have been subjected to constant evaluation over the years.

The number of operations performed each year in the USA rose from 15,000 in 1971 to 107,000 in 1985 [1] at a total cost in excess of one billion dollars [2]. The rationale for this increase arose from the findings of the Joint Study of Extracranial Arterial Occlusion, which showed that approximately 45% of the 500,000 Americans who suffered a stroke each year had a surgically accessible carotid artery stenosis [3].

The causes of stroke are, however, multifactorial, and the link between asymptomatic carotid lesions or minor degrees of carotid stenosis and stroke had not yet been elucidated. At the end of the 1980s there was considerable uncertainty about the value of carotid endarterectomy [4]. There had been improvements in medical management and considerable geographical variation was recognised in the number of carotid endarterectomies performed [5], with striking differences in the rates of postoperative stroke and death. Mature reflection led to the conclusion that the indications for operation were inappropriate in one third of patients and equivocal in a further third [6]. Clearly, there was a need for large-scale, randomised trials to examine the relationship between degree of carotid stenosis and medical or surgical treatment for both symptomatic and asymptomatic patients.

Symptomatic carotid artery disease

The European Carotid Surgery Trial (ECST) and the North American Symptomatic Carotid Endarterectomy Trial (NASCET) published their interim results in 1991 [7, 8] (Table 1). Patients who had suffered a non-disabling stroke, hemispheric (carotid territory) transient ischaemic attack (TIA), or an episode of fleeting monocular blindness (amaurosis fugax) were included in the trials. Randomisation was either to carotid endarterectomy or best medical management. The degree of internal carotid artery stenosis in both trials was measured by carotid angiography. ECST stratified patients into three groups: mild stenosis (0-29%), moderate stenosis (30-69%) and severe stenosis (70-99%). NASCET randomised only those with moderate or severe stenosis, using the same percentage categories as ECST.

Table 1. Symptomatic trial results.

Methodology	ECST	NASCET
Years of study	1981 - 1991	1987 - 1990
Geographical origin	Europe	North America
No. randomised	2518	1212
Population	Men and women	Men and women (median age 66 years)

	ECST 70 - 99%		ECST 50 - 69%		ECST 30 - 49%		ECST 0 - 29%		NASCET 70 - 99%	
Stenosis range	Surgical	Medical	Surgical	Medical	Surgical	Medical	Surgical	Medical	Surgical	Medical
30-day outcome										
Death	9.9%	12.7%	1.4%		0.8%		11.4%	7.7%		
Death+ ipsilateral stroke	0.7%	2.2%					0	0		
Death+ any stroke	7.5%	3%	7.9%		8%		2.3%	1.3%	5.8%	3.3%
Death+ disabling stroke	3.7%									
Late outcome										
2-year ipsilateral stroke (+operative risk)									9%	26%
3-year ipsilateral stroke (+operative risk)	9.3%	16.8%								
2-year disabling +fatal stroke (+operative risk)									2.5%	13.1%
3-year disabling +fatal stroke (+operative risk)	4.8%	8.4%								
5-year ipsilateral stroke			15.7%	22.2%						

Severe (70-99%) internal carotid artery stenosis

Both trials showed a clear benefit in avoiding any ipsilateral stroke, or ipsilateral disabling or fatal strokes, in patients with a severe stenosis who had carotid endarterectomy **(Ib/A)**. The incidence of any peri-operative stroke or death was 7.5% in ECST and 5.8% in NASCET. In ECST there was an additional 2.8% risk of postoperative ipsilateral stroke at three years after surgery compared with 16.8% after medical management (control group). The most important events to prevent are disabling or fatal strokes, and in ECST the rate of ipsilateral fatal or disabling stroke was 3.7% after surgery, with an additional 1.1% risk over three years. This compared with 8.4% in the control group at three years. The risk of fatal or disabling stroke in the medically managed patients was greatest in the first year after the onset of symptoms, and so if operation was delayed the benefits of carotid endarterectomy might be lost.

The results of NASCET were similar, with a 9% incidence (including peri-operative strokes) of any ipsilateral stroke at two years in the surgery group, compared with 26% in the control group. The corresponding figures for fatal or disabling ipsilateral stroke were 2.5% (surgery) and 13.1% (medical). The yearly incidence of ipsilateral stroke in the medically treated groups was approximately 6% in ECST, and 10% in NASCET, although the rate of stroke appeared to plateau after three years.

The final results from ECST were published in 1998 and included a longer follow-up (mean 6.1 years) [9]. Carotid endarterectomy could be expected to benefit men with a symptomatic carotid stenosis >80%, and women with a stenosis >90% **(Ib/A)**. Long-term results from NASCET have confirmed the continuing benefit for surgery in patients with a severe (>70%) carotid stenosis [10]. At eight years follow-up, the incidence of any ipsilateral stroke was approximately 14% after surgery compared with 27% in the medical group **(Ib/A)**.

The initial ECST report identified duration of surgery (<1 hour) and a systolic blood pressure >160mmHg as factors increasing the risk of operative stroke. Further risk factors have been highlighted by multiple regression analysis of ECST data [11]. The risks of peri-operative stroke are increased in patients with cerebral symptoms compared with ocular symptoms, in women, in patients with a systolic blood pressure >180mmHg, and in those with peripheral vascular disease. Operative risk did not differ between groups with different degrees of stenosis [12]. No difference in operative risk was demonstrated for patients with established stroke compared to those with TIA, or for patients with established carotid territory stroke or TIA compared to those with non-hemispheric events. There was a trend to higher operative risk in urgent surgery (for stroke in evolution or crescendo TIAs), but for stable patients no excess operative risk accrued from operating early compared with delaying surgery for four to six weeks [13].

Moderate (30-69%) stenosis

Surgery cannot be justified in symptomatic patients with moderate internal carotid artery stenosis **(Ib/A)**. While some benefit could not be ruled out in the very long term, no benefit from carotid endarterectomy would be gained within four to five years for stenoses of 50-69%, and within six to seven years for stenoses of 30-49% [10, 14]. NASCET assessed patients with stenoses of <50% and stenoses from 50-69% for moderate stenosis [10]. Operation was clearly not beneficial in the former group. A marginal benefit from carotid endarterectomy was reported in patients with stenoses from 50-69%; the five-year rate of any ipsilateral stroke was 15.7% in the surgery group compared with 22.2% in the medical group (p=0.045). This means that 15 patients would have to undergo carotid endarterectomy to prevent one stroke in five years. This degree of stenosis corresponds to an ECST stenosis of 70-80%, and the marginal benefit of surgery reported reflects the similar benefit shown for 70-79% stenoses in the final ECST results [9].

Mild (0-29%) stenosis

Surgery cannot be justified in symptomatic patients with mild internal carotid artery stenosis **(Ib/A)**. Only ECST randomised patients with this degree of stenosis. The risk of ipsilateral stroke in the medical group was negligible and so surgery could only prove to be detrimental due to the early peri-operative mortality and morbidity [7].

Conclusions from ECST and NASCET

For the first time these two large, randomised trials have clarified the indications for carotid endarterectomy in symptomatic patients and quantified the expected benefit or lack of benefit for surgery, depending on the degree of carotid stenosis **(Ib/A)**. Many of the discrepancies between the two studies have been ironed out by re-measuring ECST angiograms using the NASCET criteria and then analysing the pooled data from the two trials using the same definitions for outcome criteria [15]. In this analysis the benefit of carotid endarterectomy for symptomatic stenosis of 70-99% was very clear **(Ia/A)**. For all outcomes benefit was apparent at one year of follow-up, was maximum at three years and still maintained to ten years. The number needed to treat to prevent one event was five for any stroke or surgical death, and ten for disabling or fatal ipsilateral carotid territory ischaemic stroke and disabling surgical stroke or surgical death.

Surgery was harmful for patients with stenosis <30% and showed no effect on outcome for patients with 30-49% stenosis. There was a borderline statistically significant reduction in the risk of any stroke or surgical death for patients with 50-69% stenosis, but no reduction in the risk of ipsilateral carotid territory ischaemic stroke and surgical stroke or death. Importantly, surgery was of no benefit in patients with near occlusion, contrary to a prevailing clinical opinion that such patients require urgent operation **(Ia/A)**.

Results of the studies apply only to patients with the symptoms specified in the trial inclusion criteria and without specific exclusion criteria; they cannot be extrapolated to patients with vertebrobasilar ischaemia, non-hemispheric symptoms or other uncommon cerebrovascular complaints, such as pulsatile tinnitus. Although reports have documented relief of these symptoms following carotid endarterectomy, they involve small numbers of non-randomised patients in retrospective reviews with historical controls. These reports offer no rationale for patient selection to ensure successful relief of symptoms and non-hemispheric symptoms remain a minor and unorthodox indication for carotid endarterectomy **(III/B)**.

Applying the results of studies to clinical practice

Trials are inevitably conducted under artificial constraints and individual doctors have to decide the relevance of trial cohorts, methods and results to their own patient population. NASCET established entry criteria for participating centres - a review of the last 50 carotid endarterectomies within the preceding 24 months had to demonstrate a peri-operative stroke and death rate of less than 6%. NASCET excluded patients older than 79 years and those with significant cardiac, pulmonary, renal or hepatic disease likely to cause death within five years. ECST randomised patients when clinicians were 'substantially uncertain' if carotid surgery was indicated; specific exclusion criteria were not given, nor were entry criteria for participating centres established. This probably means that the results of ECST are more applicable to clinical practice than those of NASCET.

Pooled data from ECST and NASCET have allowed subgroup analysis to inform selection of patients for carotid endarterectomy who would benefit most [16]. Benefit from surgery was greater in men than women and in those >75 years old; it decreased with time since the last symptom **(IIb/B)**. This last factor is crucial in the organisation of services to deliver carotid surgery. While current clinical guidelines state that surgery should occur within six months of the presenting event [17, 18], the subgroup analysis showed maximal benefit for those operated on within two weeks, with considerable reduction of benefit after a lapse of 12 weeks from the presenting event. This suggests that the current guidelines should be revised.

NASCET and ECST used different methods of measurement to assess the degree of carotid stenosis from biplanar angiography and controversy about this has raged ever since. Furthermore, duplex ultrasonography is now widely used to assess carotid stenosis and angiograms are performed infrequently, but duplex imaging does not always detect distal internal carotid artery disease. Duplex criteria for classifying stenoses vary across the UK, and many departments do not validate their own criteria against angiographic measurements [19]. The European Carotid Surgery Trialists' Collaboration has recommended the universal adoption of the NASCET criteria for measuring stenosis on angiography. Ultrasound criteria have been established to allow diagnosis of a carotid stenosis equivalent to 70% or greater on an angiogram measured using the NASCET formula [20].

Best medical treatment also merits consideration. The introduction of statins, lipid-lowering agents, since the start of all the major carotid trials means that the medical arms of these trials are now out of date. Repeating the studies with the medically treated patients receiving a statin might well produce a different result.

Asymptomatic carotid artery stenosis

Population studies have shown the prevalence of carotid stenosis greater than 50% (almost all asymptomatic) to rise from 0.5% in people in their 50s to about 10% in those over 80 [21, 22]. The risk of stroke for those with asymptomatic internal carotid artery stenosis is about 2% per year, significantly less than for those with symptomatic disease [23, 24]. Under these circumstances the balance between benefit and harm from prophylactic surgery is much finer. Conclusive evidence of the benefit of carotid endarterectomy would be required before prophylactic operation in an asymptomatic subject could be recommended.

Asymptomatic carotid surgery trials (Table 2)

Two early American randomised trials were too small to provide any useful information on outcome [25, 26]. One of these was also stopped prematurely because of the high incidence of myocardial infarction in the surgical group, who were not prescribed aspirin [26].

The Carotid Artery Stenosis with Asymptomatic Narrowing - Operation versus Aspirin (CASANOVA) study [27] randomised patients with a carotid stenosis between 50-90%. No difference was found in the rates of stroke or death in the surgical and medical groups. However, the study design was unusual in that those with a stenosis greater than 90% were thought to require operation and were excluded from randomisation. Patients in the non-surgery group also had a carotid endarterectomy if a stenosis progressed to greater than 90%, if bilateral stenoses >50% developed (operation on the more severe side), or if the patient suffered a TIA with a >50% stenosis related to the symptomatic side. In total, 118 endarterectomies were performed on the 204 patients randomised to the medical arm. Data from this study are, consequently, largely discredited.

The Veterans Affairs Cooperative Study Group trial did, however, show a significant difference in the rate of ipsilateral neurological events (TIA, amaurosis fugax, or stroke) between its medical and surgical groups (8.0% surgery versus 20.6% medical at a mean follow-up of 47.9 months) [28]. However, the overall incidence of ipsilateral stroke, and the combined incidence of all strokes and death, were the same in both groups. Half of the deaths in each group were attributable to cardiac events, reflecting the elderly male population studied. In the presence of such a high mortality rate from other causes, it would be difficult for the effect of less frequent events, such as strokes, to be detected. The higher incidence of TIAs in the medical group was largely irrelevant as the affected patients could be offered surgery as they became symptomatic, when the benefits of operation are more clearly defined [7, 8].

The value of carotid endarterectomy in reducing the risk of stroke has been demonstrated by the Asymptomatic Carotid Atherosclerosis Study (ACAS) [24], a meta-analysis in 1998 of data then available from randomised trials [29] and the Asymptomatic Carotid Surgery Trial (ACST) [30]. ACAS randomised patients with an asymptomatic carotid stenosis greater than 60% on angiography (equivalent to about 75% stenosis measured by the 'European' method). After a median follow-up of 2.7 years the trial was stopped. Actuarial estimated five-year risk of stroke was 5.1% after surgery versus 11.0% in the medical group. This represented an absolute risk reduction of 5.9% or a relative risk reduction of 53%. The primary endpoints of ipsilateral stroke and peri-operative stroke or death showed a statistically significant advantage for surgery at three years, with the medical and surgical survival curves crossing at ten months. The secondary endpoints of any stroke or death and ipsilateral TIA with or without stroke showed results which tended to favour the surgical group.

The meta-analysis analysed data from five trials available at that time. Data from CASANOVA were excluded due to the large number of patients in the medically treated group undergoing operation. There

Table 2. Asymptomatic trial results.

	CASANOVA	Veterans		ACAS		ACST	
Methodology							
Years of study	1982-1988	1983 - 1991		1987 - 1993		1993 - 2003	
Geographical origin	Germany	United States		North America		Europe, North and South America, North Africa	
No. randomised	410	444		1662		3120	
Population	Men + women Mean 64 yrs ± 8.6	Men 64.5 yrs (± 6.7)		Men + women (40-79 years)		Men + women	
Degree of stenosis	50-90%	>50%		>60%		>60%	
30-day outcome		Surgical	Medical	Surgical	Medical	Surgical	Medical
Death		1.9%	0.9%			0.9%	0.01%
Death + any stroke		4.7%	0.9%	2.3%	0.4%	2.5%	
Late outcome							
4-year ipsilateral TIA + stroke		8%	20.6%				
4-year ipsilateral stroke + death		41.2%	44.2%			2.7% excluding events	9.5% peri-operative
						6.4% including events	11.8% peri-operative
5-year ipsilateral stroke				5.1%	11%		
Final outcome	Completed, but largely disregarded today	Completed		Stopped 2.7 years, significance achieved		Completed	
Comments	Included surgical patients in both arms so data cannot be simplified for this table			9% did not receive assigned treatment; 1.2% angiogram complication rate in surgical group			

was a significant reduction in ipsilateral stroke and combined stroke and death in patients undergoing surgery compared with best medical treatment (OR 0.62, 95% CI 0.44-0.86). However, given the modest advantage confirmed by surgery, the authors did not recommend operation in this setting until high-risk subgroups could be identified **(Ia/A)**.

ACST, a multicentre study, involved 30 countries worldwide. Excluding peri-operative events, five-year all-stroke risks were 3.8% in its surgical group and 11% in its medically-treated group. This advantage was mostly due to decreased numbers of ipsilateral ischaemic strokes. Benefits were recorded for both men and women, for all degrees of carotid stenosis and for patients up to 74 years of age. No benefit was demonstrated in older patients due to the high death rate for unrelated causes similar to the findings of the Veterans study **(Ib/A)**.

Applying the results of studies to clinical practice

The benefit of carotid endarterectomy in asymptomatic patients is extremely small, as shown by the meta-analysis referenced above. Data from the meta-analysis indicate that 50 people would need to have a carotid endarterectomy to prevent one stroke over a three-year interval. If the risk of stroke in the group who did not have surgery continues beyond three years, then the benefit of surgery could accrue for more than three years and the number needed to treat might be less [31].

The data from ACAS (used in the American guidelines on carotid surgery [32]), with an absolute risk reduction of 5.9%, are problematic in terms of clinical practice. Centres participating in ACAS were rigorously selected to control peri-operative stroke and death rates. If the angiographic stroke rate (1.2%) was largely avoided by the use of duplex ultrasonography, the overall peri-operative stroke and death rate in the surgical group would have been 1.1%. It must be appreciated, however, that patients were carefully selected and about 25 were screened for every one entered into the trial; non-whites represented only 5% of those enrolled [33]. Furthermore, data from the trial were projected from

2.7 years of follow-up to five years by actuarial analysis.

These points should be borne in mind when considering the available data on carotid endarterectomy for asymptomatic stenosis. Undoubtedly there are asymptomatic patients who would benefit from carotid endarterectomy, either because they are at low risk of peri-operative stroke or, more likely, because they are at high risk of stroke without operation. Although ACST has gone some way to clarify the situation, once again it must be remembered that even in this study best medical treatment changed during the trial period, with the introduction of statins in the latter years.

Combined carotid and cardiac surgery

There is no evidence from randomised trials to guide clinicians on whether carotid endarterectomy and coronary artery bypass should be performed as a combined procedure, or separately. It is suggested that where both lesions are symptomatic a combined operation is appropriate [34]. A systematic review has shown a higher mortality rate, and higher combined death and stroke rate after synchronous carotid endarterectomy and coronary artery bypass [35]. This review contained little randomised data **(III/B)**. The multifactorial nature of stroke in association with coronary surgery, and the paucity of quality randomised data in this area, mean that the selection of patients for carotid endarterectomy to reduce stroke risk at coronary surgery, remains at the whim of the individual surgeon.

Conclusions

There is strong evidence that carotid endarterectomy prevents strokes in patients with symptomatic internal carotid artery stenosis of 70-99%. Appropriate symptoms are amaurosis fugax, retinal infarction, carotid territory TIAs and non-disabling stroke. Symptomatic patients with mild (0-29%) or moderate (30-69%) stenosis should not undergo carotid endarterectomy **(Ia/A)**. Carotid endarterectomy confers the greatest benefit in men, in the elderly and in those patients operated on rapidly after their presenting event **(IIb/B)**. Younger asymptomatic patients with stenoses greater than 70% may benefit from carotid endarterectomy, the risk of stroke at five years being halved.

Further data are required before firm conclusions can be drawn in a number of areas. No data from randomised trials exist to evaluate the role of carotid endarterectomy for other cerebral symptoms, such as those of vertebrobasilar ischaemia; the same is true for non-hemispheric symptoms and eye signs other than amaurosis fugax. There are no data from randomised trials to support combined carotid endarterectomy and coronary artery bypass for symptomatic cardiac and carotid disease, or to guide in the selection of patients who would benefit from carotid endarterectomy before coronary bypass surgery.

Key points	Evidence level
◆ Patients with symptomatic ipsilateral carotid stenosis >70% benefit from carotid endarterectomy (five operations will prevent one stroke). Patients with near occlusion do not benefit from surgery.	Ia/A
◆ There is no advantage from surgery over best medical therapy in patients with symptomatic ipsilateral carotid stenosis <70%.	Ia/A
◆ Carotid endarterectomy must be performed as rapidly as possible after the presenting event. Benefit is substantially reduced if the surgery takes place more than 12 weeks after the initial symptoms.	IIb/B
◆ Younger patients with asymptomatic carotid stenosis >70% have reduced risk of stroke after carotid endarterectomy. This is only valid if the peri-operative stroke and death rate remains low (<2.8%).	Ib/A

References

1.   Pokras R, Dyken M. Dramatic changes in the performance of endarterectomy for diseases of the extracranial arteries of the head. *Stroke* 1988; 19: 1289-90.
2.   Dyken M. Carotid endarterectomy studies: a glimmering of science. *Stroke* 1986; 17: 355-8.
3.   Fields W, Maslenikov V, Meyer J, *et al.* Joint study of extracranial arterial occlusion. *JAMA* 1970; 211: 1993-2003.
4.   Warlow C. Carotid endarterectomy: does it work? *Stroke* 1984; 15: 1068-76.
5.   Chassin M, Brook R, Park R, *et al.* Variations in the use of medical and surgical services by the Medicare population. *N Engl J Med* 1986; 314: 285-90.
6.   Winslow C, Solomon D, Chassin M, *et al.* The appropriateness of carotid endarterectomy. *N Engl J Med* 1988; 318: 721-6.
7.   European Carotid Surgery Trialists' Group. MRC European Carotid Surgery Trial: interim results for symptomatic patients with severe (70-99%) or with mild (0-29%) carotid stenosis. *Lancet* 1991; 337: 1235-43.
8.   North American Symptomatic Carotid Endarterectomy Trial Collaborators. Beneficial effect of carotid endarterectomy in symptomatic patients with high-grade stenosis. *N Engl J Med* 1991; 325: 445-53.
9.   European Carotid Surgery Trialists' Collaborative Group. Randomised trial of endarterectomy for recently symptomatic carotid stenosis: final results of the MRC European Carotid Surgery Trial. *Lancet* 1998; 351: 1379-87.
10.   North American Symptomatic Carotid Endarterectomy Trial Collaborators. Benefit of carotid endarterectomy in patients with symptomatic moderate or severe stenosis. *N Engl J Med* 1998; 339: 1415-25.
11.   Bond R, Narayam SK, Rothwell PM, Warlow CP, on behalf of the European Carotid Surgery Trialists' Collaboration Group. Clinical and radiographic risk factors for operative stroke and death in the European Carotid Surgery Trial. *Eur J Vasc Endovasc Surg* 2002; 23: 108-16.
12.   Rothwell PM, Eliasziw M, Gutnikov SA, *et al* for the Carotid Endarterectomy Trialists' Collaboration. Analysis of pooled data from the randomised controlled trials of endarterectomy for symptomatic carotid stenosis. *Lancet* 2003; 361: 107-16.

13. Bond R, Rerkasem K, Rothwell PM. Systematic review of the risk of carotid endarterectomy in relation to the clinical indication for and timing of surgery. *Stroke* 2003; 34: 2290-303.

14. European Carotid Surgery Trialists' Collaborative Group. Endarterectomy for moderate symptomatic carotid stenosis: interim results of the MRC European Carotid Surgery Trial. *Lancet* 1996; 347: 1591-3.

15. Rothwell PM, Gutnikov SA, Warlow CP, for the European Carotid Surgery Trialists' Collaboration. Reanalysis of the final results of the European Carotid Surgery Trial. *Stroke* 2003; 34: 514-23.

16. Rothwell PM, Eliasziw M, Gutnikov SA, *et al*, for the Carotid Endarterectomy Trialists' Collaboration. Endarterectomy for symptomatic carotid stenosis in relation to clinical subgroups and timing of surgery. *Lancet* 2004; 363: 915-24.

17. The Intercollegiate Working Party for Stroke. National clinical guidelines for stroke. London: Royal College of Physicians, 2000.

18. Moore WS, Barnett HJM, Beebe HG, *et al*. Guidelines for carotid endarterectomy: a multidisciplinary consensus statement from the ad hoc committee, American Heart Association. *Stroke* 1995; 26: 188-201.

19. Perkins JMT, Galland RB, Simmons MJ, Magee TR. Carotid duplex imaging: variation and validation. *Br J Surg* 2000; 87: 320-2.

20. Grant EG, Benson CB, Moneta GL, *et al*. Carotid artery stenosis: gray-scale and Doppler ultrasound diagnosis: Society of Radiologists in Ultrasound Consensus Conference. *Radiology* 2003; 229: 340-6.

21. O'Leary DH, Polak JF, Kronm RA, *et al*. Distribution and correlates of sonographically detected carotid artery disease in the Cardiovascular Health Study. *Stroke* 1992; 23: 1752-60.

22. Prati P, Vanuzzo D, Casaroli M, *et al*. Prevalence and determinants of carotid atherosclerosis in a general population. *Stroke* 1992; 23: 1705-11.

23. European Carotid Surgery Trialists' Collaborative Group. Risk of stroke in the distribution of an asymptomatic carotid stenosis. *Lancet* 1995; 345: 209-12.

24. Executive Committee for the Asymptomatic Carotid Atherosclerosis Study. Endarterectomy for asymptomatic carotid artery stenosis. *JAMA* 1995; 273: 1421-8.

25. Clagett GP, Youkey JR, Brigham RA, *et al*. Asymptomatic cervical bruit and abnormal ocular pneumoplethysmography: a prospective study comparing two approaches to managment. *Surgery* 1984; 96: 823-9.

26. Mayo Asymptomatic Carotid Endarterectomy Study Group. Results of a randomised controlled trial of carotid endarterectomy for asymptomatic carotid stenosis. *Mayo Clin Proc* 1992; 67: 513-8.

27. CASANOVA Study Group. Carotid surgery versus medical therapy in asymptomatic carotid stenosis. *Stroke* 1991; 22: 1229-35.

28. Hobson R, Weiss D, Fields W, *et al*, for the Veterans Affairs Cooperative Study Group. Efficacy of carotid endarterectomy for asymptomatic carotid stenosis. *N Engl J Med* 1993; 328: 221-7.

29. Benavente O, Moher D, Pham B. Carotid endarterectomy for asymptomatic carotid stenosis: a meta-analysis. *Br Med J* 1998; 317: 1477-80.

30. MRC Asymptomatic Carotid Surgery Trial (ACST) Collaborative Group. Prevention of disabling and fatal strokes by successful carotid endarterectomy in patients without recent neurological symptoms: randomised controlled trial. *Lancet* 2004; 363: 1491-502.

31. Warlow CP. Carotid endarterectomy for asymptomatic carotid stenosis. *Br Med J* 1998; 317: 1468.

32. Biller J, Feinberg WM, Castaldo JE, *et al*. Guidelines for healthcare professionals from a special writing group of the Stroke Council, American Heart Association. *Stroke* 1998; 29: 554-62.

33. Mayberg MR, Winn HR. Endarterectomy for asymptomatic carotid artery stenosis. *JAMA* 1995; 273: 1459-61.

34. Hertzer NR. Basic data concerning associated coronary artery disease in peripheral vascular patients. *Ann Vasc Surg* 1987; 1: 616-20.

35. Naylor AR, Cuffe RL, Rothwell PM, Bell PRF. Systematic review of outcomes following staged and synchronous carotid endarterectomy and coronary artery bypass. *Eur J Vasc Endovasc Surg* 2003; 25: 380-9.

Chapter 3

Optimising the results of carotid endarterectomy

Michael J Gough MB ChB ChM FRCS, Consultant Vascular Surgeon
Leeds Vascular Institute, The General Infirmary at Leeds, Leeds, UK

Introduction

The aim of carotid endarterectomy (CEA) is the long-term abolition of neurological sequelae attributable to an internal carotid artery (ICA) stenosis while minimising any neurological or cardiopulmonary complications associated with the procedure. Although effective control of cardiovascular risk factors certainly influences the durability of the intervention, this chapter focuses specifically on peri-operative strategies that may influence outcome. As published results of CEA describe a 30-day stroke and death rate between 1.6-9.9% [1, 2], there seems to be scope for improving outcomes in some centres.

Although surgical and anaesthetic factors influence outcome, certain patient characteristics are also relevant. Adverse outcome is known to be associated with female gender, hypertension, coexistent peripheral arterial disease, stroke as the indication for CEA, contralateral carotid stenosis ≥50% and active coronary artery disease [3]. Clearly only some of these can be corrected pre-operatively.

Cardiac mortality

Severe, correctable, but often silent, coronary artery disease (CAD) is present in a third of patients with carotid atherosclerosis, resulting in an annual cardiac-related mortality of 6.5% in patients with >75% carotid stenosis [4]. Although CEA does not cause the volume-dependent haemodynamic disturbances that accompany aortic surgery, changes in cardiac rhythm and blood pressure often occur during, and immediately after, operation. In particular, locoregional anaesthesia (LA) is associated with peroperative hypertension, and altered carotid sinus nerve or baroreceptor function may lead to either hyper- or hypotension in the early postoperative period. These changes may precipitate myocardial ischaemia, myocardial infarction or cardiac dysrrhythmia, which account for most of the deaths following CEA [5], particularly in patients with pre-existing cardiac disease or in those requiring peri-operative vasopressor drugs. Careful cardiac assessment before CEA is, therefore, essential.

Ideally, patients with occult CAD should be identified pre-operatively (dipyridamole-thallium scan, exercise ECG), although most institutions do not have the resources for this and the benefit of pre-operative screening is still debated. In practice, a careful history and examination, resting ECG and a transthoracic cardiac echocardiogram are used to either exclude significant CAD or to select patients who require coronary angiography. This leaves an intermediate group for whom screening may be justified. A small group of patients with severe coexisting CAD and carotid disease will be identified who may benefit from synchronous CEA and coronary revascularisation [6] **(III/B)**.

Anaesthetic technique

CEA may be performed under either general anaesthesia (GA) or LA and there is evidence that cardiac risk is reduced with the latter [7], despite greater blood pressure instability and higher catecholamine levels. It has been suggested that peri-operative β–adrenergic blockade may protect the myocardium against these adverse effects and this is supported by studies that suggest β–blockade may reduce operative mortality [8, 9].

An ideal anaesthetic allows maintenance of normal PaO_2 and $PaCO_2$ tensions, control of arterial pressure and preservation of cerebral autoregulation. Anaesthetic agents can have both adverse and beneficial effects on cerebral perfusion and oxygenation. For instance, barbiturates reduce cerebral metabolic rate and cerebral oedema, while propofol may protect against certain biochemical effects of reperfusion and offer greater haemodynamic stability on emergence from anaesthesia. The widely used volatile anaesthetic agents (halothane, isoflurane) may increase cerebral blood flow but suppress cerebral autoregulation and increase cerebral lactate concentration; all volatile agents and nitrous oxide may increase intracranial pressure. Not surprisingly, the overall effect of GA is to some degree unpredictable, although GA does allow effective control of PaO_2 and $PaCO_2$, and of blood pressure. Finally, it should be noted that alterations in $PaCO_2$, which may influence vasomotor tone, do not appear to enhance cerebral blood flow.

In contrast, LA (superficial and deep cervical plexus block) preserves autoregulation and improves cerebral oxygenation during carotid clamping, which induces a reflex rise in systemic blood pressure [10]. This, and its ability to identify patients who require a shunt (awake testing), has resulted in the increasing popularity of LA in the UK. Drawbacks are that LA may result in hurried and technically imperfect surgery, stress for both patient and surgeon, and an unsatisfactory environment for training junior surgeons.

Preservation of cerebral autoregulation, reduced need for shunting, and a possible reduction in cardiac morbidity and mortality have led to the hypothesis that LA may be associated with lower stroke and death rates than those of GA. This issue is currently being examined by the GALA trial (GA versus LA for CEA), a multicentre, international, randomised controlled trial that will complete recruitment in 2007. Until its results become available, the only evidence to guide the choice of anaesthesia comes from a systematic review [11] in which the risk of stroke, myocardial infarction and death was examined in 25,622 patients from 41 non-randomised studies and 554 patients from seven randomised trials. Meta-analysis of the non-randomised studies suggested that LA was associated with significant reductions in the risk of death (OR 0.67 [0.46-0.97], p=0.04), stroke (OR 0.56 [0.44-0.70], p=0.001), stroke or death (OR 0.61 [0.48-0.77], p=0.001), myocardial infarction (OR 0.55 [0.39-0.79], p=0.001) and pulmonary complications (OR 0.31 [0.15-0.63], p=0.001) within 30 days of surgery. However, data from non-randomised studies must be viewed with caution; methodological issues, differences in patient characteristics, absence of independent outcome assessment and reporting bias make their conclusions unsafe. This is particularly so as meta-analysis of data from the randomised studies found no evidence of a reduction in the odds of peri-operative stroke, and reductions in the myocardial infarction, and stroke and death rates were not statistically significant. However, these trials and the number of outcome events were too small to allow any reliable conclusions. Thus, the results of the GALA trial will provide valuable information and are eagerly awaited.

On current evidence CEA under LA appears safe and effective, and the technique also provides a period of postoperative analgesia. However, some patients may be unsuitable for LA, either because of difficulty in performing awake neurological testing (previous stroke with dysphasia or hemiplegia) or because of anxiety. For these patients GA is preferred. There is no convincing evidence upon which to base a choice of anaesthetic method. The evidence in favour of local anaesthetic surgery is extremely limited **(IV/C)**.

Surgical technique

Although specific interventions that influence the outcome of CEA are discussed below, the author believes that certain aspects of technique, which cannot be subject to critical assessment, are important. These include:

- careful positioning of the patient to avoid excessive rotation or extension of the neck that may compromise cerebral blood flow during carotid clamping;
- minimal manipulation of the carotid arteries ('no-touch' technique) during dissection to reduce the risk of embolism. This is facilitated by sharp dissection of vessels and the use of pointed bent-on-flat scissors to create a tissue plane for the passage of vessel loops;
- early clamping of the ICA in patients with transcranial Doppler (TCD) evidence of peroperative embolism and in those likely to have unstable plaques (e.g. crescendo TIAs);
- the use of magnifying loupes for endarterectomy, removal of residual fragments, and vessel repair;
- the use of sharp bent-on-flat scissors for clean transection of the proximal endarterectomy limit, and appropriate use of proximal and distal tacking sutures;
- careful flushing of debris and air with heparinised saline and continuous ICA back-bleeding during final closure of the arteriotomy;
- initial reperfusion of the external carotid artery.

Endarterectomy technique and patching

Endarterectomy technique

Of the techniques described for CEA, standard endarterectomy through a longitudinal arteriotomy (sCEA) is the most widely used. Eversion endarterectomy (eCEA), which obviates the need for patching and is associated with shorter clamp times, is used by a minority of surgeons. Interposition grafting should be reserved for revisional operations.

The relative safety and efficacy of sCEA and eCEA have been examined in a number of relatively small RCTs. The potential benefits of eCEA can be gleaned from a systematic review of randomised trials of eCEA versus sCEA [12]. This examined the combined outcomes of five RCTs, the largest of which was the EVEREST trial [13]. The findings, which are summarised in Table 1, show no significant differences between the techniques for the main outcome measures of stroke or death. Although late restenosis or occlusion may be less frequent after eCEA, this advantage could not be confirmed because a number of patients were lost to follow-up. The potential impact of this is shown in Table 1. Paradoxically, the review found that the late ipsilateral stroke rate for eCEA was higher than that for sCEA, despite the possible reduction in restenosis with the former method. The incidence of myocardial infarction, neck haematoma and cranial nerve injury was similar for both techniques.

Table 1. Frequency (%) of main outcomes in systematic review of eversion versus standard CEA [12]. *Reproduced with permission from BIBA Medical Ltd. More Vascular and Endovascular Controversies. Greenhalgh RM, Ed. BIBA Medical Ltd., 2006.*

	Eversion CEA	Standard CEA	Odds ratio (95% CI)
Peri-operative stroke/death	1.7	2.6	0.44 (0.10-1.82)
Peri-operative death	0.6	0.7	0.86 (0.31-2.37)
Peri-operative stroke	1.4	2.0	0.70 (0.38-1.29)
Peri-operative ipsilateral stroke	1.5	1.7	0.92 (0.44-1.93)
Early carotid occlusion	0.7	1.0	0.62 (0.24-1.58)
Late occlusion/restenosis >50% (best) *	2.5	5.2	0.48 (0.32-0.72)
Late occlusion/restenosis >50% (worst) **	4.1	5.2	0.78 (0.54-1.13)
Ipsilateral stroke during follow-up	1.0	0.5	2.16 (0.73-6.45)

* best: assume that no 'arteries' lost to follow-up developed stenosis/occlusion
** worst: assume all eversion CEA 'arteries' lost to follow-up developed stenosis/occlusion

Data from other observational studies only add to the confusion regarding the impact of eCEA on restenosis. While some suggest a possible benefit, two report recurrent stenosis rates of 9% [14] and 36% [15], respectively. For comparison, 6% of patients having sCEA in this latter study developed a >50% stenosis, while late occlusion rates were 4% for eCEA and 1% for sCEA. This suggests that the potential benefits of eCEA might not be realised in everyday vascular surgical practice.

Some authors believe that not all patients are suitable for eCEA, particularly if the atheromatous plaque extends >1.5-2cm into the ICA. Under these circumstances it becomes difficult to assess the distal limit of the endarterectomy and insert tacking sutures, if required. It is interesting that in the EVEREST trial, in which randomisation was performed after vessel dissection, 579 of 1932 patients were excluded from the study [13]; 62% were considered unsuitable for eCEA, either for anatomical reasons or because of concern about difficulty in shunt insertion and/or retention.

Advocates of eCEA say that completion imaging can identify technical defects at the distal endarterectomy limit, allowing surgical revision when necessary. In the EVEREST trial, plaque extending for >2cm into the ICA was a positive predictor for the identification of defects [13] and revision was associated with a significantly higher peri-operative ipsilateral stroke rate [16]. These findings question the wisdom of using eCEA for such plaques. A further report by Osman and Gibbons [17] indicated that completion imaging led to a decision to undertake revision in 10% of patients having eCEA.

In summary, although there is no evidence to support the preferential use of either sCEA or eCEA, the greater technical demands of eCEA for plaques of >2cm length, difficulties with shunt insertion and retention, and the need for obligatory completion imaging argue against its routine use.

Patching

Patch angioplasty following sCEA may reduce the risk of early ICA thrombosis and late restenosis, thereby reducing both early and long-term stroke

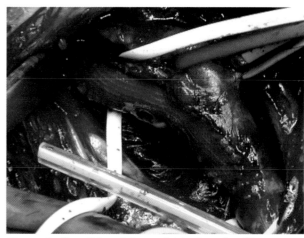

Figure 1. Carotid patch angioplasty using Dacron.

rates (Figure 1). However, potential drawbacks are an increase in carotid clamp time and the risk of patch-related complications (rupture, false aneurysm, sepsis).

A meta-analysis of seven randomised trials of patching versus primary repair has been performed by the Cochrane Stroke Review Group [18]. The results are summarised in Tables 2 and 3. Based on these data, the authors calculated that for every 1000 CEAs performed, routine patching would prevent 40 ICA occlusions within 30 days of surgery and a further 50 occlusions or restenosis >50% during follow-up. This would prevent 30 ipsilateral peri-operative strokes and result in 75 fewer strokes or deaths during overall follow-up. While this is persuasive evidence to support patching, the data are potentially flawed by the number of patients lost to follow-up and biases from inadequate methods of randomisation/blinding in some trials.

At least two of the trials included in the review excluded patients with small ICAs (<4 or 5mm in diameter) from randomisation but, even so, the apparent benefit of patching remained, suggesting that it is independent of vessel size. This argues against the view of those who advocate selective patching on the basis that the complications of direct repair are greater when the ICA diameter is 5mm or less, particularly in women in whom the mean diameter of the ICA (4.9±0.6mm) is 8-15% less than in men (5.3±0.7mm) [19, 20]. Although the randomised trials do not support this view, a non-randomised

Table 2. Benefit of routine patching: outcomes within 30 days of operation [18].

	Peto odds ratio (95% CI)	p
Any peri-operative stroke	0.33 (0.15-0.70)	0.004
Ipsilateral peroperative stroke	0.31 (0.15-0.63)	0.0008
Peri-operative stroke and/or death	0.39 (0.20-0.78)	0.007
Peri-operative ipsilateral ICA occlusion	0.15 (0.06-0.37)	0.00004

Table 3. Benefit of routine patching: outcomes during long-term follow-up (minimum one year) including events during the first 30 days [18].

	Peto odds ratio (95% CI)	p
Any stroke	0.32 (0.17-0.63)	0.0009
Fatal stroke	0.27 (0.05-1.6)	0.15
Ipsilateral stroke	0.32 (0.16-0.63)	0.001
Any stroke or death	0.59 (0.42-0.84)	0.004
Occlusion or restenosis greater than 50%	0.20 (0.13-0.29)	0.00001

study has reported a lower incidence of residual/recurrent ICA stenosis when selective patching was applied in this way [21]. The issue of patching is clearly important. Ideally, it should be investigated in a large multicentre, randomised trial, but this would need to enrol at least 3000 patients to confirm a 50% reduction in stroke or death rates. Finally, it must be appreciated that other factors also influence the incidence of late restenosis (smoking, elevated serum lipid level, female sex) [22], although these are not relevant to the early benefits of patching.

There has been some discussion about the choice of patch material; autologous long saphenous vein (LSV), Dacron, polytetrafluoroethylene (PTFE) and autologous cervical vein (facial, internal and external jugular) all have their advocates. Cervical vein may be preferred to LSV when CEA is performed under LA but, if selected, it should be invaginated to expose the intima and a double thickness used to compensate for its thin wall. The putative advantages of vein patches include low thrombogenicity, better handling characteristics, good haemostasis and superior resistance to infection. However, early patch rupture, suture line disruption with haemorrhage and false aneurysm formation have been reported in 0-4% of

patients, particularly when the external jugular vein or LSV from the ankle are used. Proponents of synthetic patches highlight their easy availability, mechanical integrity and higher resistance to aneurysm formation. However, the risk of patch sepsis is greater and, for PTFE, haemostasis is more difficult to achieve.

In the first edition of this book three studies examining the relative benefits of different patch materials were considered; since then, a further five randomised controlled trials have been published. An updated meta-analysis shows that trials comparing vein and Dacron contain too few outcome events to detect a difference between the two materials [23] in respect of stroke, death, ICA occlusion or restenosis. These findings are consistent with a previous meta-analysis that found similar outcomes for PTFE and vein [24]. However, an alternative analysis of six studies (two randomised trials, one prospective audit and three retrospective reviews) showed a trend to a lower peri-operative stroke rate when vein was preferred to Dacron or PTFE [19]. A further trial [25], which was included in the most recent meta-analysis [23], compared PTFE and Dacron, and found an increased combined risk of stroke and TIA (p=0.03) and restenosis at 30 days (p=0.01) with Dacron.

In five trials that followed patients for over a year the only difference between synthetic or vein patches was that fewer pseudo-aneurysms occurred with the former (OR 0.09, CI 0.02-0.49) but, as none of these ruptured, their clinical significance is uncertain. As in the other analyses, the number of outcome events was small, making it difficult to reach any firm conclusion.

An observational study by Verhoeven et al [26] reported an increase in TCD-detected micro-emboli following clamp release and during wound closure when Dacron rather than vein was used, although there were no differences in the frequency of peri-operative neurological complications. This study also found that late restenosis was more common with Dacron. This latter finding is supported by another study in which patients undergoing bilateral CEA had one artery patched with vein and the other with Dacron, thus removing the influence of systemic risk factors [27].

Although there are no clear differences in major outcome events associated with patch type, meta-analysis reveals that haemostasis takes longer when PTFE is used, particularly when compared to Dacron. PTFE is also associated with a higher re-operation rate, usually for wound haemorrhage. Wound haematoma is also more common with synthetic patches as a whole.

In summary, although there is evidence to support routine patching, there is no clear evidence as to the superiority of any one patch type. While synthetic patches avoid the morbidity associated with vein harvesting and preserve the vein for future use, both PTFE and Dacron appear to be associated with a higher risk of peri-operative haemorrhage and early thrombosis. The clinical impact of these differences is, however, small. It seems reasonable that the choice of patch material be left to individual preference.

Current evidence suggests that the best outcomes from CEA are achieved following standard endarterectomy and obligatory patching **(Ia/A)**.

Cranial and cervical nerve injury

Several cranial and cervical nerves are at risk during CEA and postoperative nerve dysfunction affects 3-27% of patients. Most nerves recover within 12 months, but 7% are permanently damaged. Even when temporary, such injuries may cause significant disability, particularly when the recurrent laryngeal or hypoglossal nerves are involved. These lesions assume even greater importance when proceeding to contralateral CEA as bilateral palsies of either nerve may result in upper airway obstruction and difficulties with speech and swallowing.

Neck haematoma, re-exploration for bleeding, shunting, patch closure, a trainee surgeon, and high carotid lesions all increase the risk of nerve palsy. While more important considerations dictate the use of shunts and patches, the integrity of cranial/cervical nerves following CEA is largely surgeon-dependent. Nerve transection should be rare, given sound anatomical knowledge, but neuropraxia may still result from stretching or retraction. Thus, adequate exposure of the carotid vessels, careful deployment of self-retaining retractors and circumspect use of diathermy are important. Key points of anatomy (Figure 2) and methods of minimising nerve injury are shown in Table 4.

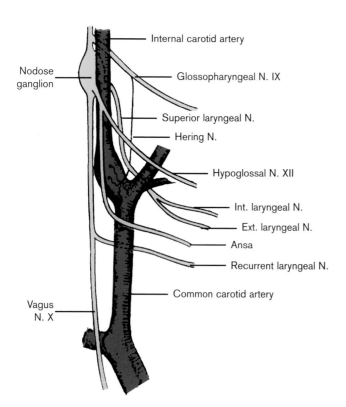

Internal carotid artery

Nodose ganglion

Glossopharyngeal N. IX

Superior laryngeal N.

Hering N.

Hypoglossal N. XII

Int. laryngeal N.

Ext. laryngeal N.

Ansa

Recurrent laryngeal N.

Common carotid artery

Vagus N. X

Figure 2. Anatomy of operative field during carotid endarterectomy.

Table 4. Anatomy, method of injury, methods of avoidance and incidence of injury to nerves at risk during CEA.

Nerve	Position	Injury	Avoidance	Incidence
Recurrent laryngeal	Tracheo-oesophageal groove. A non-RLN may leave vagus at level of bifurcation or distal CCA and cross medially, posterior to the CCA to enter the larynx	Retraction Clamping Dissection	Minimise circumferential dissection CCA, ICA, ECA. Be aware of a non-RLN. Direct laryngoscopy prior to staged contralateral CEA	1-25%
Superior laryngeal	Vertical in the carotid sheath behind ICA and ECA close to superior thyroid artery where it divides into internal (sensory) and external (motor) branches	Stretch Retraction Clamping	As for RLN and control superior thyroid artery at junction with CCA (external branch). Care with clamps on ECA	Not known
Vagus	Posterolateral to CCA/ICA in carotid sheath. May occupy anteromedial position	Clamping Dissection	Care with clamping CCA/ICA, close dissection of CCA	Not known
Hypoglossal	Crosses ICA and ECA 2-4cm above bifurcation. Tethered by the descendens hypoglossi/ansa and sternomastoid artery and vein. Can be as low as bifurcation and adherent to posterior surface of the anterior facial vein	Stretch Retraction Ligation	Careful mobilisation of nerve with division of tethering structures. Do not separate fused vagus and hypoglossal	1-13.5%
Marginal mandibular branch of facial nerve	Lies inferior and parallel to the ramus of the mandible deep to the platysma	Incision Stretch Retraction	Avoid excessive hyperextension of the neck (nerve is pulled down closer to the operative field). Curve superior extent of skin incision posteriorly. Avoid retracting onto mandible	0.5-15 %
Greater auricular and transverse cervical nerves	GAN crosses the uppermost portion of transverse incision. TCN crosses lower end of the standard neck incision	Incision	Properly placed skin incision if possible though many patients complain of numbness over ear lobe/angle of jaw (GAN) or in submental or submandibular area (TCN)	1.1-60%

CCA = common carotid artery
ECA = external carotid artery
ICA = internal carotid artery
RLN = recurrent laryngeal nerve
GAN = greater auricular nerve
TCN = transverse cervical nerve

Shunting and intra-operative monitoring

The use of shunts during CEA has attracted considerable debate; three approaches have evolved. Some surgeons shunt all patients, believing that the risk of ischaemic stroke is thereby reduced and that additional time is gained, particularly for patching or training a junior colleague. Others never use shunts, believing that they may cause neurological complications through platelet and air emboli, intimal damage, late restenosis and arterial dissection. Shunts may also kink, dislodge and reduce access to the operative field. Finally, some surgeons deploy shunts selectively when peroperative monitoring shows evidence of cerebral ischaemia after carotid clamping.

Counsell et al reviewed the trials comparing routine shunting with no shunting [28] and found trends toward fewer strokes, stroke-related deaths and lower 30-day mortality in shunted patients. However, the number of outcome events was small and the trials varied in their method of randomisation, risk stratification, surgical technique and the frequency of patching between shunted and non-shunted patients. There is, therefore, no conclusive evidence to support either routine shunting or no shunting. Although Counsell et al suggested that a multicentre prospective randomised trial was required to answer this question definitively, a more recent review [29] confirms that no such study has yet been performed and so the evidence for shunting is unchanged.

The logical approach to safe CEA is reliable detection of peroperative cerebral ischaemia, which occurs in up to a third of patients, and selective use of a shunt (Figure 3). The search for a suitable monitoring technique has proved difficult. Potential methods include physiological tests reflecting cerebral perfusion (electro-encephalography, measurement of somatosensory evoked potentials [SSEP]), assessment of cerebral blood flow (stump pressure, transcranial Doppler [TCD], cerebral oximetry) or neurological examination (awake testing during LA surgery). The relative merits of these are summarised in Table 5. No test is perfect, but it seems reasonable to believe that awake neurological testing is the best available.

Monitoring techniques with a high false positive rate result in unnecessary shunt deployment, diminishing any benefit of selective shunting. Conversely, techniques with a significant false negative rate increase the risk of ischaemic stroke. Thus, monitoring techniques require validation to establish their sensitivity and specificity (Table 5). This is almost impossible during GA CEA, although it has been suggested that different methods could be calibrated against the need for a shunt in patients having LA surgery. This concept is flawed because LA preserves cerebral autoregulation while GA does not; physiological indicators of cerebral ischaemia cannot be extrapolated from LA to GA [10]. At present, only awake testing appears able accurately to identify those patients who require a shunt. Of the others, measurement of SSEP seems the most promising, as it is continuous, relatively easy to perform and applicable to all patients.

There is minimal evidence to suggest the most appropriate policy for shunt use and assessing the risk of intra-operative cerebral ischaemia. If it is accepted that selective shunting is of potential benefit then it is logical to combine this with LA CEA and awake testing. However, the current level of evidence for such a policy can only be graded as **IV/C**.

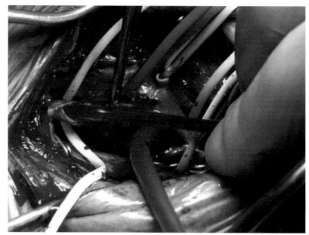

Figure 3. Javid shunt *in situ* during CEA.

Table 5. Methods of cerebral monitoring and criteria for selective shunt insertion.

Technique	Suggested criteria	Comments	False +ve	False -ve
Stump pressure	<50mmHg (other criteria 'established' during LA CEA not reliable)	Cheap, universally available. No continuous monitoring. Changes in blood pressure, $PaCO_2$, PaO_2 may affect Circle of Willis flow during CEA	High	0-23%
Cerebral blood flow (xenon [133] washout)	<18-20ml/100gm/min	Limited availability, expensive, radiation hazard. Technician required	?	?
Transcranial Doppler	Variously stated as >50%->70% decrease in middle cerebral artery velocity	Expensive, trained technician, 10% of patients do not have an acoustic window Affected by change in $PaCO_2$, BP	Depends on cut off	Up to 17% if >70% fall used as criterion
Near infra-red spectroscopy	Decrease in cerebral O_2 saturation of >10%	Expensive, research tool Uncertain contribution of extracranial perfusion	50%	4%
Local anaesthesia (awake testing)	Altered neurological function	Cheap, reliable and continuous monitoring	0%	0%
Electro-encephalography	Decreased amplitude, slowing, loss of fast activity	Continuous. Need trained technician Assesses superficial cortex >deeper tissue, affected by diathermy, some types of GA, $PaCO_2$ and previous stroke	8-13%	5-50%
Somatosensory evoked potentials	>50% decrease in amplitude of complex or >1ms increase in central conduction time following median nerve stimulation	Moderate cost. Easier than electro-encephalography. Technician required Influenced by some types of GA and analgesics Assesses internal capsule viability (unlike electro-encephalography)	0-17%	1-17% (<1% in most studies)

CEA = carotid endarterectomy
LA = local anaesthesia
GA = general anaesthesia

Anticoagulation and heparin reversal during CEA

While anticoagulation with heparin is universally used during CEA, the dose administered varies considerably. There is no evidence to suggest that such variations influence stroke or death rates, but it has been suggested that heparin reversal with protamine may increase the risk of peri-operative stroke [29-31]. A randomised prospective study by Fearn et al [29] investigated the effect of protamine on wound haematoma and reported two strokes in patients receiving protamine and none in those who did not. The study was discontinued early, prompted in part by the publication of a retrospective study of 350 patients by Mauney et al [30], in which a significantly greater risk of stroke was associated with protamine use. A further retrospective study by Levison et al [31] found a non-significant risk of stroke following protamine administration. The value of these reports is limited as only one was randomised and there were variations in shunt use and patch angioplasty in all three studies. Indeed, in one report all strokes occurred in non-patched patients [30], while in another the frequency of primary closure was 50% higher in the protamine group [29].

Stroke risk notwithstanding, protamine administration appears to reduce wound drainage and the risk of wound haematoma [29, 31, 32]. Furthermore, two retrospective studies examining processes of care and outcome following CEA did not find an association between protamine administration and adverse outcomes [33, 34]. This view is also supported by data from 2158 patients participating in the GALA trial. In summary, it seems unlikely that protamine administration adversely affects the outcome of CEA.

Other factors that may influence the outcome of CEA

A number of other factors may affect the results of CEA but it is important to understand that these have not been tested in randomised trials. They include:

♦ Hospital and surgeon clinical volume.

Studies from the USA have shown that stroke and death are more likely when CEA is performed by surgeons undertaking five or fewer procedures per year, and in institutions carrying out <100 endarterectomies per year [35, 36]. This suggests a benefit when CEA is performed in specialist units, although this is far from proven (IV/C).

♦ Adjuvant pharmacological therapy.

Pharmacological neuroprotection is an attractive concept, although little explored. It is reported that thiopentone administration before carotid clamping, in doses sufficient to suppress EEG burst activity, allows surgery to be undertaken without a shunt, with a combined stroke and death rate of 0-1.4% [37]. EEG monitoring is mandatory to confirm that the desired effect is achieved and recovery from anaesthesia is prolonged, with patients often requiring postoperative ventilation.

Several authors have reported that up to 5% of TCD-monitored patients experience multiple middle cerebral artery emboli (>50/hour) during the first few hours after CEA and that 60% progress to carotid thrombosis and stroke [38, 39]. This may reflect a technical error during arteriotomy closure, enhanced thrombogenicity of the endarterectomised vessel or patch, or altered platelet function. While re-exploration of the carotid vessels may be useful if there is a correctable abnormality, the Leicester group, which has a rigorous policy of quality assessment on completion of CEA, have reported that incremental doses of dextran 40 (20-40ml/hour) abolish embolic events and prevent stroke [38]. This promising finding requires corroboration. Although Lennard et al [38] continued TCD monitoring for up to six hours after surgery, a recent study has suggested that patients with high and increasing numbers of micro-emboli who progress to stroke can be identified when monitoring is confined to the second postoperative hour [40].

Finally, pre-operative colloid volume expansion with 500-1000ml 6% hetastarch appears to reduce the frequency of ischaemic EEG changes following application of carotid clamps. There are no data to assess its impact on stroke and death rate [41].

♦ Quality control.

TCD can be used during surgery to monitor shunt performance and detect embolisation during dissection. Following CEA, angioscopy, completion angiography and duplex imaging have all been used to examine the adequacy of the repair. However, the rate of detection of apparent defects is greater than the anticipated stroke rate without assessment. Both angioscopy [42] and arteriography [43] demonstrate abnormalities requiring further intervention in around 12% of patients. Furthermore, the risk of embolic complications or vessel damage following angiography or angioscopy should be considered.

Duplex ultrasonography has also been used to identify residual stenosis, intimal flaps and intraluminal thrombus following ICA repair. A recent study has confirmed that residual anatomical defects positively predict late restenosis, although there was no relationship between this and further neurological events during a one-year follow-up [44].

Although some surgeons believe that completion quality control is valuable, no randomised trials are available to confirm any benefit. Furthermore, there is no consensus about which abnormalities warrant surgical revision.

Conclusions

Although 15 years have elapsed since the landmark trials confirmed the clinical benefit of CEA for significant, symptomatic carotid disease, little has been achieved in terms of confirming the optimum method of performing surgery. The author's own interpretation of the available evidence is that a standard endarterectomy performed under local anaesthetic with selective shunting (awake testing) and closure with a vein patch is likely to prove safe and effective. The evidence for TCD monitoring and completion quality control is lacking, particularly given the additional expense and logistic difficulties that these policies confer.

Key points	Evidence level

On the basis of current knowledge, best practice for CEA might include:

◆ Full pre-operative cardiac assessment.	III/B
◆ Standard endarterectomy with patch closure.	Ia/A
◆ Surgery performed under local anaesthesia.	IV/C
◆ Selective shunting on the basis of awake testing.	IV/C
◆ Surgery by an experienced surgeon working in a specialist unit.	III/B

Measures requiring or undergoing further evaluation:

◆ The risk/benefit of local and general anaesthesia.
◆ The benefit of completion quality control methods.
◆ The benefit of per- and postoperative transcranial Doppler monitoring.
◆ The benefit of postoperative dextran therapy.

Subjects unlikely to be evaluated further:

◆ A comparison of eversion endarterectomy with patch angioplasty.
◆ A comparison of synthetic and venous patches.
◆ Policies for shunt deployment.
◆ The use of protamine for heparin reversal.

References

1. Hertzer NR, O'Hara PJ, Mascha EJ, *et al.* Early outcome assessment for 2228 consecutive carotid endarterectomy procedures: the Cleveland Clinic experience from 1989 to 1995. *J Vasc Surg* 1997; 26: 1-10.
2. CAVATAS Investigators. Endovascular versus surgical treatment in patients with carotid stenosis in the Carotid and Vertebral Artery Transluminal Angioplasty Study (CAVATAS): a randomised trial. *Lancet* 2001; 357: 1729 -37.
3. Halm EA, Hannan EL, Rojas M, *et al.* Clinical and operative predictors of outcomes of carotid endarterectomy. *J Vasc Surg* 2005; 42: 420-8.
4. Norris JW, Zhu CZ, Bornstein NM, Chambers BR. Vascular risks of asymptomatic carotid stenosis. *Stroke* 1991; 22: 1485-90.
5. Riles TS, Kopelman I, Imparato AM. Myocardial infarction following carotid endarterectomy: a review of 683 operations. *Surgery* 1979; 85: 249-52.
6. Mackey WC. Carotid and coronary disease: staged or simultaneous management? *Semin Vasc Surg* 1998; 11: 36-40.

7. Tangkanakul C, Counsell C, Warlow CP. Local versus general anaesthesia in carotid endarterectomy: a systematic review of the evidence. *Eur J Vasc Surg* 1997; 13: 491-9.

8. Kertai MD, Boersma E, Westerhout CM, *et al*. A combination of statins and beta-blockers is independently associated with a reduction in the incidence of perioperative mortality and nonfatal myocardial infarction in patients undergoing abdominal aortic aneurysm surgery. *Eur J Vasc Endovasc Surg* 2004; 28: 343-52.

9. Stevens RD, Burri H, Tramer MR. Pharmacologic myocardial protection in patients undergoing noncardiac surgery: a quantitative systematic review. *Anesth Analgesia* 2003; 97: 623-33.

10. McCleary AJ, Dearden NM, Dickson DH, *et al*. The differing effects of regional and general anaesthesia on cerebral metabolism during carotid endarterectomy. *Eur J Vasc Surg* 1996; 12: 173-81.

11. Rerkasem K, Bond R, Rothwell PM. Local versus general anaesthesia for carotid endarterectomy. *Cochrane Database of Systematic Reviews* 2004; CD000126.

12. Cao PG, De Rango P, Zannetti S, *et al*. Eversion versus conventional carotid endarterectomy for preventing stroke. *Cochrane Database of Systematic Reviews* 2000; CD001921.

13. Cao PG, De Rango P, Zannetti S, *et al*. Eversion versus conventional carotid endarterectomy: late results of a prospective multicenter randomized trial. *J Vasc Surg* 2000; 31: 19-30.

14. Szabo A, Brazda E, Dosa E, *et al*. Long-term re-stenosis rate of eversion endarterectomy of the internal carotid artery. *Eur J Vasc Endovasc Surg* 2004, 27: 537-9.

15. Brothers TE. Initial experience with eversion carotid endarterectomy: absence of a learning curve for the first 100 patients. *J Vasc Surg* 2005; 42: 429-34.

16. Zannetti S, Cao P, De Rango P, *et al*. Collaborators of the EVEREST study group. Intraoperative assessment of technical perfection in carotid endarterectomy: a prospective analysis of 1305 completion procedures. Eversion versus standard carotid endarterectomy. *Eur J Vasc Endovasc Surg* 1999; 18: 52-8.

17. Osman HY, Gibbons CP. Completion angioscopy following carotid endarterectomy by the eversion technique or the standard longitudinal arteriotomy with patch closure. *Ann R Coll Surg Eng* 2001; 83: 149-53.

18. Bond R, Rerkasem K, AbuRahma AF, *et al*. Patch angioplasty versus primary closure for carotid endarterectomy. *Cochrane Database of Systematic Reviews* 2004; CD000160.

19. Archie JP. Patching with carotid endarterectomy: when to do it and what to use. *Semin Vasc Surg* 1998; 11: 24-9.

20. Schneider JR, Droste JS, Golan JF. Carotid endarterectomy in women versus men: patient characteristics and outcome. *J Vasc Surg* 1997; 25: 890-8.

21. Golledge J, Cuming R, Davies AH, Greenhalgh RM. Outcome of selective patching following carotid endarterectomy. *Eur J Vasc Surg* 1996; 11: 458-63.

22. Gelabert HA, Sherif EM, Moore WS. Carotid endarterectomy with primary closure do not adversely affect the rate of recurrent stenosis. *Arch Surg* 1994; 129: 648-54.

23. Bond R, Rerkasem K, Naylor R, Rothwell PM. Patches of different types for carotid patch angioplasty. *Cochrane Database of Systematic Reviews* 2004; CD000071.

24. Counsell C, Salinas R, Naylor AR, Warlow CP. A systematic review of the randomised trials of carotid patch angioplasty in carotid endarterectomy. *Eur J Vasc Surg* 1997; 13: 345-54.

25. AbuRahma A, Hannay S, Khan JH, *et al*. Prospective randomised study of carotid endarterectomy with polytetrafluoroethylene versus collagen-impregnated Dacron (Hemashield) patching: perioperative (30-day) results. *J Vasc Surg* 2002; 35: 125-30.

26. Verhoeven BA, Pasterkamp G, de Vries JP, *et al*. Closure of the arteriotomy after carotid endarterectomy: patch type is related to intraoperative microemboli and restenosis rate. *J Vasc Surg* 2005; 42: 1082-8.

27. Archie JP. Restenosis after carotid endarterectomy in patients with paired vein and Dacron patch reconstruction. *Vasc Surg* 2001; 35: 419-27.

28. Counsell C, Salinas R, Naylor AR, Warlow CP. Routine or selective carotid artery shunting during carotid endarterectomy and the different methods of monitoring in selective shunting (Cocharne Review). *The Cochrane Library* 1998; Issue 3: 1-12.

29. Fearn SJ, Parry AD, Picton AJ, *et al*. Should heparin be reversed after carotid endarterectomy? A randomised prospective trial. *Eur J Vasc Surg* 1997; 13: 394-7.

30. Mauney MC, Buchanan SA, Lawrence WA, *et al*. Stroke rate is markedly reduced after carotid endarterectomy by avoidance of protamine. *J Vasc Surg* 1995; 22: 264-70.

31. Levison JA, Faust GR, Halpern VJ, *et al*. Relationship of protamine dosing with postoperative complications of carotid endarterectomy. *Ann Vasc Surg* 1999; 13: 67-72.

32. Treiman RL, Cossman DV, Foran RF, *et al*. The influence of neutralizing heparin after carotid endarterectomy on postoperative stroke and wound haematoma. *J Vasc Surg* 1990; 12: 440-6.

33. Hannan EL, Popp AJ, Feustel P, *et al*. Association of surgical specialty and processes of care with patient outcomes for carotid endarterectomy. *Stroke* 2001; 32: 2890-7.

34. Kresowik TF, Bratzler DW, Kresowik RA, *et al*. Multistate improvement in processes and outcomes of carotid endarterectomy. *J Vasc Surg* 2004; 39: 372-80.

35. Cebul RD, Snow RJ, Pine R, *et al*. Indications, outcomes, and provider volumes for carotid endarterectomy. *JAMA* 1998; 279: 1282-7.

36. Hannan EL, Popp AJ, Tranmer B, *et al*. Relationship between provider volume and mortality for carotid endarterectomies in New York State. *Stroke* 1998; 29: 2292-7.

37. Frawley JE, Hicks RG, Horton DA, *et al*. Thiopental sodium cerebral protection during carotid endarterectomy: perioperative disease and death. *J Vasc Surg* 1994; 19: 732-8.

38. Lennard N, Smith J, Dumville J, *et al*. Prevention of postoperative thrombotic stroke after carotid endarterectomy: the role of transcranial Doppler ultrasound. *J Vasc Surg* 1997; 26: 579-84.

39. Levi CR, O'Malley HM, Fell G, *et al*. Transcranial Doppler detected cerebral microembolism following carotid endarterectomy: high microembolic signal loads predict postoperative cerebral ischaemia. *Brain* 1997; 120: 621-9.

40. Van der Schaaf IC, Horn J, Moll FL, Ackerstaff RGA. Transcranial Doppler monitoring after carotid endarterectomy. *Ann Vasc Surg* 2005; 19: 19-24.

41. Gross CE, Bednar MM, Lew SM, *et al*. Preoperative volume expansion improves tolerance to carotid artery cross-clamping during endarterectomy. *Neurosurg* 1998; 43: 222-8.

42. Gaunt ME, Smith JL, Ratliff DA, *et al*. A comparison of quality control methods applied to carotid endarterectomy. *Eur J Vasc Surg* 1996; 11: 4-11.

43. Sala F, Hassen-Khodja R, Bouillanne PJ, *et al*. Importance of a arteriography for intraoperative quality control during carotid artery surgery. *Ann Vasc Surg* 2002; 16: 730-5.

44. Padayachee TS, Arnold JA, Thomas N, *et al*. Correlation of intra-operative duplex findings during carotid endarterectomy with neurological events and recurrent stenosis at one year. *Eur J Vasc Endovasc Surg* 2002; 24: 543-9.

Chapter 4

Carotid angioplasty

A Ross Naylor MD FRCS, Professor of Vascular Surgery

Leicester Royal Infirmary, Leicester, UK

Introduction

It seems ironic that despite the largest evidence base for treating a single pathology (which includes over 90 papers and secondary analyses from ECST, NASCET, ACAS and ACST alone), arguments about which patients benefit most from intervention in carotid disease continue. The reasons are multifactorial, but should be borne in mind when interpreting contemporary data regarding the respective roles of carotid endarterectomy (CEA), carotid angioplasty and/or stenting (CAS) and best medical therapy (BMT).

First, despite guidelines being based on evidence, neurologists and stroke physicians still question the appropriateness of a significant proportion of interventions by clinicians who undertake CEA and CAS. Second, practitioners of both CEA and CAS have been somewhat blind to the implication of advances in the modern concept of BMT. Third, protagonists in the debate (on both sides) have continued to select bits of evidence from the trials that best suit their practice, while ignoring some of the more unpalatable ones. Fourth, is the habit of only reading the headlines from abstracts rather than actually reading the paper describing a trial; often, it goes unnoticed that apples are being compared with oranges. Fifth, and most controversial, are the

evolving inter-disciplinary turf wars regarding who should be performing CAS (surgeons, interventionists, cardiologists or neuroradiologists). These represent a conflict of interest that most commentators prefer to ignore, but they have served to divert debate away from optimising the complementary roles of CEA, CAS and BMT.

Appropriateness of interventions

Carotid surgeons have been subject to retrospective reviews of whether their decision to operate was appropriate. It is an uncomfortable exercise that has, as yet, never been applied to practitioners of CAS (Figure 1). One recent example was a review of 3,360 CEAs performed in four Canadian provinces between 2000-2001 [1]. Adjudicators included: vascular surgeons, neurosurgeons, stroke neurologists, neuroradiologists, general physicians and family doctors, a broad spectrum of stakeholders within a health system that is not generally viewed as being overly aggressive regarding carotid interventions. They concluded that 48% of decisions to operate were of either uncertain appropriateness or were inappropriate. The latter comprised 10% of the overall study group and was most commonly encountered in patients undergoing intervention for asymptomatic disease (18% of treatments deemed inappropriate) compared with 5%

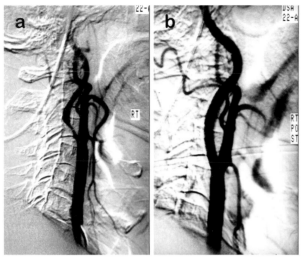

Figure 1. Symptomatic carotid stenosis a) before and b) after carotid angioplasty and stenting.

of procedures in symptomatic patients. The commonest reasons for undertaking inappropriate CEA in symptomatic patients was operating on individuals with a <50% stenosis or with a chronically occluded ICA. The most common reason in asymptomatic individuals was treating stenoses <50%. Most worrying, was the observation that inappropriate interventions were most likely to occur in hospitals and by surgeons who performed the highest volume of procedures.

Improvements in best medical therapy

It is beyond the remit of this chapter to review the potential effect of improvements in the modern concept of BMT [2]; however, they could have a considerable impact on the respective future roles of CEA and CAS. These improvements are less likely to influence decisions in symptomatic patients, as there is an inevitable lag-phase for statins, dual antiplatelet therapy and blood pressure control to take effect. The principal advantage of CEA (and by inference CAS) is the immediate benefit it confers. However, improvements in BMT could have an important impact on decisions in asymptomatic patients. Using the ACST BMT data as a guide, if CEA (or CAS) were performed on 1000 asymptomatic patients with a 30-day death/stroke rate of 2.8%, only 53 strokes will be

prevented at five years [3]. Because of the current uncertainty, there have been calls for the asymptomatic trials to be repeated, but with three limbs: BMT, CEA and CAS [4]. It would not be surprising if the overall benefits conferred by CEA or CAS in asymptomatic patients were not so pronounced.

Which evidence to remember?

The Carotid Endarterectomy Trialists' Collaboration (CETC) combined all of the data from ECST, NASCET and the VA study, having first remeasured all of the pre-randomisation angiograms using the NASCET method [5]. This enabled construction of a comprehensive database comprising 5,893 patients. The principal conclusion was that symptomatic patients gained benefit from CEA if they had a 50-99% stenosis, with the maximum benefit being in patients with the most severe disease (70-99%). Not surprisingly, this has often been translated to mean that all symptomatic patients with 50-99% stenoses benefit from CEA, and thus, by implication, CAS **(Ia/A)**.

CETC identified that the benefits of CEA were closely linked to the timing of surgery after the most recent neurological event and gender; however, little attention is directed to considering these when planning care. Maximum benefit was observed if CEA was undertaken within two to four weeks, especially if the stenosis severity was severe **(Ia/A)**. However, for those with moderate disease (50-69%), the benefit conferred by CEA disappeared if more than 12 weeks had elapsed **(Ia/A)**. More importantly, there was little or no evidence to support offering CEA (and thus, by inference, CAS) to symptomatic women with 50-69% stenoses if four weeks had elapsed since their most recent TIA/stroke [6]. With regard to asymptomatic patients, ACAS showed no evidence that women benefited from CEA [7], but despite this there is little evidence that women are treated any differently from men in the USA. ACST, however, reported that women did gain benefit from CEA [3] and this has been used as justification for treating asymptomatic women without any further consideration. In fact, when the 30-day ACST death/stroke rate was included, CEA did not confer any benefit in women, and when the data from the two trials were combined, the lack of overall benefit from surgery in women is compelling [8]. Clinicians who undertake CEA and CAS must, therefore, be more critical in applying trial results to clinical practice; in the future, CEA and CAS should probably be reserved for younger asymptomatic women (perhaps <70 years) and there is currently no evidence to support labelling any asymptomatic woman as being high risk for stroke **(Ib/A)**.

Read the paper, not just the abstract

An illustrative example refers to the definition of operative risk, a crucial component in determining long-term benefit. Traditionally, the long-term risk of stroke should include the initial risk (death/stroke). It may be assumed that the 30-day risk is standard across all of the principal randomised studies. Nothing could be further from the truth:

◆ as alluded to above, ACST presented a number of secondary analyses which did not include the operative risk;
◆ ECST did not consider permanent visual loss after CEA to be an operative stroke, but NASCET did;
◆ ECST and CAVATAS only considered neurological deficits persisting at seven days to be procedural strokes, all of the other studies used 24 hours as the threshold;
◆ ECST, ACST, WALLSTENT, CAVATAS and EVA-3S reported the operative risk as being the 30-day death/any stroke rate, while ACAS, NASCET, Leicester and LEXINGTON I reported death/ipsilateral stroke rates at 30 days.

The large stent registries are similarly guilty. The German Stent Registry [9] only reports in-hospital rates of death/stroke after CAS (rather than the 30-day risk), while only major stroke/death is documented in another very large stent registry of centres with high-volume CAS throughput [10].

Turf wars

This is one of the most controversial issues facing clinicians today. It would seem that rather than endeavour to see which patient might benefit from which treatment (CEA or CAS or even BMT), some doctors have already concluded that unless they learn how to do CAS, a large part of their clinical practice will be lost in a multidisciplinary battle that includes surgeons, neuroradiologists, interventionists and cardiologists. This debate has been fuelled by research stating that CAS is equivalent to surgery in high-risk patients and that it should be the preferred intervention in these situations [11]. As will be seen, the concept that CAS is equivalent or superior to CEA in high-risk patients is largely unfounded. This is unfortunate as it is a really important question to answer and one in which CAS could probably triumph over CEA, should the trial be done properly [12].

The evidence

The best evidence is derived from randomised trials. This section will review the available data from the randomised trials in symptomatic and asymptomatic patients and will highlight areas of misinformation, controversy, consensus and future goals for research. Registries and personal series undoubtedly represent a large amount of work, but are generally confounded by the lack of independent scrutiny, an accusation that was also levelled at surgeons in the 1980s.

CEA vs CAS in symptomatic patients

Table 1 summarises the principal results from the six randomised trials that have reported outcomes so far [13-18]. As will be seen, meaningful interpretation requires the reader to be aware of the evolving technology associated with CAS since the first trial was published in 1998 (development of dedicated carotid stents, cerebral protection devices). Two (Leicester and LEXINGTON I) were single-centre studies, one (WALLSTENT) was a commercially funded trial, while three (CAVATAS, EVA-3S and SPACE) were nationally funded studies from the UK/Europe, France and Germany/Austria, respectively. Two others (ICSS and CREST) are currently recruiting from Europe and North America.

Table 1. Summary of published results from the six randomised trials in symptomatic patients (CEA vs CAS).

	LEICESTER		WALLSTENT		CAVATAS		LEXINGTON I		EVA-3S		SPACE	
Methodology												
Year published	1998		2001		2001		2001		2004		2006	
No randomised	CEA=10		CEA=112		CEA=253		CEA=53		CEA=263		CEA=595	
	CAS=7		CAS=107		CAS=251		CAS=51		CAS=264		CAS=605	
Stenosis range	70-99%		60-99%		50-99%		70-99%		70-99%		50-99%	
Stent used	WALLSTENT		WALLSTENT		22% stented		WALLSTENT		Yes, type unknown		Yes, type unknown	
CPD used	None available		None available		None available		None available		73% used CPD		26%	
30-day outcomes	CEA	CAS	CEA	CAS	CEA	CAS	CEA	CAS	CEA	CAS	CEA	CAS
Death	0/10	0/7			2%	3%	1.9%	0.0%			0.9%	0.7%
Death/ipsilateral stroke	0/10	5/7					1.9%	0.0%			6.3%	6.8%
Death/any stroke	0/10	5/7	4.5%	12.1%	9.9%	10.0%	1.9%	0.0%	3.8%	9.5%	6.5%	7.7%
Death/disabling stroke	0/10	3/7			5.9%	6.4%	1.9%	0.0%			3.8%	4.7%
Cranial nerve injury	0/10	0/7			8.7%		8.0%					
Wound/access complications	0/7			4.0%	6.7%	1.2%	1.9%	7.8%				
Late outcomes												
1-year ipsilateral CVA (+operative risk)	3.6%	12.1%					1.9%	0.0%				
1-year restenosis (>70%)					5.0%	19%	0.0%	0.0%				
2-year ipsilateral CVA (+operative risk)							1.9%	0.0%				
2-year restenosis (>70%)							0.0%	0.0%				
3-year any CVA (+operative risk)					14%	14%						
Final outcome	Abandoned		Abandoned		Completed		Completed		Abandoned Restarted Abandoned		Stopped early	

CPD = cerebral protection device

Principal findings from the randomised trials

- They are a very heterogeneous group of trials using different CAS technology as it evolved.
- Most were done before cerebral protection devices (CPD) were available.
- None required the obligatory use of a CPD. CREST and ICSS (ongoing) are awaited.
- Some were undertaken before optimisation of antiplatelet therapy (dual treatment).
- Three stenosis subgroups were used (ECST or NASCET based?).
- Different definitions of operative risk (and stroke definitions) were used.
- 30-day death/stroke rates were relatively high in most studies (especially after CAS).
- Two were abandoned (excess risk in CAS group: Leicester, WALLSTENT).
- EVA-3S was suspended because of excess risk in the CAS group (later restarted but suspended again).
- SPACE was stopped early because of recruitment and potential funding problems.

◆ Very little late follow-up data were available (to date only in CAVATAS).

◆ Following successful CAS, long-term stroke rates were similar to CEA (CAVATAS).

◆ No other specific conclusions can be drawn; there is no evidence of superiority for CAS or CEA.

Specific studies

The three most important studies are CAVATAS, EVA-3S and SPACE. They were all large, nationally-based trials. The latter two being contemporary sets them apart from the older and much criticised CAVATAS. Notwithstanding the extremely high complication rates in CAVATAS (which would have been higher had they used a 24-hour definition for stroke), the most important finding was that after successful CAS, the three-year cumulative stroke risk was the same as after CEA [15] **(Ib/A)**. This is an important observation, suggesting that the key to optimising long-term stroke prevention is the reduction of initial risk. CAVATAS has now been superseded by the ICSS study that requires the obligatory use of stents and CPDs in a larger cohort of patients.

SPACE is the largest trial published to date and was powered to demonstrate that CAS was 'not-inferior' to CEA [18]. This was not demonstrated (Table 1). The 30-day death/stroke rate after CAS was 7.7%, compared with 6.5% following CEA. Somewhat predictably, an alternative conclusion has begun to emerge publicly, that while the trial failed to show non-inferiority for CAS, no statistically significant difference really existed between the two treatment modalities.

EVA-3S was also important, but for completely different reasons [17]. This French equivalent of CAVATAS was suspended in 2003 because of an excess procedural stroke risk in the CAS group. The Data Monitoring Committee thereafter decided that the trial be restarted with the recommendation that a CPD was employed routinely. The trial resumed, but was again suspended in October 2005 after recruiting 527 patients. The trial was suspended again by the safety committee after the stroke and death rate at 30 days was found to be 9.6% after

CAS and 3.9% after CEA. This study is an important challenge to current opinion, largely generated from registry data, that CPDs will significantly improve outcomes after CAS [11].

CEA vs CAS in asymptomatic patients

Table 2 summarises the very limited data from the two randomised trials in asymptomatic patients and instantly raises two controversies. The first is that LEXINGTON II somehow managed to devise a power calculation requiring only 85 patients to be randomised [19]. It is baffling how this was accepted by an Ethics Committee. Using no CPDs (just like its sister symptomatic trial), not one patient in either arm of the study suffered a stroke, either during the peri-operative period or the four years of follow-up. Moreover, not one patient in either limb of either study developed a significant restenosis during follow-up. It remains difficult to put the LEXINGTON trials in context, but neither has really contributed towards a

Table 2. Summary of the published results from the randomised trials in asymptomatic patients (CEA vs CAS).

	LEXINGTON II	SAPPHIRE
Methodology		
Year published	2004	2004
No randomised	n=85	CEA=121
		CAS=117
Stenosis range	80-99%	80-99%
Stent used	WALLSTENT	SMART/PRECISE
CPD used	NO	ANGIOGUARD

30-day outcomes	CEA	CAS	CEA	CAS
Death	0.0%	0.0%		
Death/ipsilateral stroke	0.0%	0.0%		
Death/any stroke	0.0%	0.0%	6.1%	5.8%
Death/disabling stroke	0.0%	0.0%		

Late outcomes				
4-year any CVA	0.0%	0.0%		
4-year restenosis (>70%)	0.0%	0.0%		

Final outcome	Completed	Stopped early

more discriminating analysis of who benefits most from CEA or CAS.

The most controversial (and yet paradoxically the most influential) study is SAPPHIRE [20]. Unlike all the other randomised trials, SAPPHIRE recruited only patients who were considered high-risk for surgical intervention and thereafter randomised them between surgery and CAS (using a stent and CPD produced by the sponsoring company). To qualify for entry, patients had to be either symptomatic with a 50-99% stenosis, or asymptomatic with an 80-99% stenosis and have at least one additional adverse risk factor (significant cardiac disease, severe pulmonary disease, contralateral occlusion, recurrent laryngeal nerve palsy, neck irradiation, recurrent stenosis after CEA or aged >80 years). The interpretation of this study hinges on the definition of high risk. Although the trial recruited asymptomatic and symptomatic patients, 71% were actually asymptomatic. Accordingly, the data from this majority subset have been presented in Table 2 in the asymptomatic section. In short, a trial comprising mostly asymptomatic patients has been used to justify practice in all high-risk patients and, by inference, symptomatic patients as well.

SAPPHIRE's primary endpoint at 30 days was death/stroke and ECG/enzyme evidence of myocardial infarction (MI). Surgeons were resentful of the inclusion of MI within the primary endpoint, but this decision was not unreasonable because there is emerging evidence that occult MI is a predictor of poor long-term cardiovascular risk. This misplaced anger, however, actually deflected attention from the fact that the trial's conclusions were totally unjustified. The SAPPHIRE results (in a predominantly asymptomatic population) have been hailed as showing that CAS was not inferior to CEA when treating patients considered high-risk for surgical intervention. Inevitably, this has evolved to elevate CAS as the preferred choice in any high-risk patient [11]. In fact, this interpretation is not at all supported by the data. Table 2 shows that both CEA and protected CAS were associated with a 6% 30-day risk of death/stroke in the asymptomatic cohort, who made up the vast majority of patients in SAPPHIRE. It is a simple fact that at this level of risk neither intervention confers any benefit regarding long-term stroke prevention **(Ib/A)**. Accordingly, it would be wrong to label any asymptomatic patient (especially a woman, or anyone over 75 years) as high risk for stroke, based on currently available data **(Ib/A)**. Once the procedural risk exceeds 4%, all long-term benefit

Table 3. 30-day outcomes from 'high-risk' carotid stent registries *.							
	ARCHeR	CHRS	SECuRITY	BEACH	CABERNET	MAVERiC	CREATE
n	437	161	305	480	454	498	419
Criteria λ	>80%A	>80%A	>50%S	>50%S	>60%A		>50%S
	>50%S	>70%S	>80%A	>80%A	>50%S		>70%A
Symptoms ∝	48%A	75%A	79%A	76%A	76%A		83%A
	52%S	25%S	21%s	24%S	24%S		17%S
Restenosis after CEA	32%	41%	21%	41%			23%
30-day death	2.3%	1.2%	1.0%	1.6%	0.5%	1.0%	1.0%
30-day stroke	5.3%	6.2%	6.9%	4.6%	3.4%	3.6%	5.5%
30-day death/ stroke	6.6%	6.8%	6.9%	5.3%	3.6%		
30-day death/ stroke/MI	7.8%	7.5%	8.5%	5.8%	3.8%	5.9%	6.2%

* none of the studies has been reported in a peer reviewed journal.

λ = stenosis thresholds for including symptomatic (S) and asymptomatic (A) patients in the registry

∝ = percentage of registry cohort who were asymptomatic (A) or symptomatic (S)

from intervention in asymptomatic patients (whether it be CEA or CAS) ceases. Remember, these patients were high risk for surgical intervention, not high risk for stroke.

High-risk registries

Although SAPPHIRE was flawed, it was nevertheless highly influential because it triggered another growth industry, the emergence of high-risk stent registries. It was the emergence of one of these registries (ARCHeR) that was cited as the principal reason for stopping SAPPHIRE early. Seven of these registries (all commercially funded) have now released their data, though none in a peer reviewed journal. All were developed to support applications for Federal approval for proprietary stents and CPDs.

Table 3 summarises the principal findings. As can be seen, most adopted SAPPHIRE inclusion criteria, most used the extended primary endpoint (including MI) and most shared the same demographic characteristics. In short, most patients were again asymptomatic, including a high proportion with recurrent stenoses after CEA. Although the composite endpoint (death/stroke/MI) was the most frequently quoted, 30-day death/stroke rates were identifiable provided the data were searched thoroughly.

The results are very similar to those found in the asymptomatic patients in SAPPHIRE. Accordingly, the main conclusions are generally the same. These patients do not represent a cohort of patients who are high risk for stroke and, accordingly, the data do not support preferential use of CAS in patients defined as high risk in this way. The inevitable conclusion is that asymptomatic patients considered high risk for CEA (as opposed to stroke) should probably be treated conservatively **(IV/C)**.

Conclusions

Symptomatic patients

The randomised comparisons of CEA and CAS have not had the same impact as the earlier symptomatic and asymptomatic trials comparing CEA with BMT. Six have reported, but most were stopped prematurely. None has demonstrated superiority for either treatment modality,

but several have raised concerns **(Ib/A)**. Hopefully, ICSS and CREST will provide better data for interpretation in the future; there is still good reason to continue randomising patients. One important piece of information has, however, emerged. In its credentialing phase, CREST found that patients over 80 years had an unacceptably high death/stroke rate after CAS (approximately 12%), and these are now excluded from the trial with a recommendation that they be treated by CEA [21]. A similar finding (excess procedural risk after CAS in patients aged >75 years) was also observed in SPACE [18].

It is likely that CAS will assume an increasing role in intermediate-risk, symptomatic patients **(IV/C)**, provided the impact of the learning curve is lessened. This may extend to 80-100 procedures [22], and yet no model has ever factored in the effect of this learning curve on the overall effectiveness of stroke prevention conferred by CAS. Paradoxically the learning curve is less of a problem with CEA.

Surgeons probably need not worry too much about erosion of their practice. The future will undoubtedly see increasing political emphasis towards treating patients with TIA/minor stroke as an emergency, largely because many suffer a stroke before being seen in the outpatient department. This group will be directed towards emergency centres that will target patients for expeditious thrombolysis, anticoagulation, or rapid intervention (within days) for patients with severe carotid disease. Inevitably, these patients will have a very high incidence of luminal thrombus and surgeons are likely to be too pre-occupied dealing with these truly high-risk patients to worry about whether their practice will diminish.

Asymptomatic patients

The least amount of quality evidence (in fact none) to guide practice exists inevitably in the cohort in whom the most controversy will develop. Two more international (randomised) trials are in the embryonic planning phase. There are methodological and conceptual differences between the two trials but, hopefully, these can be reconciled so that everyone can collaborate in a single (extremely) large study. In the interim, the available evidence cannot support the uncritical use of CAS in asymptomatic patients outwith randomised trials.

Key points	Evidence level

Recently symptomatic 50-99% (NASCET) stenosis

◆ In the low/intermediate-risk patient (for CEA), there is still no randomised trial evidence that CAS is superior to CEA. **Ia/A**

◆ Until evidence of equivalence or non-inferiority for CAS is established, most patients should still be considered for randomisation in ICSS or CREST. **Ia/A**

◆ Centres with established CAS programmes for low/intermediate-risk symptomatic patients can continue to offer this service, provided independently audited procedural risks are comparable to those accepted for carotid surgery. **Ia/A**

◆ CAS is, however, an appropriate alternative to CEA in patients deemed high risk for surgery, provided the patient is recently symptomatic, and the independently audited procedural risks are ≤8%. Patient selection is a balance of risk and benefit. Maximum benefit is observed in patients with 70-99% stenoses who are (i) male, (ii) aged >75 years with (iii) plaque irregularity or (iv) contralateral occlusion. Females and patients with moderate stenoses are at relatively low risk of stroke in the long term. **IIa/B**

Asymptomatic 70-99% (NASCET) stenosis

◆ In the low/intermediate-risk patient (for CEA), there is currently no evidence that CAS is superior or even equivalent to CEA, largely because CEA and CAS have never been subjected to randomised comparison. Accordingly, unless CAS is undertaken with an independently audited procedural risk of <4%, CAS cannot be recommended as an alternative to CEA in low/intermediate-risk patients outwith randomised trials. **IV/C**

◆ In the high-risk (for CEA) patient, there is no systematic evidence that CAS confers any reduction in long-term stroke risk over best medical therapy alone, unless the independently audited procedural risk is <4%. There is no evidence to support raising this threshold for risk in asymptomatic patients at high risk for CEA. **IV/C**

References

1. Kennedy J, Quan H, Chali WA, Feasby TE. Variations in rates of appropriate and inappropriate carotid endarterectomy for stroke prevention in four Canadian Provinces. *CMAJ* 2004; 171: 455-9.

2. Naylor AR. Does the modern concept of 'best medical therapy' render carotid surgery obsolete? *Eur J Vasc Endovasc Surg* 2004; 28: 457-61.

3. Asymptomatic Carotid Surgery Trial Collaborators. The MRC Asymptomatic Carotid Surgery Trial (ACST): carotid endarterectomy prevents disabling and fatal carotid territory strokes. *Lancet* 2004; 363: 1491-502.

4. Gaines PA, Randall MS. Carotid artery stenting for patients with asymptomatic carotid disease (and news on TACIT). *Eur J Vasc Endovasc Surg* 2005; 30: 461-3.

5. Rothwell PM, Eliasziw M, Gutnikov, *et al,* for the Carotid Endarterectomy Trialists' Collaboration. Endarectomy for symptomatic carotid stenosis in relation to clinical subgroups and timing of surgery. *Lancet* 2004; 363: 915-24.

6. Rothwell PM, Eliasziw M, Gutnikov, *et al,* for the Carotid Endarterectomy Trialists' Collaboration. Sex difference in the effect of time from symptoms to surgery on benefit from carotid endarterectomy for transient ischaemic attack and non-disabling stroke. *Stroke* 2004; 35: 2855-61.

7. Executive Committee for the Asymptomatic Carotid Atherosclerosis Study. Endarterectomy for asymptomatic carotid artery stenosis. *JAMA* 1995; 273: 1421-8.

8. Rothwell PM. ACST: which subgroups will benefit most from carotid endarterectomy? *Lancet* 2004; 364: 1122-3.

9. Zahn R, Mark B, Niedermaier N, *et al.* Embolic protection devices for carotid artery stenting: better results than stenting without protection. *Eur Heart J* 2004; 25: 1550-8.

10. Bosiers M, Peeters P, Deloose K, *et al.* Does carotid artery stenting work on the long run: 5-year results in high-volume centers (ELOCAS Registry). *J Cardiovasc Surg* 2005; 46: 241-7.

11. Roubin GS, Iyer S, Halkin A, *et al.* Realizing the potential of carotid artery stenting: proposed paradigms for patient selection and procedural technique. *Circulation* 2006; 113: 2021-30.

12. Naylor AR, Golledge J. High risk plaque, high risk patient or high risk procedure? *Eur J Vasc Endovasc Surg* 2006; in press.

13. Naylor AR, Bolia A, Abbott RJ, *et al.* Randomized study of carotid angioplasty and stenting versus carotid endarterectomy: a stopped trial. *J Vasc Surg* 1998; 28: 326-34.

14. Alberts MJ, WALLSTENT. Results of a multicenter prospective randomized trial of carotid artery stenting versus carotid endarterectomy (abstract). *Stroke* 2001; 32: 325.

15. CAVATAS Investigators. Endovascular versus surgical treatment in patients with carotid stenosis in the Carotid and Vertebral Artery Transluminal Angioplasty Study (CAVATAS): a randomised trial. *Lancet* 2001; 357: 1729-37.

16. Brooks WM, McClure RR, Jones MR, *et al.* Carotid angioplasty and stenting versus carotid endarterectomy: randomized trial in a community hospital. *J Am Coll Cardiol* 2001; 38: 1589-95.

17. EVA-3S Investigators. Carotid angioplasty and stenting with and without cerebral protection: clinical alert from the endarterectomy versus angioplasty in patients with symptomatic severe carotid stenosis. *Stroke* 2004; 35: e18-e20.

18. SPACE Collaborative Group. 30-day results from the SPACE trial of stent-protected angioplasty versus carotid endarterectomy in symptomatic patients: a randomised non-inferiority trial. *Lancet* 2006; in press.

19. Brooks WH, McClure RR, Jones MR, *et al.* Carotid angioplasty and stenting versus carotid endarterectomy for treatment of asymptomatic carotid stenosis: a randomised trial in a community hospital. *Neurosurgery* 2004; 54: 318-24.

20. Yadav JS, Wholey MH, Kuntz RE, *et al,* for the SAPPHIRE Investigators. Protected carotid artery stenting versus endarterectomy in high-risk patients. *N Engl J Med* 2004; 351: 1493-1501.

21. Hobson RW, Howard VJ, Roubin GS, *et al,* for the CREST Investigators. Carotid artery stenting is associated with increased complications in octogenarians: 30-day stroke and death rates in the CREST lead-in phase. *J Vasc Surg* 2004; 40: 1106-11.

22. Ahmadi R, Willfort A, Lang W, *et al.* Carotid artery stenting: effect of learning curve and intermediate-term morphological outcome. *J Endovasc Ther* 2001; 8: 539-46.

Chapter 5

Risk factor management in peripheral arterial disease

Cliff Shearman BSc MB BS FRCS MS, Professor of Vascular Surgery

University of Southampton, Southampton General Hospital, Southampton, UK

Introduction

Atherosclerotic peripheral arterial disease (PAD) affects an estimated 27 million people in Europe and North America [1]. The disease may remain asymptomatic or manifest as intermittent claudication or critical leg ischaemia (CLI). The Edinburgh Artery Study surveyed a population aged between 55 and 74 years and found that 4.5% had symptomatic claudication, 8.0% had major asymptomatic disease and a further 16.6% had abnormal haemodynamic variables indicative of PAD [2]. Over a five-year follow-up the development of new symptoms of claudication was confined to those who previously had asymptomatic disease [3]. This is encouraging as it suggests there is a window of opportunity to prevent disease progression. CLI is another daunting problem, with an annual incidence of 500-1000 patients per million of the population and an annual cost to the NHS of over £200 million [4].

PAD not only affects quality of life, it is also a powerful marker of cardiovascular risk. Patients with PAD are six times more likely to die from cardiovascular disease (CVD) within ten years than those with no PAD [5]. The accrued mortality risk of those with PAD is 30% within five years, rising to 78% within 15 years (compared to 22% in subjects with no PAD) [6, 7]. To put this into context, five years after diagnosis the death rate for a patient with PAD is twice that of a patient with breast cancer [1]. In fact PAD ranks alongside angina, diabetes and even previous myocardial infarction and stroke in importance as a risk factor for CVD [1, 3]. The outlook for someone with CLI is even worse - one in five will be dead from CVD within a year of diagnosis.

Ankle brachial pressure index (ABPI) is a major progressive marker of cardiovascular risk. An ABPI of ≤0.9 is 95% sensitive in detecting angiographically defined disease and, importantly, can predict an increased risk of mortality or major cardiovascular morbidity [2]. Although symptomatic patients fare worse, even asymptomatic PAD is associated with much lower survival rates than in healthy individuals [5].

It has become apparent that atherosclerosis is not a slowly progressive disease, but can undergo periods of intense biological activity resulting in intra-plaque haemorrhage or rupture. These sudden changes either occlude a vessel or expose the highly thrombogenic subintimal surface, promoting platelet adherence and activation. This process is termed atherothrombosis and most clinical vascular events (such as myocardial infarction) are associated with such acute changes in the plaque. Plaque instability is strongly associated with inflammatory changes, both locally and systemically. These observations have prompted renewed interest in exploring ways to reduce the clinical sequelae of PAD [8].

Based on the above observations, a major component of the treatment of PAD should include measures to reduce the excessive associated cardiovascular mortality and morbidity, as well as to attenuate the progression of arteriosclerosis. Several factors that increase cardiovascular risk have been identified (Table 1). This chapter examines the prevalence of these factors and the evidence of benefit that might accrue from their modification.

Table 1. Risk factors associated with cardiovascular disease.

Fixed	Modifiable	Lifestyle
Age	Smoking	Exercise
Gender	Cholesterol	Antiplatelet drugs
Diabetes (Type 1)	Diabetes (Type 2)	Diet
Family history	Hypertension	Vitamins/antioxidants
Genotype	Metabolic syndrome	

Risk factors

The large Interheart Sudy found that over 90% of the risk of myocardial infarction could be determined from the following factors [9] **(IIa/B)**:

- abnormal lipids;
- smoking;
- hypertension;
- diabetes;
- abdominal obesity;
- psychosocial factors;
- diet (regular consumption of fruit, vegetables and alcohol);
- regular exercise [9].

The REACH (Reduction of Atherothrombosis for Continued Health) Registry is a multinational registry of patients with established coronary artery disease (CAD), cerebrovascular disease or PAD (or patients with at least three risk factors for atherosclerosis) [10]. The Registry consists of 63,814 patients and the aim is to observe the burden of disease in those with atherosclerosis and to monitor the outcome over at least two years. Of the 7,663 patients with symptomatic PAD, 37% had PAD alone, 40% also had CAD, 9% also had cerebrovascular disease and 14% had all three manifestations of atherothrombosis. In this Registry those with PAD alone had a high prevalence of associated risk factors: 39% were diabetic, 73% were hypertensive, 59% had hypercholesterolaemia, 46% were former smokers and 31% were current smokers. Disappointingly, only 32% of these individuals were receiving adequate treatment (Table 2).

Smoking

Cigarette smoking is the leading cause of preventable death in the Western World; one in five of all deaths are attributable to cigarettes [11]. It is also the single most important risk factor for PAD, associated with a three-fold increased risk of developing the disease [12]. Clinically significant disease progression is also more likely in persistent smokers, subsequent intervention is less likely to succeed and amputation is more common compared to non-smokers [13]. Active cigarette smoking is associated with an 80% risk of cardiovascular disease, but even passive smokers, with about one hundredth of the exposure, experience a 30% increased risk [14] **(Ia/A)**.

It remains unclear precisely how cigarette smoke causes damage and whether it is dose-related. Both nicotine and carbon monoxide in smoke appear to cause harm in a number of ways, including affecting other risk factors. Smoking increases blood pressure and total serum cholesterol, reduces oxygen carriage, increases vascular resistance and vasospasm (which may cause plaque rupture), and adversely affects vascular endothelium, platelets and thrombotic mechanisms. Free radical-mediated oxidative stress seems to be of particular importance, and this may play a central role in all of the above events [13].

There are short-term and long-term benefits from stopping smoking. Nicotine levels fall by half within eight hours and carbon monoxide levels return to

Table 2. The findings of the Reach Registry (Reduction of Atherothrombosis for Continued Health). The Registry consists of 63,814 patients with peripheral arterial disease (PAD), coronary artery disease (CAD) or cerebrovascular disease (CVD). *Modified from* [10].

Patients with PAD (n=7663)		Associated risk factors in PAD Group	
PAD alone	37.1%	Diabetes	38.7%
PAD + CAD	39.6%	Hypertension	73.3%
PAD + CVD	9.3%	Dyslipidaemia	58.7%
PAD + CAD + CVD	14.1%	Smoking	
		Current	31%
		Ex	46%

normal in 24-48 hours; oxygen carriage and blood pressure take longer to normalise. Evidence of the benefit of stopping smoking has never been established in a randomised controlled trial, but several large cohort studies have shown clearly that smoking cessation produces cardiovascular benefit [15]. The excess cardiovascular risk is halved within one year and the risk is the same as for non-smokers within 5-15 years. After surgical intervention the benefit of stopping smoking is still apparent. In the Coronary Artery Surgery Study (CASS) those who had undergone coronary artery bypass surgery and given up smoking had a significantly better survival rate at ten years (84% v 68%) and less re-intervention than those who continued to smoke [16]. Several observational studies have identified an improvement in walking distance in patients with claudication and a reduced risk of amputation in those who gave up cigarettes.

Persuading patients to stop smoking is notoriously difficult - success rates as low as 2% are reported. However, this can be improved to 27% with the support of nicotine patches, counselling and behaviour modification [17]. Legislation also seems to have a marked effect, not only on smoking habits but probably also on the associated CVD [18]. It is estimated that smoking-related diseases cost the health service in the UK £1.4 billion per year and that smoking cessation is highly cost-effective [19]. The large benefit from stopping smoking and the large numbers of people at risk mean that even a modest reduction in the number of smokers has a big impact.

Diabetes

Insulin resistance is a common finding in diabetic and non-diabetic patients with PAD and seems to play a key role in atherogenesis [20]. Those with Type 2 diabetes have a 3-5 times increased risk of developing PAD compared to non-diabetics. Intensive blood glucose control does not appear to reduce the risk of developing macrovascular disease or prevent amputation [21]. However, development of the complications of diabetes is strongly associated with previous episodes of hyperglycaemia reflected by HbA1C levels. A reduction of 1% in HbA1C is associated with a 21% reduction in complications [22]. Also, associated risk factors seem to be amplified in patients with diabetes and optimising them gains more benefit than in non-diabetics [23] **(Ia/A)**.

Cholesterol

That elevated cholesterol levels increase the risk of ischaemic heart disease in a linear manner is well established [24]. Although the relationship is more complex for PAD, there is evidence of a strong association [25]. Attempts at reducing cholesterol levels by diet are generally disappointing, producing only modest reductions of 5-10% and requiring considerable patient encouragement. The statin class of drugs (HMG-CoA reductase inhibitors) produce reductions in serum cholesterol of around 25-30% and appear safe. Several large, prospective primary intervention studies (West of Scotland Coronary Prevention Study [26], Air Force/Texas Coronary

Atherosclerosis Prevention Study [27]) and secondary intervention studies (Scandinavian Simvastatin Survival Study [28], Cholesterol and Recurrent Events Study [29]) have demonstrated a significant reduction in cardiovascular events associated with cholesterol-lowering therapy using statins. Cholesterol was lowered by about 25% with a risk reduction of about 30%, the benefits being greatest in those with the highest cardiovascular risk **(Ia/A)**.

The Heart Protection Study randomised 20,536 adults with cholesterol >3.5mmol/l who were considered to be at increased cardiovascular risk to simvastatin (40mg day) or placebo for five years. For the 2701 patients with PAD, the major cardiovascular event rate was 24.7% in the treatment group compared to 30.5% in the placebo group [30]. This resulted in an event rate of 247/1000 per five years for those taking simvastatin compared to 300/1000 per five years for those taking placebo. During the study there was also an overall 24% reduction in the need for re-vascularisation procedures (cardiac and peripheral) in the simvastatin group. Simvastatin also appeared safe; this very large study found no difference in terms of reported muscle pain or ache between the groups **(Ib/A)**.

A number of previous small studies had suggested that statins might have a direct effect on atherosclerotic plaque. The Asteroid Study used intravascular ultrasonography to demonstrate a reduction in coronary artery plaque volume in patients taking a high dose of rosuvastatin (40mg/day) over a 24-month interval [31]. Although encouraging, further work is needed to determine whether this translates into clinical benefit.

Hypertension

Elevated blood pressure is very common - it has been estimated that up to 24% of the adult population may be hypertensive. It is not only a strong independent predictor of CVD, especially stroke and ischaemic heart disease, but is also associated with an approximately three-fold increased risk of PAD [32]. Clear benefit through treating hypertension has been demonstrated in a number of studies **(Ia/A)**. The stroke rate can be reduced by 38%, cardiovascular

deaths by 14%, and other cardiovascular events by 26%; these effects are also apparent in elderly patients. In the Heart Outcomes Prevention Evaluation Study, normotensive patients with PAD treated with ramapril had a significant reduction in cardiovascular events [33].

Metabolic syndrome

Metabolic syndrome is a cluster of conditions that include obesity, dyslipidaemia, hypertension and hyperinsulinaemia [34]. Obesity is the dominant factor and it is increased visceral fat, in particular, that seems to be important. Waist circumference alone is very effective in identifying those affected, but a more accurate diagnosis requires any three of the following five features:

- waist circumference >102cm (men); >88cm (women);
- high density lipoprotein cholesterol <1.04mmol/l (men); <1.29mmol/l (women);
- triglyceride >1.69mmol/l;
- blood pressure >130/85mmHg;
- fasting glucose >6.1mmol/l.

Patients with metabolic syndrome have a 20% increased risk of CVD and, as obesity has become so common in the USA and Europe, it is likely that this condition will become one of the commonest identifiable risk factors. The obvious solution is weight reduction and increased exercise, but patient compliance is poor. A number of drugs are now being marketed to aid weight loss, either by acting on central receptors to suppress appetite or on fat cells directly.

Exercise

A sedentary lifestyle is a major risk for CVD. Those who undertake even a moderate amount of exercise on a regular basis, such as walking 30 minutes a day, have half the cardiovascular mortality rate of those who rarely exercise. Increasing physical activity in previously inactive adults is beneficial, but the effect is lost if the individual returns to their previous lifestyle. Exercise combined with weight loss is associated with a reduction in cholesterol and blood pressure; several studies suggest clinical benefit.

Exercise may also improve the walking ability of patients with PAD and a meta-analysis of 21 studies has suggested an improvement in walking distance of 124% [35]. Walking for 30 minutes a day, three times a week for six months, appears to produce the greatest benefit. Although some form of walking is better, upper limb exercises also seem to confer benefit, presumably by improving cardiovascular fitness. The optimal method and frequency of exercise therapy, and whether it needs to be supervised, has not been established **(IIa/B)**.

Numerous mechanisms have been proposed for this improvement, including muscle fibre-type transformation, metabolic adaptation, increased muscle capillary blood flow, reduction in blood viscosity and simply using non-ischaemic muscles. On balance, exercise is essential for patients with PAD, as it not only improves the primary problem in the leg, but also reduces cardiovascular risk. The main challenge remains making it attractive to patients.

Antiplatelet agents

Platelets show evidence of increased activation in patients with PAD. Atheromatous plaque rupture may lead to further platelet activation and aggregation at the site of disruption. This can cause occlusion of the vessel or sudden increase in plaque volume, resulting in a clinical event. Aspirin irreversibly blocks platelet cyclo-oxygenase-mediated production of thromboxane A2, a powerful promoter of platelet aggregation. Experimentally, low doses of 40-80mg are effective at blocking cyclo-oxygenase for the ten-day life span of the platelet, while higher doses may have an adverse effect on cyclo-oxygenase in the vascular endothelium and are more likely to cause bleeding complications.

The Antithrombotic Trialists' Collaboration meta-analysis of 2002 assessed 287 reports involving 135,000 patients in studies of an antiplatelet agent versus placebo and 77,000 patients in comparison studies of other antiplatelet agents [36]. Overall, they found that antiplatelet agents reduced the risk of serious cardiovascular events by approximately 25%. Unlike a previous meta-analysis from 1994, the 2002 paper described more patients with PAD (9214) and found that they had a significant reduction of 23% for serious cardiovascular events. Aspirin was the most widely used agent and benefits outweighed the risks of bleeding complications; 75-150mg was as effective as higher doses. For every 1000 patients with PAD treated with aspirin, it is likely that 10-20 vascular events would be prevented each year, but one to two patients would suffer a major gastrointestinal bleed [37].

Up to 20% of people cannot take aspirin or are resistant to it at normal doses. Furthermore, for those at high risk, aspirin alone may not be enough. Clopidogrel is a theopyridine derivative that blocks adenosine diphosphate-induced platelet activity. The CAPRIE Study, a large randomised study of 19,185 patients at increased cardiovascular risk, compared aspirin 325mg daily to clopidogrel 75mg daily [38]. There was a significant reduction in cardiovascular events in both treatment groups compared to what would have been expected if the patients had received no treatment. Clopidogrel was found to be more effective than aspirin, with a reduction in relative risk of 8.7%. From these data it was estimated that 1000 patients with arterial disease who did not receive aspirin would suffer 77 cardiovascular events in one year. Treatment with aspirin would reduce this by 19 events, but clopidogrel would reduce it by 24 events. On subgroup analysis, patients with PAD gained more benefit than those who had myocardial infarction or stroke, with a relative risk reduction of 23.8%. While clopidogrel is at least as safe as aspirin it is more expensive.

In the recent Charisma Study, clopidogrel combined with aspirin appeared not to have any advantage over aspirin alone in patients at increased cardiovascular risk. In fact, in low-risk patients, with risk factors alone, the combination appeared to do harm and increased the risk of bleeding [39] **(Ia/A)**.

Homocysteine

There have been several reports of a strong relationship between elevated serum homocysteine and PAD. In particular, elevated homocysteine is strongly associated with early onset atheroma. The mechanism of homocysteine-induced atheroma is multifactorial but probably involves impaired endothelial production of nitric oxide. Proliferation of smooth muscle cells can be reduced by dietary supplementation with folic acid, and vitamins B12 and B6. There have been no randomised controlled trials of this treatment, but there are preliminary claims that it can slow atherosclerotic plaque progression.

Antioxidants and vitamins

Oxidative damage seems to play a significant role in the genesis and progression of atherosclerosis. Patients with claudication have less antioxidant capacity, supporting the hypothesis that is has been mopped up by continued oxidant activity. It is possible then that antioxidants, such as vitamins C and E, ß carotene and selenium, could be used to reduce the risk of CVD. Although appealing, and probably safe, there is no evidence to support the use of these vitamins as a protection against atherosclerosis. Omega-3 fatty acids (fish oils) have been shown to reduce re-infarction rate after myocardial infarction and may reduce inflammation in atherosclerotic plaque. Preliminary results suggest that they may also improve walking in PAD, but at present the evidence is not conclusive.

Oestrogen

CVD is the commonest cause of death in post-menopausal women. Several observational studies have suggested a reduction in cardiovascular death in women taking hormone replacement therapy, promoting the suggestion that oestrogen may be cardioprotective. However, a recent study that randomised women after myocardial infarction to placebo or oestrogen treatment failed to show any benefit from hormone replacement therapy, largely due to the increased thrombotic complications in the group receiving oestrogen.

Conclusions

In risk factor identification and reduction, any potential benefit must be weighed against the risk of intervention and the cost of identifying and treating the risk factor. There is overwhelming evidence to suggest that active risk factor intervention significantly reduces cardiovascular mortality in patients with PAD. In general, most of the interventions discussed above are safe, or at least of low risk. They are highly cost-effective. Despite the evidence, in the UK over 50% of patients with PAD do not receive optimum treatment; this is the real challenge.

In the past, most patients with PAD were treated either by a vascular surgeon or a general practitioner. Increasingly, in the UK at least, specialist nurses are taking on this role. The essence of risk factor management lies in having well-developed protocols and good relationships with other relevant medical teams, such as diabetic physicians. Patients need to comply with these protocols, and this is another challenge. To date, the most successful clinical programmes have employed intervention at several different levels and tend to be part of a community-based health awareness campaign. Although not easy, tackling some of the reversible causes of PAD could have as much impact on patient survival and quality of life as revascularisation procedures.

Key points	Evidence level
◆ PAD affects over 25% of adults over 55 years of age.	IIa/B
◆ Patients with PAD have three to four times risk of dying from cardiovascular disease.	IIa/B
◆ Modification of risk factors reduces cardiovascular mortality and morbidity in patients with PAD. This includes:	
• smoking cessation;	Ia/A
• treatment of hypertension;	Ia/A
• reduction of cholesterol;	Ia/A
• statin therapy;	Ib/A
• good glycaemia control in diabetes;	Ib/A
• antiplatelet therapy;	Ia/A
• exercise;	IIa/B
• weight loss if obese;	IIa/B
◆ Risk factor reduction is highly cost-effective.	IIa/B
◆ Many patients with PAD currently receive inadequate treatment.	IIa/B

References

1. Belch J, Topol E, Agnelli G, Bertrand M. Critical issues in peripheral arterial disease detection and management. *Arch Int Med* 2003; 163: 84-92.

2. Fowkes FG, Housley E, Cawood EH, *et al.* Edinburgh Artery Study: prevalence of symptomatic and asymptomatic peripheral arterial disease. *Int J Epidemiol* 1991; 20: 384-92.

3. Leng GC, Lee AJ, Fowkes FGR, *et al.* Incidence, natural history and cardiovascular events in symptomatic and asymptomatic peripheral arterial disease in the general population. *Int J Epidemiol* 1996; 25: 1172-81.

4. Hart WM, Guest JF. Critical limb ischaemia the burden of illness in the UK. *Br Med Econ* 1995; 8: 211-21.

5. Criqui MH, Langer RD, Fronek A, *et al.* Mortality over a period of 10 years in patients with peripheral arterial disease. *N Engl J Med* 1992; 326: 381-6.

6. Dormandy JA, Rutherford RB. Management of peripheral arterial disease (PAD) TACS Working Group. TransAtlantic Intersociety Consensus (TASC). *J Vasc Surg* 2000; 31(1 Pt2): S1-S296.

7. Tierney S, Fennessy F, Hayes DB. ABC of arterial and vascular disease. Secondary prevention of peripheral vascular disease. *Br Med J* 2000; 320: 1262-5.

8. Libby PGeng YJ, Aikawa M, *et al.* Macrophages and atherosclerotic plaque stability. *Curr Opin Lipidol* 1996; 7: 163-73.

9. Yusuf S, Hawken S, Ounpuu S, *et al*, on behalf of the INTERHEART Study Investigators. Effect of potentially modifiable risk factors associated with myocardial infarction in 52 countries (the INTERHEART study): case-control study. *Lancet* 2004; 364: 937-52.

10. REACH Registry. http://reachregistry.org/.2005.

11. Centres for disease control and prevention. Cigarette smoking - attributable mortality and years of potential life lost - United States, 1990. *Morb Mort Wkly Rep* 1993; 42: 645-9.

12. Hiatt WR, Hoag S, Hamman RF. Effect of diagnostic criteria on the prevalence of peripheral arterial disease. The San Luis Valley Diabetes Study. *Circulation* 1995; 91: 1472-9.

13. Hirch AT, Hoag S, Hamman RF. The role of tobacco cessation, antiplatelet and lipid-lowering therapies in the treatment of peripheral arterial disease. *Vasc Med* 1997; 2: 243-51.

14. Ambrose JA, Baruna RS. The pathophysiology of cigarette smoking and cardiovascular disease. An update. *JACC* 2004; 43: 1731-7.

15. Doll R, Peto R, Wheatley K, Gray R, Sutherland I. Mortality in relation to smoking: 40 years' observations on male British doctors. *Br Med J* 1994; 309: 901-11.

16. Cavender JB, Rogers WJ, Fisher LD, *et al.* Effects of smoking on survival and morbidity in patients randomised to medical or surgical therapy in the coronary artery surgery study (CASS): 10-year follow-up. *J Am Coll Cardiol* 1992; 20: 287-94.

17. Joseph AM, Norman SM, Ferry LH, *et al.* The safety of transdermal nicotine as an aid to smoking cessation in patients with cardiac disease. *N Engl J Med* 1996; 335: 1792-8.

18. Sargent RP, Shepard RM, Glantz SA. Reduced incidence of admissions for myocardial infarction associated with public smoking ban: before and after study. *Br Med J* 2004; 328: 977-80.

19. Parrott S, Godfrey C. The economics of smoking cessation. *Br Med J* 2004; 328: 947-9.

20. Uutisupa MIJ, Niskanen LK, Siitonen O, *et al*. The incidence of atherosclerotic vascular disease in relation to general factors, insulin level and abnormalities in lipoprotein composition in non-insulin-dependent diabetic and non-diabetic subjects. *Circulation* 1990; 82: 27-36.

21. UK Prospective Diabetes Study (UKPDS) Group. Intensive blood glucose control with sulphonureas or insulin compared with conventional treatment and risk of complications in patients with type 2 diabetes (UKPDS 33). *Lancet* 1998; 352: 837-53.

22. Stratton IM, Adler AI, Neil HAW, *et al*. Association of glycaemia with macrovascular and microvascular complications of type 2 diabetes (UKPDS 35): prospective observational study. *Br Med J* 2000; 321: 405-12.

23. Stamler J, Vaccaro O, Neaton JD, Wentworth D. Diabetes, other risk factors, and 12-yr cardiovascular mortality for men screened in the multiple risk factor intervention trial. *Diabetes Care* 1993; 16: 434-44.

24. Consensus Conference from the Office of Medical Applications of Research, National Institutes of Health, Bethesda, MD. Lowering blood cholesterol to prevent heart disease. *JAMA* 1985; 253: 2080-6.

25. Murabito JM, D'Agostino RB, Sibershatz H, Wilson WF. Intermittent claudication. A risk profile from the Framingham Heart Study. *Circulation* 1997; 96: 44-9.

26. Shepherd J, Cobbe SM, Ford I, *et al*, for the West of Scotland Coronary Prevention Group. Prevention of coronary heart disease with pravastatin in men with hypercholesterolemia. *N Engl J Med* 1996; 333: 1301-7.

27. Downs JR, Clearfield M, Weiss S, *et al*. Primary prevention of acute coronary heart disease with lovastatin in men and women with average cholesterol. *JAMA* 1998; 279: 1615-22.

28. Scandinavian Simvastatin Survival Study Group. Randomised trial of cholesterol lowering in 4444 patients with coronary heart disease: the Scandinavian Simvastatin Survival Study (4S). *Lancet* 1994; 344: 1383-9.

29. Sacks FM, Pfeffer MA, Moye LA, *et al*, for the Cholesterol and Recurrent Events Trial Investigators. The effect of pravastatin on coronary events after myocardial infarction in patients with average cholesterol levels. *N Engl J Med* 1996; 335: 1001-9.

30. Heart Protection Study Group Collaborative Group. MRC/BHF Heart Protection Study of cholesterol lowering with simvastatin in 20,536 high-risk individuals: a randomised placebo-controlled trial. *Lancet* 2002; 360: 7-22.

31. Nissen SE, Nicholls SJ, Sipahi I, *et al*, for the Asteroid Investigators. Effect of very high-intensity statin therapy on regression of coronary atherosclerosis. *JAMA* 2006; 295: 1556-65.

32. Hiatt WR. Medical treatment of peripheral arterial disease and claudication. *N Engl J Med* 2001; 344: 1608-21.

33. The Heart Outcomes Prevention Evaluation Study Investigators. Effects of an angiotensin-converting enzyme inhibitor, ramapril, on cardiovascular events in high-risk patients. *N Engl J Med* 2000; 342: 145-53.

34. Khunti K, Davies M. Metabolic syndrome. *Br Med J* 2005; 331: 1153-4.

35. Leng GC Fowler B, Ernst E. Exercise for the treatment of intermittent claudication. In: *The Cochrane Library*, 2002; Issue 3. Oxford: Update Software.

36. Antithrombotic Trialists' Collaboration. Collaborative meta-analysis of randomised trials of antiplatelet therapy for the prevention of death, myocardial infarction, and stroke in high-risk patients. *Br Med J* 2002; 324: 71-86.

37. Baigent C. Aspirin for everyone older than 50? For and against. *Br Med J* 2005; 330: 1442-3.

38. CAPRIE steering committee. A randomised, blinded, trial of clopidogrel versus aspirin in patients at risk of ischaemic events (CAPRIE). *Lancet* 1996; 348: 1329-39.

39. Bhatt DL, Fox KA, Hacke W, *et al*, for the Charisma Investigators. Clopidogrel and aspirin versus aspirin alone for the prevention of atherothrombotic events. *N Engl J Med* 2006; 354: 1706-17.

Chapter 6

Management of intermittent claudication

Peter Lamont MD FRCS, Consultant Vascular Surgeon
Bristol Royal Infirmary, Bristol, UK

Introduction

The management of intermittent claudication remains one of the most controversial areas in vascular surgery. Scientific studies are confounded by the natural tendency of the symptoms to improve spontaneously. Clear guidelines are lacking and only a few good randomised studies in selected patient populations are available. The clinician can run the gamut from masterly inactivity, through drug treatment, to exercise training, to balloon angioplasty or even bypass surgery, without serious fear of criticism. Evidence in favour of any one of these therapies can be produced from the literature, although consensus on which is the most appropriate can be more difficult to elicit.

Claudication is, in itself, a relatively benign condition that need not produce major disability and patients may be content to accept the limitations imposed on their lifestyle. The first step in managing claudication is to decide whether it needs management at all, other than modification of risk factors (Chapter 5). Many patients seek treatment in the fear that their claudication is a harbinger of imminent gangrene and subsequent limb loss. Often simple reassurance about the natural history of the condition is all that is required. A prospective study of nearly 2,000 untreated claudicants followed for one year was reported by Dormandy and Murray in 1991; symptoms deteriorated to the extent of needing intervention in only 111 patients (5.5%) and 32 (1.6%) suffered a major amputation [1]. In the longer term, McAllister's study showed over six years that a patient with claudication had a 50% chance of improving spontaneously, a 30% chance of remaining unchanged and a 20% chance of deterioration, with seven of 100 patients losing a leg (six of whom had severe diabetes) [2] **(III/B)**.

Sufficient time, usually three months, must have passed from the onset of claudicant symptoms to ensure that the need for treatment will not be pre-empted by spontaneous improvement. If no improvement occurs, then both clinician and patient should come to a view about the effect of the claudication on quality of life. What exactly is the patient unable to do that he or she really wants to do and is there some lifestyle modification that would reduce the disability? If the patient remains keen for some form of treatment after examining these issues, what form of management is most appropriate?

Exercise training

Simple advice to take lots of exercise and walk at least a mile a day is laudable, but this has little effect on the quality of life as measured by an SF-36 questionnaire [3]. To this extent, Dr. Housley's treatment of claudication in five words "Stop smoking and keep walking" [4] is unlikely to improve matters much on its own. What regular exercise alone may achieve is a reduction in the annual rate of decline in walking distance, with non-exercisers declining at almost double the rate of those who walk for exercise three or more times a week [5]. In order to have a positive impact on walking distance and quality of life, exercise needs to be supervised initially, well structured and continued at home indefinitely [6] **(Ib/A)**.

Insufficient research has been done to specify the ideal exercise programme, but it is clear that some form of initial supervision in an exercise class is important to motivate the patient; most successful trials have used three supervised sessions a week for 12 weeks [7] **(Ia/A)**. After a period in a supervised environment the patient may well become self-motivated as the resulting improvement in walking distance becomes evident.

In a meta-analysis of exercise rehabilitation programmes for claudication, Gardner and Poehlman analysed those factors producing the greatest improvements in pain-free walking distance [8]. These factors included exercise continued for more than 30 minutes per session, at least three exercise sessions per week, walking used as the mode of exercise, near maximal pain during training used as the claudication pain endpoint and a programme lasting at least six months **(Ia/A)**.

Systematic review of randomised trials on the effects of exercise on claudication shows remarkably consistent results. All ten good quality trials identified in one review demonstrated an unequivocal improvement in pain-free and maximum walking distance/time ranging from 28-210% (mean 105%, SD 55.8%) [9]. Five of these trials had an untreated control group, and in all five studies the exercise training programme arm had better results than the untreated controls. A Cochrane database review has evaluated supervised exercise therapy compared to non-supervised exercise therapy [7]. The non-supervised group were advised to walk at least three times a week as opposed to no exercise at all. The review concluded that supervision produced a

significant and clinically relevant improvement in maximum walking distance, amounting to about 150m at three months. There seems little doubt that supervised exercise programmes have a place in the management of intermittent claudication [10] **(Ia/A)**.

Intermittent pneumatic compression

Recent randomised studies have reported improvement in walking distance using the technique of intermittent pneumatic compression of the calf and foot, compared to advice to exercise alone. Compression is applied for 2-2.5 hours per day, and both initial and absolute claudication distances have been shown to improve significantly, by around 200% after five months in one study [11] and by over 100m at one year in another [12]. The technique may be of value in patients unable to comply with a supervised exercise programme, although comparative studies are lacking **(Ib/A)**.

Drug therapy

Poor design of drug trials and the natural history of spontaneous improvement in claudiction make the value of drug treatment difficult to assess. In a meta-analysis of drug therapy for claudication, 75 different trials of 33 different pharmacological agents were analysed and deficiencies were found in 57 (76%) of them [13]. A significant inverse relationship between sample size and response in these studies suggested a bias produced by non-publication of negative results and the authors concluded that the information available did not establish convincingly that any drug consistently improved exercise performance in claudication **(Ia/A)**.

Two drugs, naftidrofuryl and cilostazol, are recommended for claudication in the UK [14]. In a meta-analysis of two French and two German placebo-controlled trials, a beneficial effect of naftidrofuryl on pain-free walking distance of claudicants was found [15]. The effects were most marked in non-smokers whose initial walking distance was over 150m before treatment commenced. After three months of treatment the mean improvement in pain-free walking distance of treated patients over controls was 54m. Two British randomised controlled trials have failed to show any overall benefit for naftidrofuryl over placebo [16, 17]. Subset analysis in the larger of these two trials showed a significant improvement in pain-free walking distance compared to initial walking distance for patients over 60 years of age who took the active agent. Patients over 60 years of age on placebo treatment did not improve their walking distance by a significant amount, but six months into the study their mean walking time to onset of pain was 155s, compared to 166s in the drug-treated group. The magnitude of any improvement from naftidrofuryl is not marked and probably not of clinical significance, making the cost-effectiveness of such treatment questionable **(Ia/A)**.

Cilostazol is a more recent introduction. Study results are variable, with improvements in maximal walking distance over placebo ranging from 21% in one large multicentre study [18], up to 50% in a meta-analysis of eight randomised, controlled trials [19]. Quality of life studies have shown some improvement in the physical well-being domain, although the drug has not been tested against supervised exercise programmes, many of which report a 100% increase in maximal walking distance **(Ia/A)**.

Few drug trials have considered whether or not their modest improvements in pain-free walking distance objectively influenced patients' quality of life, or if the agent studied would prove cost-effective if used in routine clinical practice. The evidence in favour of drug treatment is weak and, if drugs are to be used at all, it seems sensible to discontinue them after two or three months to assess if any improvement is dependent on drug ingestion or whether it is a result of spontaneous improvement. There is little sense in continuing drug therapy for more than a couple of months if symptoms are not improving.

The mainstay of drug therapy in claudicants is in the field of secondary prevention of coronary and cerebrovascular arterial disease. Although prescribed for secondary prevention rather than to treat claudication itself, both ramipril and atorvastatin have been noted to improve walking distances in claudicants. Non-hypertensive, non-diabetic patients treated with ramipril improved their maximal walking times by over six minutes compared to those receiving placebo, with a significant improvement in walking impairment questionnaire scores [20] **(Ib/A)**. Although atorvastatin did not improve maximal walking distance or quality of life scores, a dose of 80mg per day did produce a modest improvement in pain-free walking time and community-based physical activity compared to placebo [21] **(Ib/A)**.

Percutaneous transluminal angioplasty

Percutaneous transluminal angioplasty (PTA) using a balloon catheter remains a popular choice in the management of intermittent claudication. Complications are low with good patient selection and an experienced radiologist. Technical failure to dilate the lesion occurs in 10-20% of patients, but the need for surgical intervention to salvage the situation after an angioplasty misadventure is now <2%, with risks of amputation and death of <0.3% and <0.17%, respectively [22] **(III/B)**.

Patients who have PTA show improvement in their quality of life scores on an SF-36 questionnaire three months after the procedure [3]. Although restenosis occurs in over 20%, it is not always associated with recurrent symptoms; only one in ten restenoses causes more severe symptoms than those present before treatment. Restenosis and disease progression above, or below the angioplasty site do, however, cause a steady longer-term risk of recurrent symptoms, such that there is only a 60% chance of continuing clinical success three years after PTA. Similarly, quality of life scores revert to pre-angioplasty levels within two years [23].

While conventional PTA is most successful for occlusions <10cm long, the technique of subintimal angioplasty can be used to treat much longer femoropopliteal lesions and has been reported in patients with intermittent claudication [24, 25]. Results vary, with one-year primary assisted patency ranging from 37-62%, although there appears to be no detrimental effect on subsequent bypass surgery. Trials are lacking to compare subintimal angioplasty against exercise training or surgery **(III/B)**.

Comparison of conventional PTA with surgical bypass procedures reveals no significant differences in terms of survival, limb loss, haemodynamic improvement (ABPI) or quality of life [26] **(Ib/A)**. As angioplasty is a less invasive procedure with less time in hospital, shorter recovery times and lower costs, there is little doubt that PTA is preferable to bypass surgery in the presence of a suitable lesion. The real controversy, however, is whether such intervention produces better results than a supervised exercise programme.

A Cochrane review of PTA versus non-surgical management for intermittent claudication [23] has identified only two appropriate studies, one from Edinburgh [27, 28] and one from Oxford [29, 30]. The Edinburgh study compared the results of PTA against simple advice to stop smoking and keep walking. After six months the angioplasty group had a significantly improved pain-free walking distance compared to the conservatively treated group (median 667m versus 172m), as well as an improved quality of life measured by the Nottingham Health Profile. However, after two years of follow-up the picture changed dramatically. There was then no difference in either pain-free walking distance (median 383m versus 333m) or quality of life between the two groups **(Ib/A)**.

The Oxford study compared PTA with a supervised exercise programme. In the angioplasty group, maximum improvement in claudication distance had occurred by three months after treatment and improved no further over the ensuing 15 months. In the exercise group (supervised classes twice a week for six months), there was a continuing and incremental improvement in claudication distance at each of 6, 9, 12 and 15-month intervals. From six months onwards the claudication distances were better in the exercise group than in the angioplasty group. In the longer-term, after a median follow-up of 70 months, only a third of the remaining exercise patients were still exercising more than twice a week and there was no longer any significant difference in the maximum walking distance between the two groups. The exercise group had deteriorated from a peak of over 400m at 15 months back down to the same level as the PTA group (around 150m) after 70 months.

Stents

Attempts have been made to maintain the patency of angioplastied lesions by placing an endovascular stent across the angioplasty site. The technique is mostly used in the iliac segment, where it is favoured for the primary treatment of occlusion and the secondary treatment of restenosis. In the femoral segment, no significant difference in the clinical or haemodynamic outcome appears to be achieved by using a stent compared to angioplasty alone [31], with one-year patencies of 62% and 74% respectively [32]. Stenting of the femoral segment can improve the initial technical success rate in those with a poor result after balloon dilatation (because of dissection or residual stenosis), but, again, there is no difference in outcome between a policy of always using a stent compared to one of only using a stent selectively after suboptimal angioplasty; failure at one year is 34% and 33%, respectively [33] **(Ib/A)** (see Chapter 7).

Even in the iliac segment the value of stent placement is controversial. Meta-analysis of six angioplasty and eight stent studies shows four-year patencies in claudicants with iliac stenoses of 65% for PTA and 74% for PTA plus stenting [34]. In iliac occlusions the patencies were 54% for PTA and 61% for PTA plus stenting. This apparent small difference in favour of stenting did not stand up to scrutiny in a randomised trial from the Netherlands [35]. In this study of 279 patients there were no differences in technical success, clinical outcomes or re-intervention rates after two years' follow-up. Two-year cumulative patency rates were 71% in the PTA plus stent group versus 70% in the PTA alone group (although selective stenting was allowed in this group where a suboptimal haemodynamic result was obtained with angioplasty alone). After five to eight years' follow-up the patients who were selectively stented had a greater improvement in symptoms than those who had primary stenting, although there was no difference in iliac patency, ABPI or quality of life [36]. Since stent placement adds significant cost, there is little evidence to support its use as a primary adjunct to PTA, although it may have a place where the angioplasty result is suboptimal **(Ia/A)**.

Surgery

Surgical reconstruction of the aorto-iliac and femoropopliteal segments can be performed with good results. The real question is not whether surgery can be successful for claudication, but whether it is appropriate in the light of the risks involved for what is essentially a benign condition. The quality of life improves after successful surgery [3], but every vascular surgeon knows of a patient who came into hospital with the moderate disability of claudication and left hospital with the major disability of amputation after a failed bypass attempt. Even if the risk of this adverse event is less than 1%, can it be justified for a condition in which the natural history is for 80% of the patients either to improve spontaneously or to have no progression of symptoms over time? [2] A pragmatic answer is that a few patients have severely disabling and progressive symptoms, which interfere with their work or leave them housebound. In this selected group with major disability, surgery might reasonably be offered. However, it is essential that the patient understands and accepts the risks involved. Furthermore, such surgery should always be preceded by a period of conservative management to ensure that spontaneous improvement in symptoms does not occur. Finally, if the patient has a lesion suitable for PTA, that should be the preferred option. Studies of patients randomly assigned to operation or balloon angioplasty show no significant difference in outcomes [26, 37]. The less invasive nature of PTA dictates its preferential use where possible **(Ia/A)**.

As there is no apparent difference in outcome between exercise training and PTA [29, 30] or between PTA and surgery [26], perhaps exercise training might produce equivalent results to operation in those with claudication. A group from Goteborg in Sweden studied this issue in 75 patients, comparing not just surgery alone to exercise training alone, but also to surgery combined with subsequent exercise training [38]. After a one-year follow-up all three study groups showed improvement in walking distance. The best results were found in patients who had the combination of surgery followed by exercise training and there is a certain logic in this finding that treatment with two different modalities might be additive and beneficial. However, as the study contained only a small number of patients and the follow-up was for only one year, the conclusions that may be drawn are limited. This is an area that would benefit from further study **(Ib/A)**.

Conclusions

There is a wealth of evidence to support regular exercise as a lifestyle change in patients with cardiovascular disease generally. In the specific instance of intermittent claudication, all patients should be advised to exercise regularly and vascular surgeons should develop supervised exercise programmes. These programmes can encourage patients and monitor compliance with what for many is a stringent regimen. Most who comply with this regimen will never need interventional treatment. Finally, there is a need to educate both patients and those involved in their care that the medium to long-term outcome is likely to be just as good with exercise as with more aggressive intervention.

Drugs are not a very effective treatment for intermittent claudication. However, in resistant disease affecting those over 60 years of age, a three-month trial of naftidrofuryl or cilostazol may produce a modest improvement in walking distance.

PTA is an effective treatment, but supervised exercise training may prove a more cost-effective option. The role of adjunctive iliac stenting after PTA is uncertain. Although it has achieved a current popularity in clinical practice that owes more to fashion than to science, stents are expensive and randomised trials do not support their routine use.

Surgery must remain restricted to the more severe and disabling end of the spectrum of claudication. Even then, those thought suitable for surgery can improve with supervised exercise training, with the chance of avoiding an operation as a consequence. More use should be made of exercise before surgery and most certainly exercise is a useful adjunct thereafter.

Key points	Evidence level

- 50% of claudicants improve spontaneously over time and 30% do not deteriorate. III/B

- Supervised exercise training is an effective method of improving symptoms in the medium term and is more effective than advice to exercise. Ia/A

- Intermittent pneumatic compression of the foot and calf is an effective method of improving walking distance. Ib/B

- Drug therapy is mostly ineffective or unproven in rigorous clinical trials. Ia/A

- Modest benefits may be obtained with naftidrofuryl, cilostazol, ramipril and atorvastatin. Ib/A

- Percutaneous balloon angioplasty with selective stenting is just as effective as primary stenting both above and below the groin. Ib/A

- Percutaneous balloon angioplasty in suitable patients is as effective, but cheaper than surgery. Ib/A

- Exercise training is a useful adjunct to surgery. Ib/A

References

1. Dormandy JA, Murray GD. The fate of the claudicant - a prospective study of 1969 claudicants. *Eur J Vasc Surg* 1991; 5: 131-3.

2. McAllister FF. The fate of patients with intermittent claudication managed non-operatively. *Am J Surg* 1976; 132: 593-5.

3. Currie IC, Wilson YG, Baird RN, Lamont PM. Treatment of intermittent claudication: the impact on quality of life. *Eur J Vasc Endovasc Surg* 1995; 10: 356-36.

4. Housley E. Treating claudication in five words. *Br Med J* 1988; 296: 1483-4.

5. McDermott MM, Liu K, Ferrucci L, *et al.* Physical performance in peripheral arterial disease: a slower rate of decline in patients who walk more. *Ann Intern Med* 2006; 144: 10-20.

6. Tisi P, Shearman C. The impact of treatment of intermittent claudication on subjective health of the patient. *Health Trends* 1999; 30: 109-14.

7. Bendermacher BLW, Willigendael EM, Teijink JAW, Prins MH. Supervised exercise therapy versus non-supervised exercise therapy for intermittent claudication. *The Cochrane Database of Systematic Reviews* 2006; 2: CD005263. DOI: 10.1002/14651858.

8. Gardner AW, Poehlman ET. Exercise rehabilitation programs for the treatment of claudication pain. A meta-analysis. *JAMA* 1995; 27: 975-80.

9. Robeer GG, Brandsma JW, van den Heuvel SP, *et al.* Exercise therapy for intermittent claudication: a review of the quality of randomised clinical trials and evaluation of predictive factors. *Eur J Vasc Endovasc Surg* 1998; 15: 36-43.

10. Leng GC, Fowler B, Ernst E. Exercise for intermittent claudication. *The Cochrane Database of Systematic Reviews* 2000; 2: CD000990. DOI: 10.1002/14651858.

11. Delis KT, Nicolaides AN. Effect of intermittent pneumatic compression of foot and calf on walking distance, haemodynamics and quality of life in patients with arterial claudication: a prospective randomized controlled study with 1-year follow-up. *Ann Surg* 2005; 241: 431-41.

12. Ramaswami G, D'Ayala M, Hollier LH, *et al.* Rapid foot and calf compression increases walking distance in patients with intermittent claudication: results of a randomized study. *J Vasc Surg* 2005; 41: 794-801.

13. Cameron HA, Waller PC, Ramsey LE. Drug treatment of intermittent claudication: a critical analysis of the methods and findings of published clinical trials, 1965-1985. *Br J Clin Pharmacol* 1988; 26: 569-76.

14. British National Formulary 2005; 49: 115.

15. Lehert P, Riphagen FE, Gamand S. The effect of naftidrofuryl on intermittent claudication; a meta-analysis. *J Cardiovasc Pharmacol* 1990; 16 (Suppl. 3): S81-S86.

16. Ruckley CV, Callam MJ, Ferrington CM, Prescott RJ. Naftidrofuryl for intermittent claudication: a double blind controlled trial. *Br Med J* 1978; 1: 622.

17. Clyne CAC, Galland RB, Fox MJ, *et al.* A controlled trial of naftidrofuryl (Praxilene) in the treatment of intermittent claudication. *Br J Surg* 1980; 67: 347-8.

18. Strandness DE Jr, Dalman RL, Panian S, et al. Effect of cilostazol in patients with intermittent claudication: a randomized, double-blind, placebo-controlled study. *Vasc Endovasc Surg* 2002; 36: 83-91.

19. Thompson PD, Zimet R, Forbes WP, Zhang P. Meta-analysis of results from eight randomized, placebo-controlled trials on the effect of cilostazol on patients with intermittent claudication. *Am J Cardiol* 2002; 90: 1314-9.

20. Ahimastos AA, Lawler A, Reid CM, et al. Brief communication: ramipril markedly improves walking ability in patients with peripheral arterial disease: a randomized trial. *Ann Intern Med* 2006; 144: 660-4.

21. Mohler ER 3rd, Hiatt WR, Creager MA. Cholesterol reduction with atorvastatin improves walking distances in patients with peripheral arterial disease. *Circulation* 2003; 108: 1481-6.

22. Lewis DR, Bulbulia RA, Murphy P, et al. Vascular surgical intervention for complications of cardiovascular radiology; 13 years experience in a single centre. *Ann R Coll Surg Eng* 1999; 81: 23-6.

23. Fowkes FGR, Gillespie IN. Angioplasty (versus non-surgical management) for intermittent claudication. *The Cochrane Database of Systematic Reviews* 1998; 2: CD000017. DOI: 10.1002/14651858.

24. Laxdal E, Jenssen GL, Pedersen G, Aune S. Subintimal angioplasty as a treatment of femoropopliteal artery occlusions. *Eur J Vasc Endovasc Surg* 2003; 25: 578-82.

25. Florenes T, Bay D, Sandbaek G, et al. Subintimal angioplasty in the treatment of patients with intermittent claudication: long-term results. *Eur J Vasc Endovasc Surg* 2004; 28: 645-50.

26. Wolf GL, Wilson SE, Cross AP, et al. Surgery or balloon angioplasty for peripheral vascular disease; a randomised clinical trial. Principal investigators and their Associates of Veterans Administration Cooperative Study Number 199. *J Vasc Interv Radiol* 1993; 4: 639-48.

27. Whyman MR, Fowkes FGR, Kerracher EMG, et al. Randomised controlled trial of percutaneous transluminal angioplasty for intermittent claudication. *Eur J Vasc Endovasc Surg* 1996; 12: 167-72.

28. Whyman MR, Fowkes FGR, Kerracher EMG, et al. Is intermittent claudication improved by percutaneous transluminal angioplasty? A randomised controlled trial. *J Vasc Surg* 1997; 26: 551-7.

29. Creasy TS, McMillan PJ, Fletcher EWL, et al. Is percutaneous transluminal angioplasty better than exercise for claudication? Preliminary reults of a prospective randomised trial. *Eur J Vasc Surg* 1990; 4: 135-40.

30. Perkins JMT, Collin J, Creasy TS, et al. Exercise training versus angioplasty for stable claudication. Long and medium-term results of a prospective randomised trial. *Eur J Vasc Endovasc Surg* 1996; 11: 409-13.

31. Cejna M, Thurnher S, Illiasch H, et al. PTA versus Palmaz stent placement in femoropopliteal artery obstructions: a multicenter prospective randomized study. *J Vasc Interv Radiol* 2001; 12: 23-31.

32. Vroegindeweij D, Vos LD, Tielbeek AV, et al. Balloon angioplasty combined with primary stenting versus balloon angioplasty alone in femoropopliteal obstructions: A comparative randomized study. *Cardiovasc Intervent Radiol* 1997; 20: 420-5.

33. Becquemin JP, Favre JP, Marzelle J, et al. Systematic versus selective stent placement after superficial femoral artery balloon angioplasty: a multicenter prospective randomized study. *J Vasc Surg* 2003; 37: 487-94.

34. Bosch JL, Hunink MG. Meta-analysis of the results of percutaneous transluminal angioplasty and stent placement for aortoiliac occlusive disease. *Radiology* 1997; 204: 87-96.

35. Tetteroo E, van der Graaf Y, Bosch JL, et al. Randomised comparison of primary stent placement versus primary angioplasty followed by selective stent placement in patients with iliac artery occlusive disease. Dutch Iliac Stent Trial Study Group. *Lancet* 1998; 351: 1153-9.

36. Klein WM, van der Graaf Y, Seegers J, et al. Dutch iliac stent trial: long-term results in patients randomized for primary or selective stent placement. *Radiology* 2006; 238: 734-44.

37. Leng GC, Davis M, Baker D. Bypass surgery for chronic lower limb ischaemia. *The Cochrane Database of Systematic Reviews* 2000; 3: CD002000. DOI: 10.1002/14651858.

38. Lundgren F, Dahlhof AG, Lundholm K, et al. Intermittent claudication - surgical reconstruction or physical training? A prospective randomized trial of treatment efficiency. *Ann Surg* 1989; 209: 346-55.

Chapter 7

Advanced endovascular intervention in the infra-inguinal region

Neil Davies MB BS FRCS FRCR, Consultant Radiologist

Antony Goode MB BS BSc MRCP FRCR, Consultant Radiologist

Dominic Yu MB BS MRCPI FRCR, Consultant Radiologist

Department of Radiology, Royal Free Hospital, London, UK

Introduction

While angioplasty is now an accepted part of the management of patients with large vessel arterial disease, it has been perceived by some to be less effective in arteries below the inguinal ligament. Recent advances in equipment, technology and training have expanded the range of interventions available, and made infra-inguinal endovascular treatment a realistic alternative to surgery.

Intervention in the superficial femoral artery

The superficial femoral artery (SFA) is a frequent site for the development of atherosclerotic disease; this is likely to remain the case despite improvements in medical management [1]. Disease confined to the SFA is likely to present with intermittent claudication, a relatively benign condition in which 80% of patients improve spontaneously, and only 20% deteriorate [2]. However, if SFA disease coexists with either proximal or distal disease then critical ischaemia is the result [3]. This is the stage at which advanced intervention is most appropriate.

The available treatment options were transformed with the introduction of percutaneous transluminal angioplasty (PTA) following the work of Dotter [4] and Gruntzig [5] in the 1960s and 1970s. It was rapidly recognised, however, that PTA had its limitations, particularly in relation to long or flush origin SFA occlusions. Variations in technique, for example with the laser to open long SFA occlusions, were tried without success and it was not until the 1990s that Bolia described the technique of subintimal angioplasty [6]. This technique has been widely adopted in the UK and Europe for long occlusions, but has taken longer to be accepted in the USA. Indeed most surgeons recommended bypass procedures for extensive SFA disease. The recent BASIL randomised trial [7] compared surgery with PTA as treatment options.

Subintimal angioplasty

The choice of a standard intraluminal PTA or a subintimal angioplasty in the SFA may be predicated on the pre-procedure imaging, but similar equipment is required for both techniques, so decisions can be changed at any time during the intervention. Generally, if there is a stenotic lesion through which a guidewire will pass, then a standard intraluminal PTA

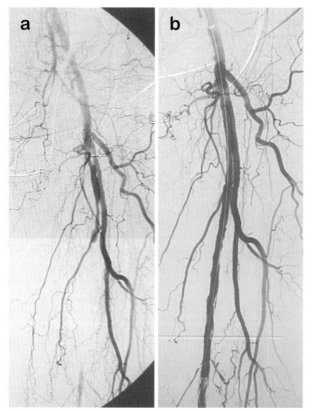

Figure 1. a) Occlusion of the left SFA with a patent profunda femoris. b) Recanalised left SFA after subintimal angioplasty.

can be performed. If one, or a combination of the following are present, then it may be more appropriate to attempt subintimal angioplasty [8] (Figure 1):

- flush SFA origin occlusion;
- long SFA occlusion;
- chronic SFA occlusion;
- diffuse SFA disease;
- heavy vessel wall calcification.

Either an antegrade or an over-the-bifurcation common femoral artery puncture is performed and a sheath inserted. Heparin (3-5,000 units) and a vasodilator such as glyceryl trinitrate (GTN) are administered before crossing the lesion. An angled catheter is used to direct the guidewire towards the wall of the artery away from any significant collateral branch. The wire is then advanced towards the occlusion, and in the majority of cases the wire passes into, and down the subintimal plane with

relative ease. The wire forms a loop within the subintimal plane and when the end of the occlusion is reached the loop in the wire should be shortened. Provided the vessel wall is not too heavily calcified the wire tends to re-enter the vessel lumen. If the wire does not re-enter the lumen then the subintimal plane may need to be extended, although not beyond any large re-constituting vessel to avoid compromising the distal run-off. Once the vessel has been re-entered, a dilatation balloon can be passed over the wire and the stenosis or subintimal plane dilated, usually to 5mm within the SFA. Aspirin 150mg daily should be given following the procedure; many interventionists add clopidogrel (75mg daily) for at least three months.

Results

The results of PTA (either standard transluminal or subintimal) are open to different interpretation. Clearly the goal should be to leave the patient mobile with a viable, pain-free leg. For example, a short-lived improvement in the blood flow to the foot is a failure in a patient with claudication, but a success if it allows time for an ulcer to heal. In addition, the underlying morphology of the lesions treated, including the length of the occlusion, has a significant effect on the outcome.

There are several case series reporting the outcome of subintimal angioplasty. Lipsitz et al [9] described 39 patients, of whom 25 had gangrene, five rest pain and nine short distance claudication. Their technical success rate was 87%, with a cumulative patency at 12 months of 74%. Of the patients with gangrene, 84% went on to heal completely following angioplasty alone. In a more recent prospective study involving 116 procedures, a primary success rate of 82% was recorded with five-year assisted patencies of 64% [10]. These excellent results were attributed to the fact that all patients entered a duplex surveillance programme resulting in early re-intervention if restenosis was detected. Combining all the available studies in 2000, the TASC publication [3] derived a one-year primary patency rate of 61% for all types of femoropopliteal angioplasty (IIa/B).

Stents in the infra-inguinal region

There has been renewed interest lately regarding the use of stents within the SFA. Intuitively they seem a good idea, with the prospect of minimising elastic recoil and residual stenoses, as well as treating flow-limiting dissection flaps. The reality has been disappointing, however, with neointimal hyperplasia (NIH) both within and around the end of the stents being a considerable problem (Figure 2). Several studies have shown no benefit from the addition of a stainless steel stent over angioplasty alone [11]. The use of more flexible, self-expanding nitinol stents has produced more promising results. Schillinger et al [12] demonstrated significantly lower restenosis rates at one year in a randomised trial that compared primary SFA stenting (37% restenosis rate) with angioplasty alone (64%). The SIROCCO trials [13] were designed to evaluate the possible benefits of drug-eluting stents to reduce NIH in the SFA. Although failing to demonstrate an advantage of sirolimus-coated stents over bare wire stents, the authors did describe excellent patency rates in both stented groups (80% patency at 18 months) **(Ib/A)**.

Clearly, further study into the long-term outcomes of stents is required. In addition, developments in stent design are needed, with particular focus on stent fracture which is well recognised to induce NIH. Other areas of research include covered stents, cryoplasty and laser angioplasty within the SFA. As yet there is no evidence that these offer any significant advantage over standard techniques.

The BASIL Trial

Severe limb-threatening ischaemia (SLI) is a significant cause of morbidity and mortality in the developed world, with an estimated incidence of 50-100 per 100,000 per year [3], and is increasing, due to aging populations and the rising incidence of diabetes mellitus. Bypass surgery and angioplasty are the two methods available for limb revascularisation. Surgery has a track record as the standard intervention, but angioplasty is less invasive, fast, carries a low risk and involves only a short hospital stay. Surgery is, however, perceived to be more durable. The aim of

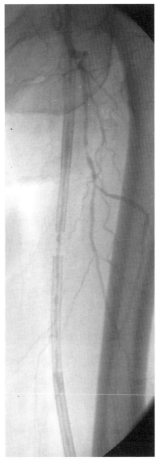

Figure 2. Angiogram showing florid neointimal hyperplasia within stents inserted in the SFA.

the BASIL trial [7] (Bypass versus Angioplasty in Severe Ischaemia of the Leg) was to compare the outcomes of bypass surgery and angioplasty in patients suitable for either treatment. In a multicentre trial that involved 27 UK hospitals, 452 patients who presented with ischaemic rest pain for more than two weeks or tissue loss of presumed arterial aetiology were recruited. The primary outcome was time to amputation of the trial leg, or death from any cause. Secondary outcomes included morbidity and mortality, re-interventions, quality of life and cost.

Patients suitable for the trial were only a fraction of all the patients that presented to the hospitals with SLI. Out of 585 patients who presented with SLI during part of the BASIL trial, 456 had infra-inguinal disease, and of these, 220 were treated without revascularisation. Therefore, 236 patients were potentially eligible for BASIL; however, only 70 (29%) were regarded as suitable for randomisation, usually because the leg was not suitable for both angioplasty and bypass surgery. Thus it remains questionable whether the results are generalisable to all patients with critical leg ischaemia due to infra-inguinal disease.

BASIL trial results

Of the 452 patients with SLI who were recruited into the trial, 228 were randomised to a surgery-first strategy, with 195 (86%) undergoing the attempted intervention, and 224 were randomised to an angioplasty-first strategy, with 216 (96%) undergoing the intervention. Forty-three angioplasty procedures (20%) were considered an immediate technical failure, compared with two of the 195 surgical procedures.

There was no significant difference in 30-day mortality between the two groups, although surgery was associated with a greater 30-day morbidity rate (57% vs. 41%). The re-intervention rate was lower after surgery (18% vs. 26%) when analysed by intention to treat. There was no significant difference between the groups for survival to the primary endpoint: at one year, survival with an intact leg was 68% after surgery, and 71% after angioplasty. The results at three years were 57% and 52%, respectively. Up to two years after intervention the results of the two treatments appeared equivalent, but after that analysis suggested an improved amputation-free survival and lower all-cause mortality after surgery, although the number of patients followed at this stage was quite small. There were no major differences in long-term quality of life, but surgery was approximately a third more expensive than angioplasty in the first 12 months after intervention (£23,322 vs. £17,419).

Surgery or angioplasty?

The BASIL trial provides the first level I evidence of the relative efficacies of bypass surgery and balloon angioplasty in patients with SLI **(Ib/A)**. The treatments were equivalent for up to two years, and it remains to be seen with more follow-up whether surgery will have an advantage in the longer term. Angioplasty has a lower early complication rate, needs a shorter hospital stay and is cheaper; it does not preclude subsequent bypass surgery if it fails. For this reason patients with a life expectancy of less than two years, or with significant comorbidity should be offered angioplasty first **(Ib/A)**. Bypass surgery may be a superior option in patients with a better long-term outlook. The life expectancy of many patients with critical leg ischaemia is limited, and the role of surgery first may not be great. It was also noted in BASIL that many patients were not receiving additional best medical therapy; many were still smoking, and drugs such as aspirin, statins and antihypertensives were underused.

Popliteal artery aneurysms

Popliteal artery aneurysms (PA) occur most commonly in elderly men and are bilateral in up to 50% (Figure 3). The aneurysm can cause

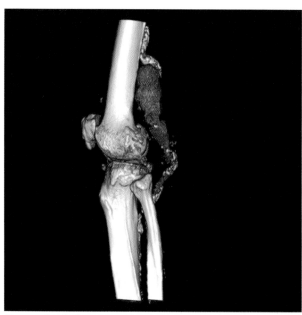

Figure 3. A 4cm popliteal aneurysm in an 84-year-old man. Unfortunately this was not suitable for endovascular repair due to size mismatch in the proximal and distal popliteal artery landing zones.

embolisation or acute thrombosis, and the five-year cumulative risk for complications has been reported to be up to 68% [14]. Acute thrombosis results in a very high rate of limb loss. Surgical ligation and bypass is the standard treatment and is advocated for asymptomatic PA over 25mm in diameter. Intra-arterial thrombolysis is a useful adjunct for the acutely thrombosed PA, but should be directed at opening the run-off vessels for subsequent bypass, rather than the aneurysm itself [15].

Marin reported the first endovascular repair of PA in 1994 [16]. Endovascular treatment is similar to aortic aneurysm repair. The inside of the popliteal artery is lined with one or more covered stent graft(s), secured with proximal and distal stents. In a recent literature review [17] the authors found a total of 106 reported procedures, with no deployment failures. It might be expected that placing a stent across the mobile knee joint could be hazardous and result in stent graft thrombosis, but this only occurred in 19/106 procedures within six months of deployment; long-term outcome data are not yet available. One-year patencies ranged from 47% to 74%, with secondary patencies of 75% to 92%.

Tielliu et al [18] reported a prospective cohort study of 57 PA in 48 patients with a two-year primary patency rate for stenting of 77% and no legs lost. There were no graft endoleaks, although one PA increased in size during follow-up. The authors added clopidogrel to aspirin for six weeks to prevent thrombosis.

Antonello et al [19] reported a prospective randomised study comparing open repair and endovascular treatment for asymptomatic PA. Twenty-six patients with 30 PA were randomised into two equal groups. The primary patency rates after 12 and 48 months were 100% and 87% for open repair, compared to 82% and 80% after endovascular repair. The authors concluded that PA can be treated safely by either method, although endovascular repair has the advantages of quicker recovery and shorter hospital stay.

These are early days, but it does appear that endovascular repair of PA is technically feasible with a reasonable primary patency rate **(Ib/A)**. It is too early

to recommend that it should replace open surgical repair, but it is a credible alternative treatment in patients who are not suitable for surgery. Long-term patency data, results from non-specialist centres and improvements in technology may open the infra-inguinal segment to covered stents for this, and other indications in future.

Infrapopliteal angioplasty

The tibial arteries have not been regarded as suitable for endovascular intervention. Yet based on technological advances from cardiac intervention, with the introduction of low-profile catheters and balloons, and steerable guidewires, infrapopliteal angioplasty has become a potential treatment option [20]. This is particularly the case for patients with critical leg ischaemia who are unsuitable for surgery, where the technical success rate is high and complication rates are low. Although long-term patency remains disappointing, the short-term improvement in blood flow may be enough to enable ulcers to heal. Several factors increase the rate of early restenosis after tibial angioplasty including diabetes, heart disease, renal disease, increased age, and high C-reactive protein levels before and after intervention [21-24].

A number of new techniques have been described to improve the success rate of infrapopliteal angioplasty. Spinosa et al [25] reported a method to improve the results of subintimal infrapopliteal angioplasty. When there is failure to re-enter the distal true lumen or when there is a limited segment of distal target artery available for re-entry, retrograde access was obtained in the distal target artery under ultrasound guidance and a retrograde subintimal channel was created. A guidewire is used to connect the antegrade and retrograde subintimal channels to create a 'flossing' wire, followed by balloon dilatation of the subintimal channel. This technique was termed subintimal arterial flossing with antegrade-retrograde intervention (SAFARI), and was highly successful in 21 legs.

Ascher et al [26] described infrapopliteal subintimal angioplasty under duplex guidance in 30 patients, achieving 95% technical success for stenotic disease and 90% for occlusive disease, and avoiding the need for contrast agent and X-rays. Stents have also been deployed in the tibial vessels. Rand *et al*[27] reported a randomised prospective study that compared angioplasty with, or without, stenting on 95 lesions in 51 patients. The stent group achieved significantly higher six-month cumulative primary patency at both the 50% and 70% restenosis threshold, compared with the angioplasty alone group.

Conclusions

In patients with critical leg ischaemia, initial treatment with balloon angioplasty has an early outcome that is as good as bypass surgery, is cheaper and has a lower morbidity **(Ib/A)**.

The results of endovascular intervention in the infra-inguinal region are improving with the introduction of new techniques and devices. Subintimal angioplasty now has an established role for long SFA occlusions that cannot be treated with intraluminal PTA **(IIb/B)**. It remains uncertain whether results could be improved further by a post-treatment surveillance programme.

The role of stents as an adjunct to PTA in the infra-inguinal region remains uncertain. Many interventionists are convinced of their benefit and there are a few supportive, usually small, randomised trials **(IIb/B)**. This is an area that needs more targeted research, including long-term outcome data, and evaluation of the role of drug-eluting stents that are so successful in the coronary arteries.

Similarly, the infrapopliteal region is becoming more accessible to treatment by endovascular means, although there are fewer large reports and the techniques are challenging **(IIb/B)**.

In a single randomised trial, endovascular repair was successful as surgery for treatment of asymptomatic popliteal aneurysm. It remains to be seen whether it will prove to be a generalisable and durable treatment, but it is currently a credible treatment for patients not fit for surgery **(Ib/B)**.

Key points	Evidence level

What is the evidence that balloon angioplasty is effective in patients with SFA disease?

◆ For patients with critical leg ischaemia, treatment with balloon angioplasty has an early outcome which is as good as that of bypass surgery, is cheaper and has a lower morbidity rate.   Ib/A

Does the use of stents improve the results of SFA intervention?

◆ Although some centres report good outcomes many studies report no advantage with SFA stents compared to balloon angioplasty alone, and no long-term data exist. New technologies, including drug-eluting stents, may result in better outcomes in the future.   IIb/B

Is endovascular repair of popliteal aneurysms an effective alternative to surgery?

◆ Endovascular repair of popliteal aneurysms has not yet been proved to be as effective as surgery, but offers a credible treatment for patients not considered surgical candidates.   IIb/B

How effective is endovascular therapy in the treatment of infrapopliteal disease?

◆ Improvements in guidewire, catheter and balloon design now mean that balloon angioplasty is an effective treatment in selected patients; however, evidence compared to surgery is lacking. Stents have yet to be shown to be effective in improving outcomes in patients with infrapopliteal disease.   IIb/B

References

1. Burns P, Gough S, Bradbury AW. Management of peripheral arterial disease in primary care. *Br Med J* 2003; 326: 584-8.
2. McAllister FF. The fate of patients with intermittent claudication managed non-operatively. *Am J Surg* 1976; 132: 593-5.
3. Management of peripheral arterial disease (PAD). TransAtlantic Inter-Society Consensus (TASC). Section D: chronic critical limb ischaemia. *Eur J Vasc Endovasc Surg* 2000; 19 Suppl A: S144-243.
4. Dotter CT, Judkins MP. Transluminal treatment of arteriosclerotic obstruction. Description of a new technique and a preliminary report of its application. *Circulation* 1964; 30: 654-70.
5. Gruntzig A, Hopff H. [Percutaneous recanalization after chronic arterial occlusion with a new dilator-catheter (modification of the Dotter technique)]. *Dtsch Med Wochenschr* 1974; 99: 2502-10, 2511.
6. Bolia A, Miles KA, Brennan J, Bell PRF. Percutaneous transluminal angioplasty of occlusions of the femoral and popliteal arteries by subintimal dissection. *Cardiovasc Intervent Radiol* 1990; 13: 357-63.
7. The BASIL Trial Participants. Bypass versus angioplasty in severe ischaemia of the leg (BASIL): multicentre, randomised controlled trial. *Lancet* 2005; 366: 1925-34.

8. Bolia A. Subintimal angioplasty in lower limb ischaemia. *J Cardiovasc Surg* (Torino) 2005; 46: 385-94.

9. Lipsitz EC, Ohki T, Veith FJ, *et al.* Does subintimal angioplasty have a role in the treatment of severe lower extremity ischemia? *J Vasc Surg* 2003; 37: 386-91.

10. Florenes T, Bay D, Sandback G, *et al.* Subintimal angioplasty in the treatment of patients with intermittent claudication: long-term results. *Eur J Vasc Endovasc Surg* 2004; 28: 645-50.

11. Becquemin JP, Favre JP, Marzelle J, *et al.* Systematic versus selective stent placement after superficial femoral artery balloon angioplasty: a multicenter prospective randomized study. *J Vasc Surg* 2003; 37: 487-94.

12. Schillinger M, Sabeti S, Loewe C, *et al.* Balloon angioplasty versus implantation of nitinol stents in the superficial femoral artery. *N Engl J Med* 2006; 354: 1879-88.

13. Duda SH, Bosiers M, Lammer J, *et al.* Sirolimus-eluting versus bare nitinol stent for obstructive superficial femoral artery disease: the SIROCCO II trial. *J Vasc Interv Radiol* 2005; 16: 331-8.

14. Dawson I, Sie R, van Baalen JM, van Bockel JH. Asymptomatic popliteal aneurysm: elective operation versus conservative follow-up. *Br J Surg* 1994; 81: 1504-7.

15. Steinmetz E, Bouchot O, Faroy F, *et al.* Pre-operative intra-arterial thrombolysis before surgical revascularisation for popliteal artery aneurysm with acute ischaemia. *Ann Vasc Surg* 2000; 14: 360-4.

16. Marin ML, Veith FJ, Pancetta TF, *et al.* Transfemoral endoluminal stented graft repair of a popliteal artery aneurysm. *J Vasc Surg* 1994; 19: 754-7.

17. Siauw R, Koh EH, Walker SR. Endovascular repair of popliteal artery aneurysms: techniques, current evidence and recent experience. *ANZ J Surg* 2006; 76: 505-11.

18. Tielliu IF, Verhoeven EL, Zeebregts CJ, *et al.* Endovascular treatment of popliteal artery aneurysms: results of a prospective cohort study. *J Vasc Surg* 2005; 41: 561-7.

19. Antonello M, Frigatti P, Battochio P, *et al.* Open repair versus endovascular treatment for asymptomatic popliteal artery aneurysm: results of a prospective randomised study. *J Vasc Surg* 2005; 42: 185-93.

20. Dorros G, Jaff MR, Dorros AM, *et al.* Tibioperoneal (outflow lesion) angioplasty can be used as primary treatment in 235 patients with critical limb ischaemia: five-year follow-up. *Circulation* 2001; 104: 2057-62.

21. Danielsson G, Albrechtsson U, Norgren L, *et al.* Percutaneous transluminal angioplasty of crural arteries: diabetes and other factors influencing outcome. *Eur J Vasc Endovasc Surg* 2001; 21: 432-6.

22. Soder HK, Manninen HI, Jaakkola P, *et al.* Prospective trial of infrapopliteal artery balloon angioplasty for critical limb ischaemia: angiographic and clinical results. *J Vasc Interv Radiol* 2000; 11: 1021-31.

23. Atar E, Siegel Y, Avrahami R, *et al.* Balloon angioplasty of popliteal and crural arteries in elderly with critical limb ischaemia. *Eur J Radiology* 2005; 53: 287-92.

24. Schillinger M, Exner M, Mlekusch W, *et al.* Endovascular revascularisation below the knee: 6-month results and predictive value of C-reactive protein level. *Radiology* 2003; 227: 419-25.

25. Spinosa DJ, Hartun NL, Bissonette EA, *et al.* Subintimal arterial flossing with antegrade-retrograde intervention (SAFARI) for subintimal recanalisation to treat chronic critical limb ischaemia. *J Vasc Interv Surg* 2005; 16: 37-44.

26. Ascher E, Marks NA, Hingorani AP, *et al.* Duplex-guided angioplasty and subintimal dissection of infrapopliteal arteries: early results with a new approach to avoid radiation exposure and contrast material. *J Vasc Surg* 2005; 42: 1114-21.

27. Rand T, Basile A, Cejna M, *et al.* PTA versus carbofilm-coated stents in infrapopliteal arteries: pilot study. *Cardiovasc Intervent Radiol* 2006; 29: 29-38.

Chapter 8

Improving the patency of femorodistal bypass grafts

Peter L Harris MD FRCS, Professor of Vascular Surgery

Robert K Fisher MD FRCS, Vascular Specialist Registrar

Regional Vascular Unit, Royal Liverpool University Hospital, Liverpool, UK

Introduction

Critical leg ischaemia has an incidence in the UK of 40 per 100,000, and affects about 20,000 patients a year with an amputation rate approaching 25% [1]. Although angioplasty is starting to make inroads into the management of this condition, open arterial reconstruction in the form of bypass to patent distal calf vessels remains the standard treatment and is often the only viable option for extensive, multi-level infra-inguinal arterial occlusion. Despite patency rates that are less than ideal [2], an aggressive approach to the application of distal bypass surgery is justified. A study by Cheshire et al in 1992 showed that although there is frequently a requirement for secondary and sometimes multiple re-intervention, arterial reconstruction is more cost-effective than primary amputation [3]. For most patients preservation of a pain-free leg is, more often than not, an absolute priority, even if this entails multiple operations.

Femorodistal bypass surgery has a history that extends back more than 50 years. During this interval a variety of bypass conduits have been developed, although interestingly the first to be used, the patient's own long saphenous vein, is still the gold standard. Despite considerable commercial investment and scientific endeavour no synthetic alternative has been found to compare with the patency rates of autologous vein. In recent years, attention has turned mainly to the evolution of adjuvant treatments designed to optimise the performance of vein graft substitutes.

The bypass graft

Autologous vein vs. prosthetic material, when both are available

The bypass conduit is one of the most important factors determining long-term patency, with autologous vein remaining the preferred choice since its introduction by Kunlin in 1949. The performance of autologous vein and prosthetic femoropopliteal bypass grafts has been compared in several randomised trials (Table 1) [4-9]. Bergan et al identified a difference between autologous vein and PTFE grafts when anastomosed to the infrageniculate popliteal artery, the patency of autologous vein being superior. There was no statistical difference between the patency of these two grafts, however, when anastomosed to the popliteal artery above the knee [7] **(Ib/A)**. The mean duration of follow-up in this study was only 30 months, and subsequent studies demonstrated that the superior performance of autologous vein becomes evident over time. Tilanus et al reported secondary patency rates of 37% for infra-

Table 1. Randomised controlled trials of vein vs. PTFE/Dacron grafts for infra-inguinal bypass.

Author	Procedure/ anastomosis		Number	Follow-up years	1⁰ patency	2⁰ patency	Limb salvage
Bergan et al [7] 1982	AK pop	vein	41		70%	--	--
		PTFE	33		72%	--	--
	BK pop	vein	50	2.5	76%	--	--
		PTFE	46		62%	--	--
	Infrapop	vein	57		50%*	--	--
		PTFE	58		20%	--	--
Tilanus et al [4] 1985	Fempop	vein	25	5	--	70%*	--
		PTFE	24		--	37%	--
Veith et al [6] 1986	AK pop	vein	85	4	61%	--	--
		PTFE	91		38%	--	--
	BK pop	vein	62	4	76%*	--	--
		PTFE	80		54%	--	--
	Combined fempop	vein	147	5	68%*	--	75%
		PTFE	171		38%	--	70%
	Infrapop	vein	106	4	49%*	--	61%
		PTFE	98		12%	--	57%
Kumar et al [5] 1995	AK pop	vein	50		73%*	90%*	--
		PTFE	49	4	47%	47%	--
		Dacron	46		54%	60%	--
Ballotta et al [9] 2003	AK pop	vein	51	5	94%	--	--
		PTFE	51		84%	--	--
Klinkert et al [8] 2003	AK pop	vein	75	5	76%*	--	--
		PTFE	76		52%	--	--

*   statistically significant results (p<0.05)

AK pop	above-knee popliteal artery
BK pop	below-knee popliteal artery
Infrapop	infrapopliteal
Fempop	femoropopliteal

inguinal PTFE and 70% for autologous vein grafts after five years (p<0.001). This study included both above and below-knee bypasses [4] **(Ib/A)**.

There are no randomised controlled trials that compare prosthetic and autologous vein grafts for femorotibial bypass. The conduct of such a trial would pose some difficulties. First, the number of distal bypasses performed, even in major centres, is relatively low. Second, randomisation between vein and prosthetic graft would present an ethical dilemma in the face of overwhelming evidence for the superiority of vein from non-randomised studies. Third, the limited life expectancy of patients with critical leg ischaemia would make long-term follow-up difficult.

Despite the lack of level I evidence it is accepted universally that autologous vein grafts achieve optimum patency in bypasses to crural vessels performed for critical leg ischaemia and that they should always be the first choice in this situation.

The case for preferential use of vein is less clear cut when the site of the distal anastomosis is above the knee [8, 9] **(Ib/A)**. There are legitimate arguments to support the use of PTFE or Dacron as first choice in this situation; the operations are less invasive, requiring a short incision at each end, the long saphenous vein is preserved for more critical situations, for example tibial and coronary artery bypass operations and, as noted above, there are data demonstrating comparable patency rates with autologous vein, at least for the first two years after operation. Whereas a recent study suggested improved patency for vein, an intriguing study of patients that needed bilateral bypass had equivocal results [8, 9] **(Ib/A)**. In fact, meta-analysis of published data suggests that preferential use of autologous vein for above-knee bypass is associated with a marginal, but significantly improved rate of limb salvage in the long term [10] **(Ib/A)**. Should in future the introduction of new technologies, for example pre-cuffed grafts, flow surface modification, heparin-bonding and drug-eluting products impact favourably upon the patency rates of prosthetic bypass, it is likely that the balance of risks could be tipped in favour of their preferential use above the knee. A study that compared end-to-end with end-to-side anastomoses in 328 procedures found similar three-year patency rates (63% vs. 55%, p=0.26), although the rate of major amputation was higher after failed bypass with end-to-end anastomosis [11] **(Ib/A)**.

In situ or reversed long saphenous vein bypass

For a time there was considerable debate about the relative effectiveness of *in situ* and reversed saphenous vein bypasses. Theory suggested that the intact vasa vasorum of *in situ* grafts would maintain nutrition to the vessel, preserving desirable properties such as endothelial secretion of plasminogen activators and thereby maintaining low thrombogenicity. It was argued also that the natural compliance of the wall of the vessel would be retained with a reduced risk of neointimal hyperplasia. It is

undeniable that the natural taper of *in situ* vein affords better matching for size between graft and artery at both proximal and distal anastomoses. Harris *et al* studied a series of 200 femoropopliteal bypasses, randomised into *in situ* or reversed vein groups. They reported no significant difference in three-year cumulative patency rates between the two groups (68% vs. 77%, respectively). Patency was affected adversely by small vein diameter (p<0.005), long grafts (p<0.01) and poor run-off (p<0.05) in both types of bypass [12] **(Ib/A)**.

A subsequent multicentre randomised trial confirmed similar results for infrapopliteal vein grafts, with secondary cumulative patency rates at three years of 68% and 66%, respectively, for *in situ* and reversed grafts [13]. Claims for superior patency of *in situ* bypasses were therefore unfounded. Both procedures are equally effective in randomised trials and the sensible approach is to use whichever seems most appropriate for circumstances that apply in individual patients. A summary of the results of published randomised trials of *in situ* and reversed vein grafts is shown in Table 2 [13-17] **(Ib/A)**.

Venous alternatives to the long saphenous vein

When there is no adequate length of healthy long saphenous vein available, autologous vein may be harvested from other sites for construction of a bypass graft. Options include the contralateral long saphenous vein, cephalic and/or basilic arm veins, the short saphenous vein and the superficial femoral vein. If one of these is of insufficient length, two or more segments may be spliced together to form a composite venous graft. However, the construction of a satisfactory long length of venous bypass from multiple short segments is technically demanding and gives good results only in skilled hands. Therefore, use of a prosthetic graft usually represents the preferable option. Composite prosthetic/autologous vein grafts can also be used [18] **(II/B)**, but the results tend towards those expected from the prosthetic rather than the venous component and for this reason it is doubtful whether they offer any worthwhile advantage over a simple prosthetic graft. When there is an isolated segment of popliteal artery, a useful

Table 2. Trials comparing patency and limb salvage rates for *in situ* and reversed autologous vein bypass.

Author	Procedure	Level of bypass	Follow-up years	1⁰ patency	2⁰ patency	Limb salvage
Wengerter *et al*[14] 1991	in situ (n=62) reverse (n=63)	Infrapopliteal	2.5	58% 61%	69% 67%	76% 87%
Moody *et al*[15] 1992	in situ (n=101) reverse (n=114)	Fempop AK/BK	5	64% 62%	-- --	-- --
Harris *et al*[13] 1993	in situ (n=82) reverse (n=80)	Infrapopliteal	3	-- --	68% 66%	78% 87%
Watelet *et al*[16] 1997	in situ (n=50) reverse (n=50)	Fempop AK/BK	10	42%** 65%	65% 70%	74% 74%
Lawson *et al*[17] 1999	in situ (n=307) reverse (n=775)	Fempop AK/BK	2	67%** 74%	85% 84%	89% 92%
	in situ (n=193) reverse (n=180)	Infrapopliteal	2	52%** 63%	74% 71%	82% 85%

* randomised controlled trial
** statistically significant p<0.05. Differences only identified in primary patency.

Fempop   femoropopliteal
AK   above knee
BK   below knee

strategy is to combine an above-knee prosthetic bypass and a popliteal to tibial autologous vein graft, if there is insufficient length of autologous vein for direct femorotibial bypass.

Contralateral saphenous vein

The contralateral long saphenous vein may be employed when the ipsilateral long saphenous vein is not available. However, in a series reported by Hölzenbein *et al*, the contralateral vein was available in just 38% of patients under these circumstances, and there was a 60% probability that the vein would be required for bypass in the donor leg within three years [19] **(III/B)**. Therefore, contralateral long saphenous vein should rarely be used, and only for specific indications such as active infection in the recipient leg.

Deep leg veins

Arterial bypass using the superficial femoral and popliteal veins was originally described as an alternative to prosthetic grafts in the absence of ipsilateral long saphenous vein. Schulman *et al* reported excellent long-term patency [20] and proceeded to undertake a randomised trial comparing saphenous vein (n=56) with deep leg veins (n=41) for primary femoropopliteal bypass. They found similar primary and secondary patency rates in the two groups at three years (60% and 63% for reversed saphenous vein, and 64% and 68% for superficial femoral vein, respectively). Although the deep leg vein operation is a more demanding surgical procedure, and postoperative leg swelling sometimes occurs, Schulman did not report any long-term disability in his series [21] **(Ib/A)**. Consequently, these authors boldly advocated the preferential use of deep leg vein as the primary conduit in femoropopliteal bypass, thereby preserving the saphenous vein. However, the relatively short length of the deep veins means they cannot be used for long distal bypasses and most vascular surgeons reserve them for replacement of infected aortofemoral or femoropopliteal prosthetic grafts.

Arm vein

Hölzenbein *et al* used arm vein in 250 patients as the primary alternative when there was no ipsilateral saphenous vein available. The grafts included cephalic vein alone (50%), cephalic and basilic vein (36%) and basilic vein alone (14%). They reported cumulative primary and secondary patency rates at one year of 70.6% and 76.9%, respectively, with a limb salvage rate of 88.2%. Cumulative primary and revised patency rates at three years were 49.5% and 52.8%, respectively, with a limb salvage rate of 80.4%. There was no statistically significant association between patency and the anatomical origin of the vein or the type of procedure performed [19]. Similar excellent outcomes have been achieved by Simms. There are, however, also reports of less promising results [22, 23] **(III/B)**. In the long term there seems to be a higher incidence of graft elongation and aneurysmal dilatation than occurs with saphenous vein. There are no randomised comparisons between arm vein, saphenous vein or prosthetic grafts.

Sequential and composite grafts

McCarthy *et al* performed 67 composite sequential bypasses using 6mm PTFE to the popliteal artery, with long or short saphenous vein extensions to crural vessels. They reported a cumulative patency rate at one year of 72%, and at three years of 48%, with a limb salvage rate at four years of 70% [18]. Similar success has been reported by other institutions [24], but this experience, however, is not ubiquitous, and one study reported five-year patency rates for composite prosthetic grafts of just 28% compared to 63% for autologous vein grafts (p=0.005) [25] **(III/B)**.

Prosthetic alternatives to long saphenous vein

In the early days of prosthetic lower limb bypass, Dacron produced relatively poor results: five-year patencies of less than 60% to the above-knee popliteal artery, and even less below the knee [26]. Kenney *et al* reported four-year patency approaching 80% for above-knee femoropopliteal Dacron grafts, which is as good as any series using PTFE [27]. Abbott *et al*, in a randomised prospective trial, were unable to demonstrate a difference in patency between Dacron and PTFE for above-knee bypass at three years [28] **(Ib/A)**. However, no randomised studies have compared PTFE and Dacron for femorotibial bypass. Despite this, PTFE is widely used as an alternative, when saphenous vein is not available. The early reports of PTFE grafts were encouraging, but the long-term patency in below-knee and distal bypasses was less good [29, 30] **(III/B)**.

The incidence of prosthetic graft infection is probably between 3-5%, with a subsequent major amputation rate of 30-70%. A particularly worrying problem is that of infection with methicillin-resistant *Staphylococcus aureus*, an organism that is often endemic in nursing homes and long-stay wards, where the typical patient with critical ischaemia is likely to be resident (Chapter 26).

Improving the patency of PTFE grafts

Many explanations have been proposed for the lower patency rates of PTFE bypasses. The mismatch in compliance between the relatively stiff prosthetic graft and the native artery, combined with iatrogenic injury caused by suturing the anastomosis, and areas of low shear stress at the heel and toe of the graft are all thought to induce neointimal hyperplasia (NIH) and therefore stenosis at the distal anastomosis. Additionally, interactions between the blood elements, particularly platelets, and the prosthetic flow surface are also likely to impact adversely upon thrombogenicity.

Interposition vein patches and cuffs

Several surgical techniques have been developed in an effort to limit anastomotic NIH. They have origin from the anastomotic vein patch described by Linton, and Siegman's venous cuff. Miller described the first widely used vein cuff in 1984 [31] and in 1995 he reported that cuffed PTFE grafts to the below-knee popliteal artery had superior patency over uncuffed grafts at 36 months (57% versus 29%) [32], a finding which was later corroborated in a randomised study by the Joint Vascular Research Group (Figure 1) [33] **(Ib/A)**. In the JVRG study, patients who had either above- or below-knee femoropopliteal bypass were randomised to cuff or control groups at the distal anastomosis. The cuff produced a significant advantage at the below-knee level, but not above the knee. It was suggested that when a cuffed PTFE graft occludes, the recipient artery may be spared, allowing the chance of further reconstruction [34]. However, recent evidence throws this observation into question [35]. Retrospective review of the Miller cuff in prosthetic bypasses to tibial vessels has demonstrated encouraging patency rates of 55% at two years and 52% at three years [36].

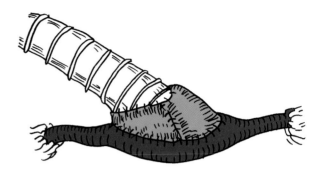

Figure 2. The St. Mary's boot.

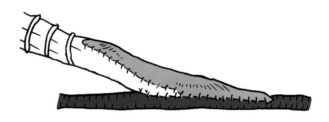

Figure 3. The Taylor patch

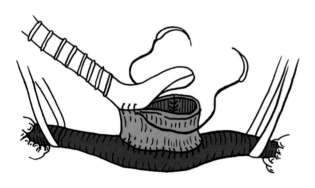

Figure 1. The Miller cuff.

The Taylor patch [37] and St. Mary's boot [38] are modifications of the distal anastomotic vein interposition technique. Both configurations have achieved patencies comparable to those of the Miller cuff, but neither has been the subject of a randomised trial (Figures 2 and 3).

Pre-cuffed PTFE grafts

Da Silva *et al* described how the configuration adopted by the Miller cuff formed a highly stable, cohesive vortex, which he speculated increased wall shear stress at critical points within the anastomosis, thereby inhibiting the accretion of NIH [39]. Although this remains an area of controversy, there is evidence that the configuration of an anastomosis impacts upon local flow dynamics and the distribution of shear stress, which is known to influence the development of NIH. Research derived from this evidence has led to the evolution of a pre-cuffed PTFE graft (Figure 4). The first to be developed was designed to modify the flow dynamics at the distal anastomosis of a femorotibial bypass, and subsequent clinical studies have confirmed the presence of the intended vortex

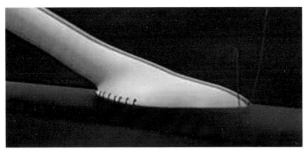

Figure 4. The pre-cuffed PTFE graft.

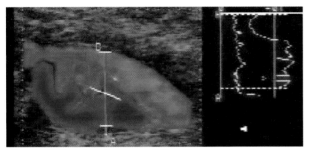

Figure 5. Duplex image of the flow vortex in a pre-cuffed graft.

(Figure 5) [40]. A multicentred randomised comparison of pre-cuffed with standard PTFE grafts with an interposition vein cuff showed comparable patency rates [41] **(Ib/A)**. Subsequently, pre-cuffed grafts with different configurations have been developed for above-knee femoropopliteal bypass and haemodialysis access grafts, where the flow dynamics differ dramatically.

Adjuvant arteriovenous fistula

The use of an arteriovenous fistula (AVF) at, or near the distal anastomosis has been advocated in order to decrease the outflow resistance and improve blood flow through the distal anastomosis (Figure 6). The combination of AVF and vein interposition for femorotibial bypass has achieved a two-year cumulative patency of 62% [42] and a three-year primary-assisted patency of 61.9% [43]. In a prospective randomised trial comparing graft patency and limb salvage rates after femorodistal prosthetic bypass with, and without adjunctive AVF, Hamsho *et al* found no significant differences between the two groups. Although the small number of patients (n=89) may have masked an early benefit in patency with AVF, any difference diminished after the first six months [44].

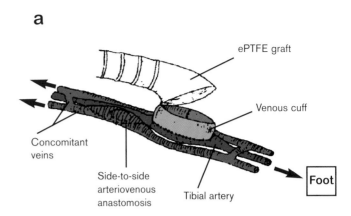

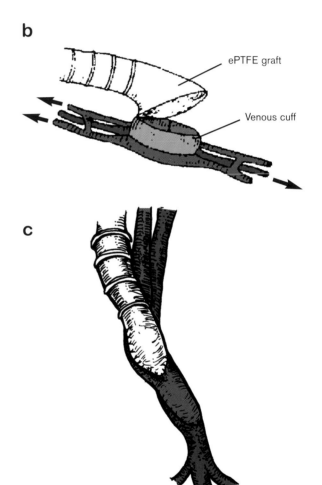

Figure 6. Types of arteriovenous fistula. a) Pre-anastomotic. b) Common ostium. c) Deep vein interposition. *Reproduced with permission from the European Journal of Vascular and Endovascular Surgery. Hamsho A, Nott D, Harris PL. Prospective randomized trial of distal arteriovenous fistula as an adjunct to femoro-infrapopliteal PTFE bypass. Eur J Vasc Endovasc Surg 1999; 17: 197-201.*

This and other trials did not show evidence of worthwhile benefit associated with AVF and there does not appear to be any indication for its routine application with prosthetic femorodistal bypass grafts [45] **(Ib/A)**.

Flow surface modification

In the 1980s and early 1990s considerable effort was expended in trying to line PTFE grafts with endothelial or mesothelial cells. The idea was to modify the flow surface in order to make it less thrombogenic. Seeding of autologous endothelial cells remained problematic, however, with forces from the flowing blood detracting from secure adherence. Potential benefits have therefore remained theoretical with little clinical impact to date.

More recently, attempts have been made to modify the flow surface chemically. Carbon-lined and heparin-bonded grafts are both commercially available, apparently with some advantages, although reliable evidence of clinical efficacy is lacking [46, 47]. In the future drug-eluting grafts with agents intended to suppress NIH may be developed.

Intra-operative quality control

Graft failure that occurs between one and 12 months after operation is usually associated with graft-related stenosis due to neointimal hyperplasia which is prone to develop either within the graft itself, or at the distal anastomosis. Disease progression either proximal or distal to the graft accounts for most later occlusions. On the other hand graft failure that occurs within the first month, is usually attributable to technical error committed at the time of the operation, or as a consequence of inappropriate selection of the patient or procedure. Early failure occurs after 5-15% of bypasses [48]. Some system of quality assessment on completion of a femorodistal bypass procedure is essential and the options, in addition to palpation of distal pulses, are insonation with Doppler ultrasound (or duplex) and angiography. A vogue for angioscopy was abandoned when it became apparent that the intraluminal manipulations of the graft that this involved did more harm than good.

Some time ago completion angiography was considered mandatory. However, Blankenstein *et al*, in a prospective study of intra-operative determinants of bypass patency, reported that continuous wave Doppler was a better indicator of technical error and concluded that intra-operative angiography could be reserved for anatomical assessment of those cases identified by Doppler as problematic [48]. In response to this and other similar studies with a similar message, angiography is employed less often, despite the ready availability of digital subtraction angiography in most operating rooms. Others have used duplex ultrasonography and other Doppler flow-derived measurements such as resistance and impedence. There is no consensus on the best method, but all agree that intra-operative quality control is an important component of distal bypass.

Drug therapy to improve patency

Adjuvant pharmacological intervention is essential not only to optimise the patency of arterial bypass grafts in the longer term but also to reduce the risk of unrelated cardiovascular events in this vulnerable population of patients. Watson *et al* published a comprehensive review of the literature to evaluate the evidence for the use of various agents in 1999 [49].

Early graft occlusion is initiated by accumulation of activated platelets at sites of endothelial denudation, with the subsequent release of myofibroblastic mitogens. Inhibition of platelets should therefore have some benefit in the prevention of NIH and improve graft patency.

Placebo controlled randomised studies have suggested that the benefit of aspirin may be greater in preventing occlusion in prosthetic than autologous vein grafts. A meta-analysis by the Antiplatelet Trialists' Collaboration provided evidence that aspirin afforded additional benefit by reducing the risk of stroke, myocardial infarction and death from other cardiovascular causes [50] **(Ib/A)**. Therefore, except when specifically contraindicated, aspirin should be prescribed for all patients who present with vascular disease, whether or not they receive interventional treatment. The preferred dose is 75mg daily.

Clopidogrel is a more potent antiplatelet agent than aspirin and causes less gastric irritation; however, its use is associated with a higher risk of bleeding complications, and it is considerably more expensive.

Clopidogrel should be reserved for those with intolerance to aspirin and for those who are considered to be at specially high risk of graft occlusion or other serious cardiovascular events.

A study by Arfvidsson et al failed to show significant difference in graft patency or limb salvage in patients given warfarin after vein and prosthetic bypass [51]. However when considering vein grafts alone, Kretschmer et al, in a series of studies, demonstrated improved graft patency and patient survival with warfarin for both short and long-term follow-up [52].

Another study that specifically examined high-risk vein grafts, defined as those with poor distal run-off, showed improved patency with the combination of aspirin and warfarin for poor quality vein, or revision procedures [53]. This was mirrored in a similar study of 831 patients where warfarin was compared with aspirin [54] **(Ib/A)**. It is fair to say that despite extensive data, larger trials often find little difference between antithrombotic regimens [55].

Postoperative graft surveillance

A decade ago postoperative surveillance of femorodistal vein grafts by duplex ultrasound imaging was considered mandatory. This was because graft failure is common, particularly in the first year after insertion. The most common cause is stenosis due to neointimal hyperplasia, either within the graft itself or within the recipient artery at, or close to the distal anastomosis. Clinically occult graft-related stenoses can easily be detected by duplex and secondary intervention to correct graft-related stenosis (angioplasty or surgery) should prevent graft failure. Because graft occlusion due to graft-related stenosis is known to occur mainly during the first year after insertion, surveillance is usually confined to this interval. A typical surveillance programme includes duplex at six weeks, three, six, nine and 12 months, although some surgeons recommend surveillance indefinitely, but with less intensity after the first year.

Detection of a graft-related stenosis is an indication for intervention. Focal lesions may be treated by percutaneous angioplasty, but secondary surgical intervention is indicated for more diffuse lesions, those that are resistant to angioplasty and those that are

relatively inaccessible, for example close to the groin anastomosis.

Two randomised controlled trials have shown a benefit associated with graft surveillance. The first by Lundell et al demonstrated improved patency of vein grafts followed by regular ultrasound surveillance, but no benefit in the case of prosthetic grafts [56]. In this and the study by Ihlberg et al, the rate of amputation was not affected significantly by the surveillance programme [56, 57] **(Ib/A)**. However, a later randomised controlled trial reported by Fasih et al showed significant benefit from surveillance of vein grafts both in terms of long-term patency and limb salvage [58] **(Ib/A)**. In both of these trials the control population was monitored by clinical examination supplemented by ankle/arm pressure measurements, which suggests that this type of surveillance alone is inadequate. More recently the Vein Graft Surveillance Trial compared duplex with clinical surveillance, and reported equivalence in terms of amputation rates and quality of life. Primary and secondary patency rates were also comparable, but clinical surveillance had a significant cost benefit over routine duplex surveillance [59]. The findings of this large, randomised trial raise doubts about the effectiveness of routine postoperative vein graft surveillance, although for many the evidence to abandon surveillance remains inconclusive. There is, however, no available evidence to support routine surveillance by duplex imaging of prosthetic femorodistal bypass grafts [56] **(Ib/A)**.

Conclusions

The evidence suggests that patency of femorodistal arterial bypass grafts is improved by:

- autologous vein;
- a cuffed configuration of distal anastomosis in the case of PTFE grafts;
- antiplatelet agents.

There is no improvement in patency rates associated with:

- reversed compared to in situ vein grafts;
- adjuvant distal arteriovenous fistulae;
- routine postoperative surveillance by duplex ultrasound imaging of prosthetic grafts.

Key points	Evidence level

- ◆ Autologous saphenous vein achieves superior patency rates to prosthetic materials, especially in femorodistal bypass. — Ia/A
- ◆ *In situ* and reversed vein graft bypasses perform equally well and the choice of technique should be based upon anatomical considerations that are specific to individual patients. — Ib/A
- ◆ In the absence of saphenous vein, no convincing studies exist to suggest the preferred prosthetic alternative. — II/B, III/B
- ◆ The patency of PTFE grafts may be improved by interposition of a vein cuff at the distal anastomosis. — Ib/A
- ◆ Patency rates associated with pre-cuffed PTFE grafts are comparable to that obtained from standard PTFE grafts with an interposition vein cuff. — Ib/A
- ◆ There is no justification for the routine use of adjuvant distal arteriovenous fistulae. — Ib/A
- ◆ Doppler ultrasound assessment is the method of choice for quality assurance on completion of the operative procedure. — II/B
- ◆ In the absence of specific contraindications, aspirin should be prescribed for all patients with peripheral vascular disease whether or not they are treated by operative or other intervention. Clopidogrel may be prescribed in those with sensitivity to aspirin and those at particularly high risk of graft failure or other adverse cardiovascular event. — Ia/A
- ◆ The use of warfarin remains controversial but is supported by evidence. — Ib/A
- ◆ Controversy remains regarding routine postoperative duplex surveillance of autologous vein grafts. Present evidence does not support routine surveillance of prosthetic bypass grafts. — Ib/A

References

1. The Vascular Surgical Society of Great Britain and Ireland. Critical limb ischaemia: management and outcome. Report of a National Survey. *Eur J Vasc Endovasc Surg* 1995; 10: 108-13.
2. Cranley JJ, Hafner CD. Revascularization of the femoropopliteal arteries using saphenous vein, polytetrafluoroethylene, and umbilical vein grafts. *Arch Surg* 1982; 117: 1543-50.
3. Cheshire NJW, Wolfe MS, Noone MA, *et al*. The economics of femorocrural reconstruction for critical limb ischaemia with and without autologous vein. *J Vasc Surg* 1992; 15: 167-75.
4. Tilanus HW, Obertop H, van Urk H. Saphenous vein or PTFE for femoropopliteal bypass. A prospective randomized trial. *Ann Surg* 1985; 202: 780-2.
5. Kumar KP, Crinnon JN, Ashley S, *et al*. Vein, PTFE or Dacron for above-knee femoro-popliteal bypass? *Int Angiol* 1995; 14: 200.
6. Veith FJ, Gupta SK, Ascer E, *et al*. Six-year prospective multicentre randomized comparison of autologous saphenous vein and expanded polytetrafluoroethylene grafts in infrainguinal arterial constructions. *J Vasc Surg* 1986; 3: 104-14.
7. Bergan JJ, Veith FJ, Bernhard VM, *et al*. Randomization of autogenous vein and polytetrafluoroethylene grafts in femoro-distal constructions. *Surgery* 1982; 92: 921-30.
8. Klinkert P, Schepers A, Burger DHC, *et al*. Vein versus polytetrafluoroethylene in above-knee femoropopliteal bypass grafting: five-year results of a randomized controlled trial. *J Vasc Surg* 2003; 37: 149-55.

9. Ballotta E, Renon L, Toffano M, Da Giau G. Prospective randomized study on bilateral above-knee femoropopliteal revascularization: polytetrafluoroethylene graft versus reversed saphenous vein. *J Vasc Surg* 2003; 38: 1051-5.

10. Mamode N, Scott RN. Graft type for femoro-popliteal bypass surgery. *Cochrane Database Syst Rev* 2000; 2: CD001487.

11. Schouten O, Hoedt MTC, Wittens CHA, *et al.* End-to-end versus end-to-side distal anastomosis in femoropopliteal bypasses: results of a randomized multicenter trial. *Eur J Vasc Endovasc Surg* 2005; 29: 457-62.

12. Harris PL, How TV, Jones DR. Prospectively randomized clinical trial to compare *in situ* and reversed saphenous vein grafts for femoropopliteal bypass. *Br J Surg* 1987; 74: 252-5.

13. Harris PL, Veith FJ, Shanik GD, *et al.* Prospective randomized comparison of *in situ* and reversed infrapopliteal vein grafts. *Br J Surg* 1993; 80: 173-6.

14. Wengerter KR, Veith FJ, Gupta SK, Goldsmith J, *et al.* Prospective randomized multicenter comparison of *in situ* and reversed vein infrapopliteal bypasses. *J Vasc Surg* 1991; 13: 189-99.

15. Moody AP, Edwards PR, Harris PL. *In situ* versus reversed femoropopliteal vein grafts: long-term follow-up of a prospective randomized trial. *Br J Surg* 1992; 79: 750-2.

16. Watelet J, Saour N, Menard J-F, *et al.* Femoropopliteal bypass: *in situ* or reversed vein grafts? Ten-year results of a randomized prospective study. *Ann Vasc Surg* 1997; 11: 510-9.

17. Lawson JA, Tangelder MJD, Algra A, Eikelboom BC, on behalf of the Dutch BOA Study Group. The myth of the *in situ* graft: superiority in infrainguinal bypass surgery? *Eur J Vasc Endovasc Surg* 1999; 18: 149-57.

18. McCarthy WJ, Pearce WH, Flinn WR, *et al.* Long-term evaluation of composite sequential bypass for limb-threatening ischaemia. *J Vasc Surg* 1992; 15: 761-70.

19. Hölzenbein TJ, Pomposelli FB, Miller A, *et al.* Results of a policy with arm veins used as the first alternative to an unavailable ipsilateral greater saphenous vein for infrainguinal bypass. *J Vasc Surg* 1996; 23: 130-40.

20. Schulman ML, Badhey MR, Yatco R, Pillari G. An 11-year experience with deep leg veins as femoropopliteal bypass grafts. *Arch Surg* 1986; 121: 1010-5.

21. Schulman ML, Badhey MR, Yatco R. Superficial femoral-popliteal veins and reversed saphenous veins as primary femoropopliteal bypass grafts: a randomized comparative study. *J Vasc Surg* 1987; 6: 1-10.

22. Hickey NC, Thomson IA, Shearman CP, Simms MH. Aggressive arterial reconstruction for critical lower limb ischaemia. *Br J Surg* 1991; 78: 1476-8.

23. Schulman ML, Badhey MR. Late results and angiographic evaluation of arm veins as long bypass grafts. *Surgery* 1982; 96: 1032-41.

24. Mahmood A, Garnham A, Sintler M, *et al.* Composite sequential grafts for femorocrural bypass reconstruction: experience with a modified technique. *J Vasc Surg* 2002; 36: 772-8.

25. Londrey GL, Ramsey DE, Hodgson KJ, *et al.* Infrapopliteal bypass for severe ischaemia: comparison of autologous vein, composite, and prosthetic grafts. *J Vasc Surg* 1991; 13: 631-6.

26. Christenson JT, Eklof B. Sparks mandril, velour Dacron and autogenous saphenous vein grafts in femoropopliteal bypass. *Br J Surg* 1979; 66: 514-7.

27. Kenney DA, Sauvage LR, Wood SJ, *et al.* Comparison of non-crimped, externally supported (EXS) and crimped non-supported Dacron prostheses for axillo-bifemoral and above-knee femoropopliteal bypass. *Surgery* 1982; 92: 931-46.

28. Abbott WA, Green RM, Matsumoto T, *et al.* Prosthetic above-knee femoropopliteal bypass grafting: results of a multicentre randomized prospective trial. *J Vasc Surg* 1997; 25: 19-26.

29. Charlesworth PM, Brewster DC, Darling RC, *et al.* The fate of polytetrafluoroethylene grafts in lower limb bypass surgery: a six year follow-up. *Br J Surg* 1985; 72: 896-9.

30. Whittemore AD, Kent KC, Donaldson MC, *et al.* What is the proper role of polytetrafluoroethylene grafts in infrainguinal reconstruction? *J Vasc Surg* 1989; 10: 299-305.

31. Miller JH, Foreman RK, Ferguson L, Faris I. Interposition vein cuff for anastomosis of prosthesis to small artery. *ANZ Surg* 1984; 54: 283-5.

32. Raptis S, Miller JH. Influence of a vein cuff on polytetrafluoroethylene grafts for primary femoropopliteal bypass. *Br J Surg* 1995; 82: 487-91.

33. Griffiths GD, Nagy J, Black P, Stonebridge PA, on behalf of the Joint Vascular Research Group. Randomized clinical trial of distal anastomotic interposition vein graft in infrainguinal polytetrafluoroethylene bypass grafting. *Br J Surg* 2004; 91: 560-2.

34. Tyrrell MR, Wolfe JHN. Myointimal hyperplasia in vein collars for ePTFE grafts. *Eur J Vasc Endovasc Surg* 1997; 14: 33-6.

35. Renwick P, Johnson B, Wilkinson A, *et al.* Limb outcome following failed femoropopliteal polytetrafluoroethylene bypass for intermittent claudication. *Br J Surg* 1999; 86: A690.

36. Wolfe JHN, Tyrrell MR. Justifying arterial reconstruction to crural vessels - even with a prosthetic graft. *Br J Surg* 1991; 78: 897-9.

37. Taylor RS, Loh H, McFarland RJ, *et al.* Improved technique for polytetrafluoroethylene bypass grafting: long-term results using anastomotic vein patches. *Br J Surg* 1992; 79: 348-54.

38. Tyrrell MR, Wolfe JHN. New prosthetic venous collar anastomotic technique: combining the best of other procedures. *Br J Surg* 1991; 78: 1016-7.

39. Da Silva AF, Carpenter T, How TV, Harris PL. Stable vortices within vein cuffs inhibit myointimal hyperplasia? *Eur J Vasc Endovasc Surg* 1997; 14: 157-63.

40. Fisher RK, Toonder I, Hoedt M, *et al.* Harnessing haemodynamics for the suppression of anastomotic intimal hyperplasia: the rationale for precuffed grafts. *Eur J Vasc Endovasc Surg* 2001; 21: 520-8.

41. Panneton JM, Hollier LH, Hofer JM. Multicenter randomized prospective trial comparing a pre-cuffed polytetrafluoroethylene graft to a vein-cuffed polytetrafluoroethylene graft for infragenicular arterial bypass. *Ann Vasc Surg* 2004; 18: 199-206.

42. Ascer E, Gennaro M, Pollina RM, *et al.* Complementary distal arteriovenous fistula and deep vein interposition: a five-year experience with a new technique to improve infrapopliteal prosthetic bypass patency. *J Vasc Surg* 1996; 24: 134-43.

43. Dardik H, Berry SM, Dardik A, Wolodiger F, *et al.* Infrapopliteal prosthetic graft patency by use of the distal adjunctive arteriovenous fistula. *J Vasc Surg* 1991; 13: 685-90.

44. Hamsho A, Nott D, Harris PL. Prospective randomized trial of distal arteriovenous fistula as an adjunct to femoro-infrapopliteal PTFE bypass. *Eur J Vasc Endovasc Surg* 1999; 17: 197-201.

45. Laurila K, Lepantalo M, Teittinen K, *et al.* Does an adjuvant AV-fistula improve the patency of a femorocrural PTFE bypass with distal vein cuff in critical leg ischaemia - a prospective randomized multicentre trial. *Eur J Vasc Endovasc Surg* 2004; 27: 180-5.

46. Devine C, McCollum C, North West Femoro-Popliteal Trial Participants. Heparin-bonded Dacron or polytetrafluorethylene for femoropopliteal bypass: five-year results of a prospective randomized multicenter clinical trial. *J Vasc Surg* 2004; 40: 924-31.

47. Kapfer X, Meichelboeck VV, Groegler F-M. Comparison of carbon-impregnated and standard ePTFE prostheses in extra-anatomical anterior tibial artery bypass. *Eur J Vasc Endovasc Surg* 2006; 32: 155-68.

48. Blankenstein JD, Gertler JP, Brewster DC, *et al.* Intraoperative determinants of infrainguinal bypass graft patency: a prospective study. *Eur J Vasc Endovasc Surg* 1995; 9: 375-82.

49. Watson HR, Belcher G, Horrocks M. Adjuvant medical therapy in peripheral bypass surgery. *Br J Surg* 1999; 86: 981-91.

50. Antiplatelet Trialists' Collaboration. Collaborative overview of randomized trials of antiplatelet therapy - II: Maintenance of vascular graft or arterial patency by antiplatelet therapy. *Br Med J* 1994; 308: 159-68.

51. Arfvidsson B, Lundgren F, Drott C, *et al.* Influence of coumarin treatment on patency and limb salvage after peripheral arterial reconstructive surgery. *Am J Surg* 1990; 159: 556-60.

52. Kretschmer GJ, Hölzenbein T, Huk I, Abela C. What is the evidence that anticoagulant treatment improves long-term patency of distal bypass? In: *Trials and Tribulations of Vascular Surgery. Evidence-based Vascular Surgery.* Greenhalgh RM, Fowkes FGR, Eds. London: Saunders,1996: 43-52.

53. Sarac TP, Huber TS, Back MR, *et al.* Warfarin improves the outcome of infrainguinal vein bypass grafting at high risk of failure. *J Vasc Surg* 1998; 28: 446-57.

54. Johnson WC, Williford WO. Benefits, morbidity, and mortality associated with long-term administration of oral anticoagulant therapy to patients with peripheral arterial bypass procedures: a prospective randomized study. *J Vasc Surg* 2002; 35: 413-21.

55. Oostenbrink JB, Tangelder MJD, Busschbach JJV, *et al.* Cost-effectiveness of oral anticoagulants versus aspirin in patients after infrainguinal bypass grafting surgery. *J Vasc Surg* 2001; 34: 254-62.

56. Lundell A, Lindblad B, Bergqvist D, Hansen F. Femoropopliteal-crural graft patency is improved by an intensive surveillance program: a prospective randomized study. *J Vasc Surg* 1995; 21: 26-33.

57. Ihlberg L, Luther M, Tierla E, *et al.* The utility of duplex scanning in infrainguinal vein graft surveillance: results from a randomised controlled study. *Eur J Vasc Endovasc Surg* 1998; 16: 19-27.

58. Fasih T, Rudol G, Ashour H, *et al.* Surveillance versus non-surveillance for femoro-popliteal bypass grafts. *Angiology* 2004; 55: 251-6.

59. Davies AH, Hawdon AJ, Sydes MR, Thompson SG, on behalf of the Vein Graft Surveillance Trialists (VGST). Is duplex surveillance of value after leg vein bypass grafting? Principal results of the vein graft surveillance randomised trial. *Circulation* 2005; 112: 1985-91.

Chapter 9

Management of critical leg ischaemia and quality of life

Shazia M Khan MRCS MSc, Specialist Registrar in Vascular Surgery
Jonathan D Beard FRCS ChM, Consultant Vascular Surgeon
Sheffield Vascular Institute, Northern General Hospital, Sheffield, UK

Introduction

The frontiers of revascularisation for critical leg ischaemia (CLI) have advanced over the last two decades. This has been due to refinement of distal bypass procedures and the development of increasingly sophisticated endovascular techniques. Such progress, inevitably, has economic consequences and it is essential to evaluate treatment strategies to determine the cost-effectiveness of revascularisation. Patients with CLI often have multiple comorbidities with a poor prognosis. This is particularly so for diabetics [1], the elderly [2] and those with end-stage renal failure [3]. Most surgical series agree that the five-year survival rate for patients with CLI is 50-60%, which emphasises the palliative nature of most treatment options for such patients [4].

Indications for primary amputation

Vascular surgeons have generally advocated reconstruction for CLI because of the poor mobility and high mortality associated with amputation [5], and the lower cost of successful reconstruction compared to that of amputation [6]. However, the high costs of both graft failure and re-intervention to maintain graft patency must be considered [7]. An aggressive policy of reconstruction for CLI can only be justified on health-economic grounds if success rates are sufficiently high. The European Consensus Document recommends that "A reconstructive procedure should be attempted if there is a 25% chance of saving a useful limb for a patient for at least one year" [8]. But a failure rate of such magnitude cannot be countenanced because of the huge cost of failed reconstruction and secondary amputation. In truth, a policy of reconstruction can only be justified on cost-effectiveness grounds if the one-year limb salvage rate is at least 75%.

Current management of CLI is confused, with large differences in practice between clinicians [9]. This is exacerbated by a lack of scientific evidence; no randomised trials of reconstruction versus amputation exist. Prospective studies comparing outcomes in these groups have, of course, been done, but, until recently, none was matched for age, sex or disease severity. At best, this represents poor level III evidence. Retrospective case series and international consensus documents can also be found, but this is only level IV evidence. Current guidelines based on this evidence are summarised in Table 1.

Table 1. Current guidelines on management of critical limb ischaemia [8, 10, 11].	
Reconstruction	**Amputation**
Attempt reconstruction if:	Primary amputation or palliative care if:
◆ patient fit enough for surgery ◆ good run-off vessel(s) ◆ suitable vein if distal anastomosis to tibial artery ◆ reasonable chance of limb salvage at 1 year ◆ likely to walk or use prosthetic leg for transferring	◆ unreconstructable arterial occlusive disease ◆ necrosis of significant weight-bearing portion of the foot ◆ severe diabetic neuropathy or foot sepsis ◆ fixed flexion contracture of the hip or knee ◆ terminal illness or very limited life expectancy because of comorbidity ◆ bed bound or dementia

Some indications for primary amputation commonly affect elderly patients. These include dementia and immobility. A demented, bed-bound patient is unlikely to benefit from arterial reconstruction. Similarly, younger patients with severe diabetic neuropathy, foot sepsis or poor run-off may be best served by a below-knee amputation rather than futile attempts at reconstruction. An infra-inguinal reconstruction that fails in the early postoperative period may adversely affect the level of amputation[12], resulting in an above-knee amputation when a primary below-knee amputation might have healed (Figure 1). While the complications and cost of reconstruction cannot be justified in these high-risk groups, percutaneous transluminal angioplasty may seem a reasonable option when there is 'nothing to lose'. Care of pressure areas and adequate analgesia rather than amputation should be provided for those who are terminally ill.

Old age alone is not an indication for amputation for CLI, but previous ability to walk and residential status should be considered. Good ambulation in the very elderly after amputation is the exception rather than the rule, whereas successful reconstruction may maintain some level of ambulation and independence at home [13]. The only other option for these patients is often a residential or nursing home, with inevitable loss of independence.

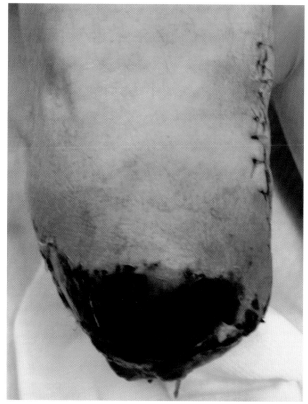

Figure 1. Failed infra-inguinal bypass with subsequent necrosis at the below-knee amputation level because of damage to the geniculate collaterals. A primary below-knee amputation would probably have healed.

Tools for assessing quality of life

Graft patency and limb salvage are crude measures of outcome; other assessments, such as treadmill walking [14] and ankle:brachial pressure index (ABPI) [15], seem irrelevant in CLI. In fact, the symptoms of limb ischaemia rather than ABPI are better predictors of the scores of two validated health-related quality of life (QoL) questionnaires (SF-36 and WIQ) [15]. QoL assessment has, therefore, become a key outcome measure in gauging the impact of arterial disease and its treatment [16]. Patients' pre-operative health perceptions have been shown to be related to surgical outcome [17]. It is also known that surgeons predict QoL less accurately than patients themselves and that perceptions may differ between colleagues [18]. This has led to a call for an objective QoL assessment tool, with particular regard to patient reported outcomes [19].

Quality of life is defined as a state of physical, emotional and social wellbeing, not just the absence of disease and infirmity [20]. The World Health Organisation QoL group has identified five major areas of importance in this regard. These are physical health, psychological health, social relationship perceptions, function and well being [21]. QoL can be assessed by either generic or disease-specific tools.

Generic tools

Generic assessment tools allow comparisons between different groups of patients by measuring the impact of any disease or treatment. They consist of global QoL dimensions, such as physical, social and psychological health. The Nottingham Health Profile (NHP) and the Medical Outcomes Short Form-36 (SF-36) both measure across the range of domains, including physical, emotional and social, and the patient's responses are scored for each domain. Currently, the SF-36 is the most appropriate generic QoL analysis tool and its use has been advocated to standardise the assessment of outcome after vascular surgery [22]. In fact both the NHP and the SF-36 have a place in assessing different aspects of vascular disease. Both have the hallmarks of a good QoL questionnaire. Both are reliable for group comparison, and exhibit construct and convergent validity [23] (Table 2). However, they are both heavily influenced by mobility and so inherently biased against amputation.

Table 2. Comparison between the Nottingham Health Profile and SF-36 questionnaires [23].

Nottingham Health Profile	SF-36

◆ Consists of two parts:
 	
   o Part 1 - pain
          - physical mobility
          - emotional reactions
          - energy
          - social isolation
          - sleep
   o Part 2 - questions concerning daily living
             problems
	◆ 36 items covering 8 health concepts:
	
	   o bodily pain
	   o physical functioning
	   o role limitation due to physical problems
	   o mental health
	   o vitality
	   o social functioning
	   o role limitation due to emotional problems
	   o general health

◆ capable of measuring changes in perceived health following different treatments	◆ responsive to changes in health status over time in patients with critical ischaemia and in claudicants
◆ 'floor' and 'ceiling' effect larger than SF-36	◆ less skewed scores than Nottingham Health Profile
◆ better discriminator of severity of ischaemia	◆ superior psychometric properties
◆ more responsive in patients with critical ischaemia	◆ more suitable for claudicants

Disease-specific tools

Disease-specific tools focus on the QoL domains affected by symptoms of the disease in question. There is no widely accepted disease-specific questionnaire for patients with CLI. However, stroke seems a fair parallel for CLI and both the Barthel Index of Self-care and the Frenchay Index of Lifestyle, which were developed for patients with stroke, are relatively independent of mobility and have been used to assess QoL in those with CLI. The first attempt at a disease-specific tool for CLI is the King's College Vascular Quality of Life (VascuQoL) questionnaire [24]. It evaluates across the whole spectrum of CLI through five domains: pain, symptoms, activities, social and emotional. Construct validity has been shown by correlation with the Fontaine classification of disease severity, treadmill walking distance and corresponding domains in the SF-36. This new tool is currently being tested further in a multicentre trial of bypass versus angioplasty in CLI [25].

It has been suggested that there should be a consensus on the most reliable QoL measure to allow a single international standard [26]. Although such a consensus has not yet been reached, the use of both generic and disease-specific QoL tools is recommended by the Transatlantic Intersociety Consensus (TASC) Group [10]. In particular, TASC recommends SF-36 as the generic health outcome measure in CLI. However, NHP has also been promoted as a preferred tool for this condition [23]. The VascuQoL tool has recently been shown to be superior to other tests for detecting changes in QoL in patients who have been treated for arterial occlusive disease [27].

Limitations of current QoL measurement

The main limitation of QoL measurement is that it frequently measures an external value system derived from group data, so a total score may bear little relationship to the experience of an individual. Events do not necessarily maintain the same meaning for individuals over time or the course of an illness, and the impact of any change is difficult to assess with a system that is confined to a few specific domains.

Many QoL tools have a 'floor' or 'ceiling' effect, i.e. limited ability to detect changes in poor or good health. For instance, the physical role in CLI frequently scores the lowest possible, so any deterioration goes undetected and any improvement must be marked to register a different score. Using any QoL tool has particular problems in the elderly because their perception of their own health is related to their peer group, and consequently their scores are usually higher than an 'objective' (younger) observer might anticipate. Individuals have different concepts of how their health state affects QoL and any deterioration in this state may not be assessed by generic QoL tools. The SF-36 is unhelpful in assessing some of the changes in health that the elderly perceive; structured interviews reveal these differences more clearly [28]. Further progress has been made using the Schedule for the Evaluation of Individual Quality of Life (SEIQOL) to assess QoL from the individual's perspective. An abbreviated form of the measure, the SEIQOL - direct weighting (SEIQOL-DW) is a simpler procedure for measuring the relative importance (weights) of the five life areas regarded as most important by the patient [29]. Using this instrument the authors have found that patients with CLI often give more weight to aspects such as family and environment than to mobility.

Current evidence for reconstruction

A growing number of studies have been published on the effects of different treatment strategies on QoL in patients with CLI. There seems to be no difference in QoL between patients operated for rest pain and those operated for tissue loss [22], but none of these studies is homogenous so it is difficult to make firm conclusions.

A multicentre, five-year follow-up study in Finland assessed the outcomes of 117 consecutive patients requiring treatment for CLI. In order to maintain mobility and independence, leg salvage by appropriate vascular reconstruction was carried out if technically feasible. There were 66 reconstructions and 51 primary amputations, with an additional 35 secondary amputations. While all patients with a successful reconstruction preserved their walking ability and independent living, only 10% of amputees could walk and only 25% could live independently [5] **(III/B)**.

The Minneapolis group used the SF-36 questionnaire before and after revascularisation in patients with CLI to assess the impact of such surgery on health-related QoL. Despite a mild improvement in physical function, overall QoL was low compared to that of age-matched controls, both at baseline and at six months after operation. The authors optimistically suggested that this was because QoL in those with CLI was slow to improve and that a longer follow-up might be necessary [30] **(IIa/B)**. In contrast, a number of uncontrolled series have reported immediate and sustained improvement up to 12 months in the SF-36 and NHP domains of physical functioning, pain, sleep, vitality and social functioning in the patients undergoing reconstruction [17, 31, 32] **(III/B)**.

A recent review has shown that the surgical ideal of an uncomplicated infra-inguinal bypass, with relief of pain, wound healing and a return to full activity without further intervention was achieved in only 16 of 112 (19%) patients [33] **(III/B)**. Paradoxically, patients with occluded grafts had improved scores in pain, vitality and social functioning, but no improvement in physical functioning or role. Those who required secondary amputation had similar improvements in pain, vitality, mental health and social functioning as those with a patent graft, and sometimes scored higher for the psychological domains [31] **(III/B)**. While this demonstrates that the time and expense incurred in revascularisation are justified for the improved QoL, it also highlights the fact that amputees may also benefit from an improvement in QoL in all except physical domains. Some report an increase in QoL because of a lack of pain or worries about their graft failing. These patients challenge the assumption that amputation reflects failure for the patient and the surgeon. The evidence suggests that mobility is the only significant difference between amputees and normal controls and that many patients remain independent despite limb loss and lack of ambulation [34] **(IIa/B)**. Despite reduction in mobility, an overall improvement in pain and anxiety scores has also been reported in amputees [35] **(III/B)**.

The Sheffield Vascular Institute has undertaken a large prospective study of QoL involving 150 consecutive patients treated for CLI [36] **(IIa/B)**. A

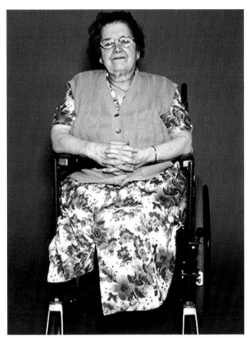

Figure 2. **Bilateral amputee with a good quality of life because of lack of pain, good wheelchair mobility, home adaptations facilitating self-care, and supportive family and friends.** *Consent obtained.*

single occupational therapist assessed the patients for pain, mobility, anxiety, depression, self-care and lifestyle at presentation, and at six and 12 months after amputation or reconstruction. The pre-operative scores were similar, suggesting that the patients were well matched. Pain and self-care both improved significantly after both treatments; mobility was better after reconstruction. There was no overall improvement in lifestyle for either group but there was a large individual variation. A good pre-operative lifestyle score was the best predictor of successful rehabilitation (Figure 2). An appropriate environment was also vital to maximise QoL.

Compared to age and sex-matched controls without CLI, successfully reconstructed patients in one study had significantly decreased independence and mobility scores, such as ability to walk, perform household tasks and bathe [37]. This is in direct contrast to the findings of the Minneapolis group [30] **(IIa/B)**. However, at four-year follow-up the patients reported that they remained well with no somatic complaints [37]. Self-perceived ambulatory function and self-perceived physical activity have been reported to outstrip objectively measured ambulation and physical activity after revascularisation in patients with CLI [38] **(III/B)**.

In a review of the treatment options available in CLI, revascularisation by angioplasty or surgical reconstruction was recognised as the treatment of choice for most patients [39]. However, primary amputation is appropriate when the benefit of surgical reconstruction appears negligible and for those in whom the chances of successful reconstruction appear small. Amputation is also appropriate for those with extensive foot necrosis, sepsis or neuropathy. Focusing on QoL helps to identify patients who might expect negligible benefit from reconstruction.

Conclusions

The decision to perform an arterial reconstruction or a primary amputation should be based on an analysis of what is best for the individual patient and not simply on technical feasibility. QoL analysis, based on a patient's own priorities rather than the preconceived notions of others, is invaluable for identifying those for whom the benefit of reconstruction would prove negligible.

Key points	Evidence level
◆ Revascularisation by angioplasty or surgical reconstruction is the treatment of choice for most patients with critical leg ischaemia but there is no level I evidence to inform that choice.	III/B
◆ Reconstruction requires a success rate of 75% at one year to become cost-effective.	III/B
◆ Only 19% of patients have an uncomplicated infra-inguinal reconstruction.	III/B
◆ Failed reconstruction may result in a higher secondary amputation level and a worse QoL than primary amputation.	IIb/B
◆ Successful reconstruction results in better mobility than primary amputation.	III/B
◆ Successful reconstruction can help to maintain independence in the elderly.	III/B
◆ Apart from mobility, there is little difference in QoL achieved between primary amputation and reconstruction.	III/B
◆ Primary amputation may be the best option for those in whom mobility is not an important factor.	III/B

References

1. Dolan NC, Liu K, Criqui MH, *et al*. Peripheral artery disease, diabetes, and reduced lower extremity functioning. *Diabetes Care* 2002; 25: 113-20.
2. Taylor SM, Kalbaugh CA, Blackhurst DW, *et al*. Preoperative clinical factors predict postoperative functional outcomes after major lower limb amputation: an analysis of 553 consecutive patients. *J Vasc Surg* 2005; 42: 227-35.
3. Redden DN, Marcus RJ, Owen WF Jr, *et al*. Long-term outcomes of revascularisation for peripheral vascular disease in end-stage renal disease patients. *Am J Kidney Dis* 2001; 38: 57-63.
4. The ICAI Group. The study group of critical chronic ischaemia of the lower extremities. Long-term mortality and its predictors in patients with critical leg ischaemia. *Eur J Vasc Endovasc Surg* 1997; 14: 91-5.
5. Luther M. Surgical treatment of chronic critical leg ischaemia. A five-year follow-up of survival, mobility and treatment level. *Eur J Surg* 1998; 164: 35-43.
6. Panayiotopoulos YP, Tyrrell MR, Owen SE, *et al*. Outcome and cost analysis after femorocrural and femoropedal grafting for critical limb ischaemia. *Br J Surg* 1997; 84: 207-12.

7. Cheshire NJW, Noone MA, Wolfe JHN. Re-intervention after vascular surgery for critical leg ischaemia. *Eur J Vasc Surg* 1992; 6: 545-50.

8. European Working Group on Critical Leg Ischaemia. Second European Consensus Document on chronic critical leg ischaemia. *Eur J Vasc Surg* 1992; 6(suppl A): 1-32.

9. Pell JP, Fowkes FGR, Lee AJ. On behalf of the Scottish and Northern Vascular Audit Group. Indications for arterial reconstruction and major amputation in the management of chronic critical lower limb ischaemia. *Eur J Vasc Endovasc Surg* 1997; 13: 315-21.

10. TASC Working Group. Management of Peripheral Arterial Disease (PAD). TransAtlantic InterSociety Consensus (TASC). *Eur J Vasc Endovasc Surg* 2000, 19 (suppl A): 1-244.

11. Apelqvist J, Bakker K, Van Houttum WH, *et al*. International Working Group on the Diabetic Foot. International consensus and practical guidelines on the management and prevention of the diabetic foot. *Diabetes Metab Res Rev* 2000, 16(suppl 1): S84-S92.

12. Evans WE, Hayes JP, Vermilion BD. Effect of failed distal reconstruction on the level of amputation. *Am J Surg* 1990; 160: 217-20.

13. Pomposelli FB, Arora S, Gibbons GW, *et al*. Lower extremity arterial reconstruction in the very elderly: successful outcome preserves not only the limb but also residential status and ambulatory function. *J Vasc Surg* 1998; 28: 215-25.

14. Barletta G, Perna S, Sabba C, *et al*. Quality of life in patients with intermittent claudication: relationship with laboratory exercise performance. *Vasc Med* 1996; 1: 3-7.

15. Long J, Modrall JG, Parker RN, *et al*. Correlation between ankle-brachial index, symptoms, and health-related quality of life in patients with peripheral vascular disease. *J Vasc Surg* 2004; 39: 723-7.

16. Humphreys W, Evans F, Williams T. Quality of life: is it a practical tool in patients with vascular disease? *J Cardiovasc Pharmacol* 1994; 23(suppl. 3): S34-S36.

17. Thorsen H, McKenna S, Tennant A, Holstein P. Nottingham Health Profile scores predict the outcome and support aggressive revascularisation for critical ischaemia. *Eur J Vasc Endovasc Surg* 2002; 23: 495-9.

18. Hicken GJ, Lossing AG, Ameli FM. Assessment of generic health-related quality of life in patients with intermittent claudication. *Eur J Vasc Endovasc Surg* 2000; 20: 336-41.

19. Chassany O, Le-Jeunne P, Duracinsky M, *et al*. Discrepancies between patient-reported outcomes and clinician-reported outcomes in chronic venous disease, irritable bowel syndrome, and peripheral arterial occlusive disease. *Value Health* 2006; 9: 39-46.

20. World Health Organisation. The constitution of the WHO. *WHO Chronicle* 1947; 1: 29.

21. WHOQOL group: Study protocol for the World Health Organisation project to develop a quality of life instrument (WHOQOL). *Quality of Life Research* 1993; 2: 153-9.

22. Chetter IC, Spark JI, Dolan P, *et al*. Quality of Life analysis in patients with lower limb ischaemia: suggestions for European standardisation. *Eur J Vasc Endovasc Surg* 1997; 13: 597-604.

23. Wann-Hansson C, Hallberg IR, Risberg B, Klevsgård R. A comparison of the Nottingham Health Profile and Short Form 36 health survey in patients with chronic lower limb ischaemia in a longitudinal perspective. *Health and Quality of Life Outcomes* 2004; 2: 9.

24. Morgan M, Crayford T, Murrin B, Fraser S. Developing the vascular quality of life questionnaire: a new disease-specific quality of life measure for use in lower limb ischaemia. *J Vasc Surg* 2001; 33: 679-87.

25. Morgan MB, Fraser SC, Bradbury A. Health Outcomes. *Eur J Vasc Endovasc Surg* 2000; 20: 316-7.

26. Beattie DK, Golledge J, Greenhalgh RM, Davies AH. Quality of life assessment in vascular disease: towards a consensus. *Eur J Vasc Endovasc Surg* 1997; 13: 9-13.

27. De Vries M, Ouwendijk R, Kessels AG, *et al*. Comparison of generic and disease-specific questionnaires for the assessment of quality of life in patients with peripheral arterial disease. *J Vasc Surg* 2005; 41: 261-8.

28. Hill S, Harries U, Popay J. Is the Short Form-36 (SF-36) suitable for routine health care for older people? Evidence from preliminary work in community-based health services in England. *J Epidemiol Community Health* 1996; 50: 4-98.

29. Hickey AM, Bury G, O'Boyle CA, *et al*. A new short-form individual quality of life measure (SEIQoL-DW): application in a cohort of individuals with HIV/AIDS. *Br Med J* 1996; 313: 29-33.

30. Tretinyak AS, Lee ES, Kuskowski MA, *et al*. Revascularisation and quality of life for patients with limb-threatening ischaemia. *Ann Vasc Surg* 2001; 15: 84-8.

31. Chetter IC, Spark JI, Scott DJA, *et al*. Prospective analysis of quality of life in patients following infrainguinal reconstruction for chronic critical ischaemia. *Br J Surg* 1998; 85: 951-5.

32. Klevsgard R, Risberg BO, Thomsen MB, Hallberg IR. A 1-year follow-up quality of life study after haemodynamically successful or unsuccessful surgical revascularisation of lower limb ischaemia. *J Vasc Surg* 2001; 33: 114-22.

33. Nicoloff AD, Taylor LM, McLafferty RB, *et al*. Patient recovery after infrainguinal bypass grafting for limb salvage. *J Vasc Surg* 1998; 27: 256-66.

34. Nehler MR, Coll JR, Hlan WR, *et al*. Functional outcome in contemporary series of major lower extremity amputations. *J Vasc Surg* 2003; 38: 7-14.

35. Nehler MR, McDermott MM, Treat-Jacobson D, *et al*. Functional outcomes and quality of life in peripheral arterial disease: current status. *Vasc Med* 2003; 8: 115-26.

36. Johnson BF, Singh S, Evans L, *et al*. A prospective study of the effect of limb-threatening ischaemia and its surgical treatment on the quality of life. *Eur J Vasc Endovasc Surg* 1997; 1: 306-14.

37. Seabrook GR, Cambria RA, Freischlag JA, Towne JB. Health-related quality of life and functional outcome following arterial reconstruction for limb salvage. *Cardiovasc Surg* 1999; 7: 279-86.

38. Gardner AW, Killewich LA. Lack of functional benefits following infrainguinal bypass in peripheral arterial occlusive disease patients. *Vasc Med* 2001; 6: 9-14.

39. Sillensen H. Conservative treatment, amputation or revascularisation for critical limb ischaemia. *Ann Chir et Gynae* 1998; 87: 159-61.

Chapter 10

Non-surgical treatment of critical leg ischaemia

Frank CT Smith BSc MD FRCS FRCSEd, Consultant Senior Lecturer in Vascular Surgery
Bristol Royal Infirmary, Bristol, UK

Introduction

Critical leg ischaemia (CLI) affects approximately one in 2,500 of the population annually and carries poor long-term prognosis [1] (Figure 1). One year after developing CLI only 56% of patients will be alive with two legs, more than 20% will have had an amputation and 10-20% will have died from concomitant coronary or cerebrovascular disease. Surgical reconstruction with, or without endovascular intervention offers the best hope of limb salvage and improved quality of life, but up to 20% of patients may not be amenable to arterial reconstruction. This chapter reviews the evidence for medical and non-surgical treatments of CLI for patients in whom surgical reconstruction is not feasible.

Drug treatment

Use of prostanoids: the rationale

More research has been undertaken into prostanoids than any other class of drugs in the medical treatment of CLI. CLI usually occurs as a result of multi-segment arterial disease. Long-standing proximal arterial stenoses or occlusions result in vasodilation and development of collateral channels which, in CLI, progressively fail to compensate

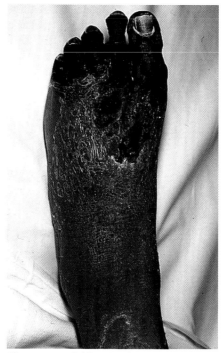

Figure 1. Critically ischaemic foot with extensive tissue necrosis

adequately for impairment of blood flow to the foot. In conjunction with disease of the larger arteries there is progressive microcirculatory impairment, largely as a result of decreased perfusion pressure. Activation of platelets and leucocytes occurs with release of growth factors, free radicals, cytokines and proteases. Vasoconstriction and endothelial cell swelling contribute to a decrease in the number of perfused capillaries. Cellular plugging of capillaries exacerbates this situation further and endothelial dysfunction is accompanied by tissue oedema. It is at this microcirculatory level that the prostanoids which have antiplatelet, anti-leucocyte, vasodilatory and cytoprotective functions exert their beneficial effects. Prostacyclin (PGI2) has a short half-life of 2-3 minutes, limiting its therapeutic potential. Research has therefore concentrated on the stable prostacyclin analogue, Iloprost, which has a half-life of approximately 30 minutes. To date, Iloprost has only been available for intravascular administration, although phase 3 trials of an oral form have now been completed and this formulation will probably be available in the near future. PGE1 has also been studied intensively in CLI, particularly in Germany.

Current prostanoid treatment regimens are labour intensive, involving strictly monitored intravenous infusions administered for up to six hours a day for several days. Gradual increases in dose to a maximum level are titrated against vasodilatory side effects that may include facial flushing, nausea, headaches and abdominal pain. With higher doses systemic hypotension and angina may occur.

Iloprost

The effects of Iloprost in CLI have been evaluated in six large European multicentre randomised controlled studies, involving more than 700 patients with Fontaine stage III (ischaemic rest pain alone) or Fontaine stage IV (gangrene) ischaemia [2-7]. These trials have been summarised in a meta-analysis by Loosemore et al [8], and reviewed by Guilmot and Boissier (1999) [9] **(Ia/A)**. Iloprost or placebo was administered intravenously at doses to a maximum of 2ng/kg/minute for six hours per day for the duration of each study which varied between two to four weeks. Overall, one third of patients had already undergone an attempt at either surgical or endovascular revascularisation. Three quarters of patients were receiving medication for heart disease and there were high prevalences of diabetes and hypertension in treatment and placebo groups in all studies. On completion of the treatment, patients were judged to be responders or non-responders according to complete pain relief in Fontaine stage III patients and healing of at least 30% of ulcer surface in patients with tissue loss (Fontaine IV). In all trials the number of responders was significantly higher in the Iloprost-treated group than in the placebo group **(Ia/A)**. In each trial patients in the placebo group also improved, presumably due to the effects of adjunctive best medical treatment. Pain relief and ulcer healing have been criticised as soft endpoints in these trials, but in the three most recent trials major amputation rates were also evaluated on an intention-to-treat basis [5-7]. Amputation rates were significantly lower in Iloprost-treated patients in UK and Scandinavian studies, and in all three trials analysed together by meta-analysis **(Ia/A)**. In the UK and Scandinavian studies mortality or major amputation occurred in 35% of Iloprost-treated patients and in 55% of the placebo group [5, 6]. The chances of a patient treated with Iloprost being alive with both legs at six-month follow-up were significantly higher than those of a patient given placebo (p<0.001) **(Ia/A)**.

Two further important studies involving Iloprost have been reported. In a European multicentre trial involving 133 patients the drug was evaluated for thrombo-angiitis obliterans (Buerger's disease), against aspirin instead of placebo [10]. An 87% response rate occurred in the Iloprost-treated group versus a 17% response rate in the aspirin group, with benefits maintained at six-month follow-up. Complete pain relief and ulcer healing occurred in 63% and 35% of Iloprost-treated patients compared to 28% and 13% of the aspirin-treated group, respectively **(Ib/A)**. In a further trial (the Hawaii Study), involving 713 patients, in which Iloprost was used as an adjunct to healing following below-knee amputation for CLI, Iloprost did not improve stump healing or re-amputation rates [11] **(Ib/A)**.

Prostaglandin E1

PGE1 suffers from a potential therapeutic disadvantage in that it is metabolised at first passage through the pulmonary circulation. Early trials therefore administered the drug by intra-arterial infusion, but this practice has largely been abandoned. In one large trial involving 267 patients that compared intravenous PGE1 to Iloprost in patients with Fontaine IV ischaemia, there was a trend towards benefit with Iloprost but this did not achieve statistical significance for survival, limb salvage, ulcer healing or relief of rest pain at six months [12]. Side effects occurred more frequently in the Iloprost group.

In a large randomised controlled trial undertaken in Italy by the ICAI Study Group (Ischemia Cronica degli Arti Inferiori), 1560 patients with CLI were randomised to receive either a daily intravenous infusion of 60µg of prostaglandin E1 in the form of alprostadil-cyclo-dextrine (n=771), or no additional treatment for up to 28 days [13]. The incidence of the combined endpoints (death, major amputation, persistence of critical leg ischaemia, acute myocardial infarction or stroke) was lower in the alprostadil group than in control patients at hospital discharge: 493 (63.9%) patients compared with 581 (73.6%); relative risk, 0.87 (95% CI, 0.81 to 0.93); p<0.001. The difference disappeared by six months: 348 of 661 (52.6%) patients compared with 387 of 673 (57.5%) patients; relative risk, 0.92 (95% CI, 0.83 to 1.01), p=0.074 **(Ib/A)**.

In a more recent double-blind, placebo-controlled randomised trial, lipo-ecraprost (Circulase) 60µg (a lipid-encapsulated prostaglandin E1 prodrug), or placebo, was administered intravenously to patients with CLI, on each of five days per week for eight weeks [14] **(Ib/A)**. The primary outcome measure was the rate of achievement of a composite endpoint of death or amputation above the ankle at 180 days. The study was terminated prematurely on the recommendation of the Data and Safety Monitoring Board after completion of a protocol-specified interim analysis for futility. At the time of termination, 383 of the planned 560 patients had been randomised and 379 had received at least one dose of medication. At six-month follow-up, of those patients available for assessment, there were 23 amputations in the 177 patients who had received placebo and 29 amputations in the 179 patients treated with lipo-ecraprost. There were ten deaths in the placebo group and 18 in the lipo-ecraprost-treated group.

Other medical treatments

Conclusive evidence of the benefit of other medical treatments of CLI is limited. Two drugs used extensively for treatment of claudication, naftidrofuryl (Praxilene) and pentoxifylline (Trental), have been evaluated. Microcirculatory benefits of naftidrofuryl, in terms of increased $TcpO_2$ in Fontaine III/IV patients have been reported [15, 16], but in a further placebo-controlled trial in patients with rest pain, no significant clinical advantage was found in the treatment group [17]. In two multicentre (Norwegian and European) trials involving 420 patients with CLI, pentoxifylline (600mg b.d.), or placebo, was administered intravenously for up to 21 days [18, 19]. Rest pain was improved by treatment in one study, but not in the other.

Other drugs used to treat CLI for which unequivocal benefits have not yet been demonstrated include antiplatelet agents, heparin, defibrinating agents (ancrod) and L-arginine, a precursor of endogenous nitric oxide (NO).

Spinal cord stimulation

Epidural spinal cord stimulation (SCS) has been described as a method for the control of chronic pain and has also been employed specifically for treatment of intractable ischaemic rest pain. This technique involves conduction of low voltage electrical impulses from a pulse generator to an electrode positioned in the epidural space and thence to the spinal cord and dorsal columns. Implantation of both stimulator and electrode involves a minor surgical procedure performed under local anaesthesia and fluoroscopic control with prophylactic antibiotic cover (Figure 2). Stimulation produces a sensation of paraesthesia in the lower limbs, more tolerable than rest pain, and the electrode is manipulated into an optimal position for pain ablation, usually at the T10 to T12 level. The pulse generator has programmable parameters for pulse width, amplitude and frequency and these are adjusted to provide maximal pain relief using either continuous or cyclical modes. The stimulator is usually controlled by the patient using magnetic switching.

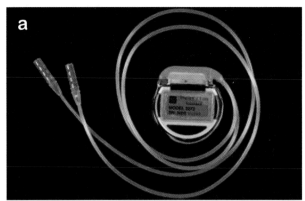
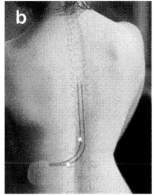

Figure 2. a) Commercially available spinal cord stimulation device, b) Diagrammatic representation of implanted SCS device.

Mechanism of SCS

The mechanism of pain relief is based on the pain gate theory described by Melzack and Wall (1965). In ischaemia both deep ischaemic and superficial pain may occur, arising from ulcers and surrounding ischaemic tissue. Nociceptive input may also be affected by neuropathy. Pain impulses are transferred by large myelinated A-type nerve fibres and C-type fibres to the cells of the substantia gelatinosa, the dorsal column fibres and to the first order communicating cells in the dorsal horn of the spinal cord. SCS induces both orthodromic and antidromic conduction of impulses. Antidromic impulses are transmitted to the dorsal horn of the spinal cord exciting the larger A-type fibres, inhibiting the first order communicating fibres and blocking nerve transmission by the smaller nociceptive C-fibres. Orthodromic impulses result in the paraesthesia perceived by the patient. Pain relief may also attenuate reflex vasoconstriction mediated through reduction in sympathetic tone, resulting in peripheral vasodilation. Roles for involvement of vasoactive neurotransmitter peptides, such as substance P, serotonin, vasoactive intestinal polypeptide (VIP), and other substances including prostaglandins and nitric oxide (NO) have also been proposed. However, there is a paucity of substantiative evidence supporting direct involvement of these substances as a consequence of SCS.

Uncontrolled trials of SCS

Outcome measures in uncontrolled clinical trials of SCS have concentrated principally on clinical assessments of pain reduction, healing of small ulcers and limb salvage. Ankle Doppler pressures, $TcpO_2$ readings, skin temperature recordings and capillary microscopy have been employed to detect changes in macro- and microcirculatory parameters.

Claims of reduction in rest pain (60-94%), healing of ulcers less than 3cm in diameter and variable limb salvage (42-88%) over follow-up intervals ranging from less than 12 months to four years have been made by various authors. In most studies SCS did not increase ankle systolic blood pressure. Improvements in $TcpO_2$ and skin temperature following treatment by SCS have been demonstrated in several studies, suggesting a beneficial microcirculatory effect. Use of $TcpO_2$ has been investigated as a means of determining potential beneficial outcome from SCS and patient selection for treatment, which has been recommended on the basis of a foot $TcpO_2$ of between 10-30mmHg [20]. Further objective evidence of microcirculatory effects has been provided by Jacobs et al, who demonstrated increased capillary density and red blood cell velocity using capillary microscopy, in patients with severe ischaemia (Fontaine stage III/IV) who responded to SCS [21] **(IIa/B)**. However, the trials described above are uncontrolled. Improvements in pain scores might well have been achieved equally with analgesia or placebo treatment and quoted ranges of limb salvage in these studies were equivalent to those described in natural history studies of CLI.

Prospective randomised trials of SCS

Data from prospective randomised controlled trials of SCS in CLI are limited to a few principal studies. Jivegård et al randomised 26 patients with inoperable severe leg ischaemia to SCS and 25 to oral analgesic treatment in a prospective study with an 18-month follow-up [22]. No significant change in ankle brachial pressure index (ABPI), toe pressures or skin temperature occurred in either group **(Ib/A)**. Using a visual analogue pain scale and semi-quantitative pain scores, significant long-term pain relief occurred in the SCS group but not in the control group. At 18 months there was no significant difference in limb salvage (62% SCS versus 45% controls). However, sub-group analysis suggested significantly lower amputation rates in normotensive patients, treated by SCS. There were eight deaths in each group.

In a prospective randomised trial with one-year follow-up reported by Claeys et al, patients with Fontaine stage IV ischaemia received 21 days of intravenous PGE1 plus SCS (n=45) or PGE1 alone (n=41) [23]. At 12 months total healing of foot ulcers had apparently occurred in 69% of the SCS group versus 17% of controls (p<0.0001). Maintained increases in $TcpO_2$ were described in the SCS group, although a baseline $TcpO_2$ level of <10mmHg was found to be prognostic for poor outcome with SCS. Pain relief was reported to be significantly better in the SCS group but there were no differences in either ABPI or amputation rates between the two groups **(Ib/A)**.

Comprehensive data have been obtained from the Dutch SCS Multi-centre Study Group (1999) [24]. One hundred and twenty patients with CLI (Fontaine III/IV) not suitable for vascular reconstruction were randomised to spinal cord stimulation in addition to best medical treatment or to best medical treatment alone, according to the intention-to-treat principle. Both groups were well matched with diabetes occurring in 37% of patients. Primary outcomes were mortality and amputation, with the primary endpoint of limb salvage at two years. Median follow-up was 605 days. Some 67% of patients who had SCS were alive at the end of the study compared to 69% of controls (p=0.96). Twenty-five major amputations were undertaken in the SCS group compared to 29 in controls (p=0.47). The risk ratio for survival at two years without major amputation in the SCS group, compared to controls was 0.96 (95% CI 0.61-1.51). In the SCS group, analgesic requirements were reduced, but there was no statistically significant difference in ulcer healing between the SCS group and controls. These results failed to demonstrate a significant clinical benefit for spinal cord stimulation over conservative medical treatment **(Ib/A)**. Subsequent cost-effectiveness studies highlighted the 26% increase in the overall cost of spinal cord stimulation over best medical treatment.

Ubbink and Vermeulen have recently undertaken a Cochrane Database Systematic Review of SCS for non-reconstructable chronic critical leg ischaemia [25] **(Ia/A)**. Six studies containing nearly 450 patients, in which SCS was compared against any form of conservative treatment, were included. Limb salvage after 12 months was significantly higher in the SCS group (relative risk 0.71, 95% CI 0.56 to 0.90; risk difference -0.11, 95%CI -0.20 to -0.02). Significant pain relief occurred in both groups but was more prominent in the SCS group, in which patients required significantly less analgesia. No significant difference in ulcer healing was noted between the groups, although significantly more patients in the SCS group reached Fontaine stage II than in the conservative treatment group. The authors noted implantation problems, a need for re-intervention and infections of the lead or pulse generator pocket in a small proportion of patients treated with SCS. Overall costs of treatment at two years were 36,500 euros for SCS-treated patients versus 28,600 euros for patients treated conservatively.

In summary, spinal cord stimulation may occasionally confer benefit for an individual patient with CLI, particularly with respect to analgesic requirements **(Ia/A)**. However, it does not reduce the risk of amputation compared to best medical treatment and potential benefits must be offset against the risk of minor complications and costs **(Ia/A)**.

Angiogenic revascularisation and gene therapy

Gene therapy

Potential advantages of revascularisation of ischaemic tissue by inducing formation of new blood vessels without recourse to angioplasty or bypass are evident. Angiogenesis involves activation of quiescent vascular endothelial cells causing sprouting of new vessels from existing ones with controlled proliferation, migration and differentiation, resulting in neovascularisation. The feasibility of using recombinant formulations of angiogenic growth factors (including vascular endothelial growth factor [VEGF], fibroblast growth factor [FGF], hypoxia-inducible factor-1 [HIF-1] and platelet-derived growth factor [PDGF]) or as DNA encoding these proteins, has recently been demonstrated in animal studies and early clinical trials.

Isner and his colleagues first administered human plasmid DNA encoding VEGF, applied to the coating of an angioplasty balloon, to stimulate popliteal collateral vessel development which was evident four weeks after gene therapy in a patient with CLI [26]. However, systemic dilution of the gene-therapy product and diffuse atherosclerotic arterial occlusion in CLI limits efficient gene transfer to the vicinity of ischaemic cells. Subsequently, the same workers employed intramuscular injections of 4000µg of naked plasmid DNA encoding phVEGF165 in an uncontrolled clinical trial involving nine patients with CLI [27]. Increases in ABPI were noted and new collateral vessel formation was documented by angiography **(IIb/B)**. Similar techniques have since been used to induce angiogenesis in patients with Buerger's disease [28].

In another uncontrolled trial that studied intramuscular injections of 400-2000µg of phVEGF 165 in 24 legs of 21 patients with CLI, Shyu et al demonstrated improvement in ABPI from 0.58 ± 0.24 to 0.72 ± 0.28 [29]. Angiography showed qualitative evidence of improved distal flow in 19 (79%) limbs. Ischaemic ulcers were reported to have improved markedly in 12 legs (75%) and rest pain was diminished in 20 legs (83%). Transient leg oedema was encountered in six patients. These findings are at odds with those of Rajagopalan et al, who conducted

a phase 2, randomised, double-blind, placebo-controlled randomised trial using intramuscular injection of a VEGF121 adenovirus [30] **(Ib/A)**. One hundred and five patients with severe intermittent claudication were randomised on a 1:1:1 basis to low dose (4 x 109 particle units), high dose (4 x 1010 particle units) or placebo. A single dose of the VEGF121 adenovirus was administered via 20 intramuscular injections to the ischaemic leg. At 12 weeks no difference was noted between the three groups in peak walking time, ABPI, claudication distance or quality of life **(Ib/A)**.

Makinen et al employed catheter-mediated VEGF gene therapy in ischaemic leg arteries after percutaneous transluminal angioplasty (PTA) [31]. Forty patients with intermittent claudication (IC) and 14 with CLI were included. Eighteen patients received 2 x 10 plaque-forming units (pfu) of VEGF-adenovirus (VEGF-Ad), 17 received VEGF-plasmid/liposome and 19 control patients received Ringer's lactate at the angioplasty site. Digital subtraction angiography (DSA) was employed to evaluate vascularity before, immediately after, and three months after PTA. Secondary study endpoints were restenosis rate, Rutherford class and ABPI after three months follow-up. DSA revealed increased vascularity in both VEGF-treated groups, distally to the gene transfer site, compared to controls. Mean Rutherford class and ABPI also showed significant improvements, although similar improvements were also noted in the control group **(Ib/A)**.

In a further uncontrolled study, Comerota et al administered increasing doses of intramuscular naked plasma DNA, encoding for fibroblast growth factor FGF Type 1 (NV1FGF), into the ischaemic thigh and calf muscles of 51 patients with CLI [32]. Arteriography was performed before treatment and at 12 weeks after treatment. Although 66 adverse events were reported, none was apparently attributed to NV1FGF. The authors described significant reduction in pain and aggregate ulcer size and an increase in transcutaneous oxygen pressure compared to baseline pre-treatment values. A significant increase in ABPI was also noted **(IIb/B)**.

An early trial of adenovirus 5-delivered FGF-4 given by intramuscular injection to patients with CLI has also been undertaken recently [33]. Thirteen patients with CLI were randomised to receive active drug and three placebo. Although there was an apparent subjective trend to larger blood vessels being observed on angiography in treated patients, conclusions with respect to clinical efficacy were impossible to draw from this small patient cohort.

Emmerich has reviewed trials of gene therapy to date and draws attention to the following caveats [34]:

- it is currently impossible to affirm whether gene therapy is an efficacious treatment in CLI because choice of endpoints varies. (The Transatlantic Conference on Clinical Trial Guidelines in Peripheral Arterial Disease recommends that complete healing of ulcers, relief from pain such that analgesic dependence ceases and amputation should be the endpoints in randomised, double-blind, placebo-controlled trials in CLI [35]);
- to date there have been no randomised treatment versus placebo studies that have demonstrated significant benefits of treatment;
- when increased collateralisation has been observed, this does not necessarily imply that blood flow is sufficient to reverse ischaemia;
- cessation of growth factor treatment has been accompanied by regression of neovascularisation [36];
- at this stage, it is also not known whether a single angiogenic growth factor is sufficient to stimulate angiogenesis reliably or whether treatment by growth factors in combination may have advantages. No such trials on combination therapy have yet been undertaken.

The conclusion drawn in the first edition of this book, that early clinical results herald the dawn of an exciting and novel vascular biological approach to the treatment of CLI, persists. However, the accompanying proviso also stands, that therapeutic gene transfer is still in its infancy and the findings from clinical studies should be interpreted with caution.

Stem cell therapy

Endothelial progenitor cells, or angioblasts, derived from bone marrow circulate in the blood. In animal models of ischaemia, heterologous, homologous and autologous endothelial progenitor cells have been shown to incorporate into sites of active angiogenesis and appear to contribute to new vessel formation. These findings suggest that endothelial cell progenitors may be useful for augmenting collateral vessel growth to ischaemic tissues (therapeutic angiogenesis) and for delivering anti- or pro-angiogenic agents, respectively, to sites of pathological or utilitarian angiogenesis.

Two main types of progenitor cells have been employed in early preclinical studies: early progenitor cells from monocytic origin (CD14+), and late, or outgrowth, endothelial cells (CD14-). These have been shown to act synergistically, both types of cell stimulating angiogenesis in animal models. Although these cells have been employed in animal models, only bone marrow-derived mononuclear cells (BMMNCs) and peripheral blood mononuclear cells (PBMNCs) have been used, after stimulation with granulocyte colony-stimulating factor (G-CSF), in clinical trials.

Tateishi-Yuyama et al have investigated the safety and feasibility of using BMMNCs injected into the gastrocnemius muscles of patients with an ischaemic leg [37]. Under general anaesthetic 500ml of bone marrow was aspirated from both iliac crests. Mononuclear cells were separated and concentrated to produce a final 30ml volume. Forty x 0.75ml aliquots of isolated BMMNCs were injected into ischaemic gastrocnemius muscles. A total of 47 patients were recruited for two studies, the first group of 25 patients receiving progenitor cells injected into ischaemic muscle, with saline injected into contralateral legs as a control. In the second 22 patients, with bilateral leg ischaemia, BMMNCs were injected into one leg and PBMNCs into the other. At four weeks, in patients in the latter group, ABPI was significantly improved in legs injected with BBMNCs (difference 0.09, 95% CI 0.06-0.11; p<0.0001). Similar improvements were described for rest pain, TcpO$_2$ measurements and pain-free walking time. These improvements appeared sustained at 24 weeks. Improvements were also recorded for the patients with PBMNCs, although there were two deaths in this group from myocardial infarction; neither was felt to be related to treatment. The authors concluded that treatment with BMMNCs appeared to be safe and effective for therapeutic angiogenesis and that the apparent benefits might be related to the ability of marrow cells to provide endothelial progenitor cells and to secrete various angiogenic factors and cytokines **(IIa/B)**.

Using a different approach, Huang *et al*, have assessed the effects of application of autologous transplantation of granulocyte colony-stimulating factor (G-CSF)-mobilised PBMNCs in the treatment of CLI in diabetic patients [38]. This study also purported to evaluate efficacy, safety and feasibility of this novel therapeutic approach. Twenty-eight patients with CLI were randomised to transplant or control groups. In the transplant group, patients were treated with subcutaneous injections of recombinant human G-CSF (600μg/day) for five days to mobilise stem/progenitor cells. Their PBMNCs were collected, concentrated (1 x 10^8 mononuclear cells/ml) and transplanted by multiple intramuscular injections into the ischaemic leg. Patients were followed-up after three months. In the transplant group, significant improvements were noted in laser Doppler assessments of lower limb perfusion (0.44 ± 0.11 to 0.57± 0.14 perfusion units, p<0.001), mean ABPI (0.50± 0.21 to 0.63 ± 0.25, p<0.001) and complete ulcer healing (77.8%), versus controls, (38.9%; p=0.016). Angiographic scores were also significantly improved in treated patients. Five controls needed a leg amputation compared to none in the treated group **(Ib/A)**. An advantage of this technique is that general anaesthesia is not needed, whereas it is required for BMMNC harvest. A disadvantage, however, is the inherent thrombogenic potential associated with use of G-CSF, which may assume particular relevance in patients with underlying systemic atherosclerosis.

The START Trial (STimulation of ARTeriogenesis) employed granulocyte-macrophage colony-stimulating factor (GM-CSF) in a double-blind randomised placebo-controlled study in 40 patients with moderate or severe intermittent claudication [39] **(Ib/A)**. Patients were treated with placebo or GM-CSF (10μg/kg) for 14 days (seven injections). GM-CSF treatment led to a strong increase in white blood cell count and C-reactive protein. Both placebo and treated groups had a similar and significant increase in walking distance at day 14 (placebo 127 ± 67 to 184 ± 87m, p=0.03; GM-CSF 126 ± 66 to 189 ± 141m, p=0.04). However, no changes in walking time, the primary endpoint, were noted between groups. There was no change in ABPI at days 14 or 90. Laser Doppler flowmetry showed a significant decrease in mirocirculatory flow reserve in the control group, but no change in the GM-CSF group. The authors concluded that the study results could not support the use of GM-CSF for treatment of patients with moderate or severe claudication **(Ib/A)**.

The studies described above represent trials of feasibility. No current gene or cell-based research has provided a definitive answer to the potential role of therapeutic angiogenesis in the treatment of CLI. Larger randomised trials with hard clinical endpoints, including amputation, are needed. A variety of important questions need to be answered. Will combined gene and cellular therapy stimulate angiogenesis more effectively than individual therapies? What are the optimum routes and durations of therapeutic delivery? Are there potential negative effects of angiogenic stimulation in the longer term? Emmerich has referred to this period as a 'prehistoric age' in the development of a fascinating and promising therapeutic armamentarium for CLI [34]. Passage of time will allow judgement of the efficacy and value of these novel treatments.

Conclusions

The best results for treatment of CLI are achieved by surgery alone, or in combination with endovascular intervention. Primary amputation may be a preferred option in a small sub-group of patients. The results of non-surgical treatment are largely disappointing, although administration of prostanoids or spinal cord stimulation may have a palliative role, particularly for the treatment of rest pain or small ulcers in patients with inoperable disease **(Ia/A)**. Early gene therapy and novel progenitor cell-based studies have demonstrated some promise with respect to stimulation of angiogenesis. However, therapeutic promise has not yet been borne out in the few randomised controlled trials.

Key points	Evidence level
◆ There are beneficial microcirculatory effects of prostanoids.	Ia/A
◆ There is an improvement in 'soft' clinical endpoints including rest pain in some patients following treatment with prostanoids or spinal cord stimulation in inoperable CLI.	Ia/A
◆ Iloprost infusion appears to reduce both risk of amputation and six-month mortality in Fontaine Stage III/IV leg ischaemia.	Ia/A
◆ SCS reduces analgesic requirements in non-reconstructable CLI, but is significantly more expensive than conservative management.	Ia/A
◆ Gene and stem cell therapy promote angiogenesis but this has not yet been demonstrated to have clinically significant beneficial effects.	

References

1. Critical limb ischaemia: management and outcome. Report of a national survey. The Vascular Surgical Society of Great Britain and Ireland. *Eur J Vasc Endovasc Surg* 1995; 10: 108-13.

2. Diehm C, Abri O, Baitsch G, *et al*. Iloprost a stable prostacyclin derivative, in stage 4 arterial occlusive disease. A placebo-controlled multicenter study. *Deutsch Med Wochenschr* 1989; 114: 783-8.

3. Brock FE, Abri O, Baitsch G, *et al*. Iloprost in the treatment of ischemic tissue lesions in diabetics. Results of a placebo-controlled multicenter study with a stable prostacyclin derivative. *Schweiz Med Wochenschr* 1990; 120: 1477-82.

4. Balzer K, Bechara G, Bisler H, *et al*. Reduction of ischaemic rest pain in advanced peripheral arterial occlusive disease. A double blind placebo controlled trial with iloprost. *Int Angiol* 1991; 10: 229-32.

5. Norgren L, Alwmark A, Angqvist KA, *et al*. A stable prostacyclin analogue (iloprost) in the treatment of ischaemic ulcers of the lower limb. A Scandinavian-Polish placebo controlled, randomised multicenter study. *Eur J Vasc Surg* 1990; 4: 463-7.

6. UK Severe Limb Ischaemia Study Group. Treatment of limb threatening ischaemia with intravenous iloprost: a randomised double blind placebo controlled study. *Eur J Vasc Surg* 1991; 5: 511-6.

7. Guilmot JL, Diot E. Treatment of lower limb ischaemia due to atherosclerosis in diabetic and nondiabetic patients with iloprost, a stable analogue of prostacyclin. Results of a French multicenter trial. *Drug Invest* 1991; 3: 351-9.

8. Loosemore TM, Chalmers TC, Dormandy JA. A meta-analysis of randomized placebo control trials in Fontaine stages III and IV peripheral occlusive arterial disease. *Int Angiol* 1994; 13: 133-42.

9. Guilmot JL, Boissier C. Medical treatment with prostanoids in patients with critical ischaemia. In: *Critical Limb Ischaemia*. Branchereau A, Jacobs M, Eds. Futura Publishing Co., 1999; 9: 63-8.

10. Fiessinger JN, Schafer M. Trial of iloprost versus aspirin treatment for critical limb ischaemia of thromboangiitis obliterans. The TAO study. *Lancet* 1990; 335: 555-7.

11. Dormandy J, Belcher G, Broos P, *et al*. Prospective study of 713 below-knee amputations for ischaemia and the effect of a prostacyclin analogue on healing. Hawaii Study Group. *Br J Surg* 1994; 81: 33-7.

12. Alstaedt HO, Berzewski B, Breddin HK, *et al*. Treatment of patients with peripheral arterial occlusive disease Fontaine stage IV with intravenous iloprost and PGE1: a randomized open controlled study. *Prostaglandins Leukot Essent Fatty Acids* 1993; 49: 573-8.

13. The ICAI Study Group (Ischemia Cronica degli Arti Inferiori). Prostanoids for chronic critical leg ischemia. A randomized, controlled, open-label trial with prostaglandin E1. *Ann Intern Med* 1999; 130(5): 412-21.

14. Brass EP, Anthony R, Dormandy J, *et al*; Circulase investigators. Parenteral therapy with lipo-ecraprost, a lipid-based formulation of a PGE1 analog, does not alter six-month outcomes in patients with critical leg ischemia. *J Vasc Surg* 2006; 43(4): 752-9.

15. Abendroth D, Sunder-Plassman L. Einfluss einer intravenosen naftidrofurylbehandlung auf die Mikrozirkulation von Patienten im Stadium III und IV einer peripheren arteriellen Verschlusskrankheit. *VASA* 1988; Suppl 24: 33-7.

16. Horsch S. Uber den Einsatz von naftidrofuryl im Stadium III/IV einer peripher arteriellen Verschlusskrankheit. *VASA* 1988; Suppl 24: 38-43.

17. Greenhalgh RM. Naftidrofuryl for ischemic rest pain: a controlled trial. *Br J Surg* 1981; 68: 265-6.

18. Intravenous pentoxifylline for the treatment of chronic critical limb ischaemia. The European Study Group. *Eur J Vasc Endovasc Surg* 1995; 9: 426-36.

19. Efficacy and clinical tolerance of parenteral pentoxifylline in the treatment of critical lower limb ischemia. A placebo controlled multicenter study. The Norwegian Pentoxifylline Multicenter Trial Group. *Int Angiol* 1996; 15: 75-80.

20. Ubbink DT, Vermeulen H. Spinal cord stimulation for critical leg ischemia: a review of effectiveness and optimal patient selection. *J Pain Symptom Manage* 2006; 31(4 Suppl): S30-5.

21. Jacobs MJ, Jorning PJ, Beckers RC, *et al.* Foot salvage and improvement of microvascular blood flow as a result of epidural spinal cord electrical stimulation. *J Vasc Surg* 1990; 12: 354-60.

22. Jivegard LEH, Augustinsson LE, Holm J, *et al.* Effects of spinal cord stimulation (SCS) in patients with inoperable severe lower limb ischaemia: a prospective randomised controlled study. *Eur J Vasc Endovasc Surg* 1995; 9: 421-5.

23. Claeys LG, Horsch S. Transcutaneous oxygen pressure as predictive parameter for ulcer healing in end-stage vascular patients treated with spinal cord stimulation. *Int Angiol* 1996; 15: 344-9.

24. Klomp HM, Spincemaille GH, Steyerberg EW, *et al.* Spinal-cord stimulation in critical limb ischaemia: a randomised trial. ESES Study Group. *Lancet* 1999; 353: 1040-4.

25. Ubbink DT, Vermeulen H. Spinal cord stimulation for non-reconstructable chronic critical leg ischaemia. *Cochrane Database Syst Rev* 2005; 3: CD004001.

26. Isner JM, Pieczek A, Schainfeld R, *et al.* Clinical evidence of angiogenesis after arterial gene transfer of phVEGF165 in patient with ischaemic limb. *Lancet* 1996; 348: 370-4.

27. Baumgartner I, Pieczek A, Manor O, *et al.* Constitutive expression of phVEGF165 after intramuscular gene transfer promotes collateral vessel development in patients with critical limb ischemia. *Circulation* 1998; 97: 1114-23.

28. Isner JM, Baumgartner I, Rauh G, *et al.* Treatment of thromboangiitis obliterans (Buerger's disease) by intramuscular gene transfer of vascular endothelial growth factor: preliminary clinical results. *J Vasc Surg* 1998; 28: 964-73.

29. Shyu KG, Chang H, Wang BW, Kuan P. Intramuscular vascular endothelial growth factor gene therapy in patients with chronic critical leg ischemia. *Am J Med* 2003; 114: 85-92.

30. Rajagopalan S, Mohler ER 3rd, Lederman RJ, *et al.* Regional angiogenesis with vascular endothelial growth factor in peripheral arterial disease: a phase II randomized, double-blind, controlled study of adenoviral delivery of vascular endothelial growth factor 121 in patients with disabling intermittent claudication. *Circulation* 2003; 108: 1933-8.

31. Makinen K, Manninen H, Hedman M, *et al.* Increased vascularity detected by digital subtraction angiography after VEGF gene transfer to human lower limb artery: a randomized, placebo-controlled, double-blinded phase II study. *Mol Ther* 2002; 6: 127-33.

32. Comerota AJ, Throm RC, Miller KA, *et al.* Naked plasmid DNA encoding fibroblast growth factor type 1 for the treatment of end-stage unreconstructable lower extremity ischemia: preliminary results of a phase I trial. *J Vasc Surg* 2002; 35: 930-6.

33. Matyas L, Schulte KL, Dormandy JA, *et al.* Arteriogenic gene therapy in patients with unreconstructable critical limb ischemia: a randomized, placebo-controlled clinical trial of adenovirus 5-delivered fibroblast growth factor-4. *Hum Gene Ther* 2005; 16: 1202-11.

34. Emmerich J. Current state and perspective on medical treatment of critical leg ischemia: gene and cell therapy. *Int J Low Extrem Wounds* 2005; 4: 234-41.

35. Dormandy JA, Rutherford RB. Management of peripheral arterial disease (PAD). TASC Working Group. TransAtlantic Inter-Society Consensus (TASC). *J Vasc Surg* 2000; 31: S1-S296.

36. Gounis MJ, Spiga MG, Graham RM, *et al.* Angiogenesis is confined to the transient period of VEGF expression that follows adenoviral gene delivery to ischemic muscle. *Gene Ther* 2005; 12: 762-71.

37. Tateishi-Yuyama E, Matsubara H, Murohara T, *et al*; Therapeutic Angiogenesis using Cell Transplantation (TACT) Study Investigators. Therapeutic angiogenesis for patients with limb ischaemia by autologous transplantation of bone-marrow cells: a pilot study and a randomised controlled trial. *Lancet* 2002; 360: 427-35.

38. Huang P, Li S, Han M, *et al.* Autologous transplantation of granulocyte colony-stimulating factor-mobilized peripheral blood mononuclear cells improves critical limb ischemia in diabetes. *Diabetes Care* 2005; 28: 2155-60.

39. van Royen N, Schirmer SH, Atasever B, *et al.* START Trial: a pilot study on STimulation of ARTeriogenesis using subcutaneous application of granulocyte-macrophage colony-stimulating factor as a new treatment for peripheral vascular disease. *Circulation* 2005; 112: 1040-6.

Chapter 11

The diabetic foot

John F Thompson MS FRCSEd FRCS, Consultant Surgeon
Andrew R Cowan FRCS, Consultant Surgeon
Exeter Vascular Service, Royal Devon and Exeter Hospitals, Exeter, UK
Peninsula Medical School, Exeter, UK

Introduction

The increasing incidence of obesity has fanned the flames of a worldwide epidemic of diabetes. Foot ulceration is one of the most sinister complications, and a fifth of diabetics will experience it during their lifetime. Foot complications are the most common reason for hospitalisation among these patients, and diabetes remains the leading risk factor for major amputation. A half of all diabetics who have a major amputation will lose their second leg within five years [1]. In addition, the one-year survival rate for diabetics with critical leg ischaemia is around 50%.

The spectrum of diabetic foot disease is wide, from asymptomatic through to life-threatening gas gangrene. The best approach to avoiding catastrophe is prevention, through minimising arterial risk factors and educating the patient and their family. This demands close co-operation between the specialist diabetic clinic and primary care **(Ib/A)** [2, 3].

The pathophysiology of the diabetic foot

In diabetes, neuropathy, ischaemia and infection contribute to the onset of ulceration, necrosis and gangrene (Figure 1).

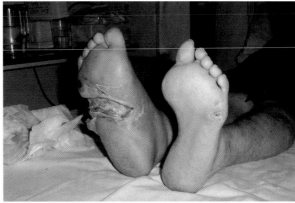

Figure 1. Diabetic feet with severe ulceration and infection due to neuropathy.

Neuropathy affects 80% of diabetics presenting with foot lesions, and can be divided into sensorimotor and autonomic.

Sensory neuropathy deprives the patient of their protective pain reflexes. Motor neuropathy affects the intrinsic muscles of the foot such that the long extensors over-ride which leads to clawing of the toes. The sesamoid bones move forwards so that weight is borne by the metatarsal heads (notably the second). The ankle is eventually thrown into equinus. Abnormal load-bearing eventually leads to pressure ulceration. Inappropriate footwear can also lead to ulceration.

Autonomic neuropathy affects skin, blood vessels and bone. This autosympathectomy leads to shunting of blood through precapillary vessels giving a paradoxically warm foot. Anhidrosis, leading to skin dehydration and fissuring, is made worse by glycosylation of keratin which reduces skin flexibility. Loss of bone mineral follows increased bony blood flow; so called mineral washout.

The combination of all these factors eventually leads to the development of a disrupted Charcot's foot, which leads to bony collapse as the patient attempts to walk on the affected leg.

Ischaemia is caused by a combination of proximal occlusive atherosclerosis and distal microcirculatory failure [4]. This is a complex process which is not simple 'small vessel disease'.

The aetiology includes:

- failure of the diabetic endothelium to respond to vasodilatation, particularly due to nitric oxide [5];
- hyperglycaemia and insulin resistance [6];
- microstructural changes in basement membranes produced by the products of glycation [7];
- impaired leucocyte migration;
- loss of local axon-mediated vasodilation.

Macrovascular disease is structurally similar between diabetic and non-diabetic patients, but the distribution is different. The femoropopliteal segment and foot vessels are relatively protected, whereas the tibial vessels are severely affected (Figure 2). Characteristically the peroneal artery is the last to occlude. This distribution enables bypass grafts to be constructed between the superficial femoral and pedal arteries. Another important feature of diabetic atherosclerosis is the prominent medial calcinosis that affects the pedal vessels and is visible on a plain X-ray.

Infection is potentially disastrous in diabetics. It can arise insidiously, usually in the sole of the foot or a nailbed (which is why diabetics are advised to use a mirror, or ask their spouses to inspect their feet regularly). The anatomical compartments of the foot's web spaces constrain pus which tracks backwards,

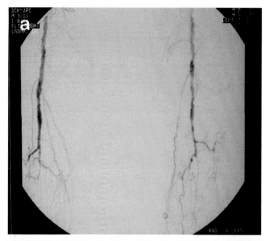

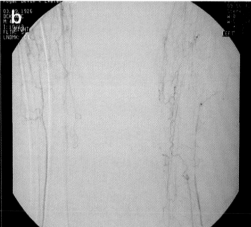

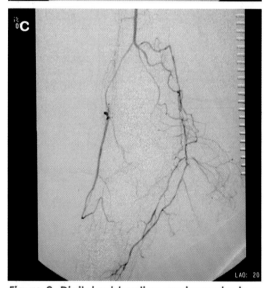

Figure 2. Digital subtraction angiography in a typical diabetic showing: a) patent but diseased superficial femoral arteries with occluded popliteals; b) severe tibial artery disease, with peroneal sparing; c) a patent distal peroneal artery feeding a patent foot arch. This patient would be suitable for a very distal bypass, if indicated.

not to the dorsum of the foot where it would be noticed. The obtunded immune response and hyperglycaemia, combined with aerobic and anaerobic commensals, can lead to synergistic infections and even gas gangrene. Established infection is a real risk to the foot, particularly in a diabetic with arterial insufficiency.

History

In a patient with an acute diabetic foot problem, the history should be directed towards the following:

- what is the reason for the acute deterioration? Infection may follow innocuous injuries or injudicious chiropody;
- is there evidence of pre-existing arterial disease in the limb?
- is there evidence of neuropathy?
- what is the realistic goal of treatment, considering the patient, their leg and social circumstances?

If an ulcer is chronic and has been present for some time (or if it has previously healed) there is likely to be underlying infection, ischaemia or pressure from an uncorrected bony deformity. Diabetic neuropathy, often compounded by ischaemic neuropathy, can mask ischaemic rest pain that would be agonising for a non-diabetic. Limitation of mobility may hide claudication pain.

Neuropathic pain differs from both of these types of pain in that although it is often worse at night, it characteristically occurs at the front of the shin and is relieved by exercise. It has a burning, tingling character and is usually associated with a well perfused foot.

The classical symptoms of underlying infection are less obvious in diabetics. General malaise, increased insulin requirements and modest increases in temperature or inflammatory markers are often the only sign of localised foot infection.

Examination

The whole foot should be carefully searched for areas of potential or actual infection. Inexperienced staff often continue to apply dressings over thickened hyperkeratotic tissue and are reluctant to remove toenails. Osteomyelitis should be excluded; there are several tell-tale signs:

- sausage-shaped swelling of the whole digit;
- a chronically discharging sinus with movement of the overlying skin relative to the deeper tissues;
- easy subluxation of the interphalangeal or metatarsophalangeal joints; air can sometimes be sucked into the joint on traction;
- visible or palpable bone on probing with a microbiological swab (deep swabs should be sent to avoid contamination with skin commensals).

Neuropathy can be assessed with either an automated machine or with 5.07 strength Semmes-Weinstein monofilaments; inability to feel the nylon brush correlates well with increased risk of ulceration [8] **(IIa/B)**.

The appearance of the ulcer is a good guide to underlying ischaemia. An indolent ulcer with little granulation tissue, that bleeds very little during debridement is a clue to poor perfusion. An easily palpable pedal pulse is the only reliable sign that the foot is adequately perfused, so an ulcer in the presence of a good pulse is either traumatic or neuropathic.

Classically, diabetic vascular disease is characterised by an easily palpable popliteal pulse, with impalpable foot pulses. This alone should alert the clinician to the diagnosis. Doppler ankle pressures can be unreliable, and may be normal because vessel wall calcification renders the pedal arteries incompressible [9]. Incompressible arteries are an independent predictor of amputation in diabetics. One prospective study found a U-shaped relationship between ankle pressure and amputation risk [10] **(IIb/B)**. The appropriate sized sphygmomanometer cuff is vital for ankle pressure measurement, especially in obese patients. An ankle brachial index below 0.6 has been accepted as the critical level in the diabetic with ulceration, but the character of the Doppler signal is potentially more informative than the absolute systolic pressure. A biphasic pedal Doppler signal is reassuring, whereas a monophasic signal implies significant proximal arterial occlusion. Toe pressures are more reliable, but the cuffs are not widely available.

Diagnostic imaging

Duplex ultrasound is the standard method of imaging the peripheral vascular tree in many centres. It is, however, operator-dependent, and can take up to an hour in a typical diabetic patient with multilevel disease. Duplex imaging can be difficult in small distal arteries, but it is helpful in identifying proximal lesions suitable for angioplasty. Treating the rare iliac artery stenosis is useful, even in the presence of severe distal disease as it can enhance inflow for a subsequent graft or improve the chances of a transtibial amputation healing.

Magnetic resonance angiography is widely available and has the advantage of avoiding a contrast load. The images are easier for the patient to understand during a consultation about treatment. They should be discussed at a multidisciplinary meeting with the radiologist because of various technical pitfalls such as mis-registration and early venous filling in diabetics with infection. Duplex imaging is occasionally required to confirm a questionable lesion and so guide management.

Conventional digital subtraction angiography is the gold standard before distal reconstruction and has the advantage that subintimal tibial angioplasty can be performed at the same sitting. In the emergency situation, on-table pre-reconstruction arteriography can identify target vessels. The potential hazard of contrast-induced nephropathy can be reduced by adequate hydration and by rendering the urine alkaline with sodium bicarbonate [11] **(Ib/A)**. The risk of nephropathy is increased in diabetic patients who take metformin.

Treatment

Initial treatment of the infected diabetic foot should involve analgesia, hydration, supplemental oxygen and control of the diabetes with an intravenous insulin infusion. Blood should be taken to eliminate electrolyte or acid base disturbance and to measure white count and C-reactive protein level. Joint care with the diabetic team is ideal.

Infection should be treated with intravenous high-dose antibiotics. Broad spectrum cover is needed before swab results are available. High-dose penicillin, flucloxacillin and metronidazole are appropriate. Several comparative studies have looked at alternative regimens such as piperacillin/ tazobactam and linezolid [12-14] **(IIb/B)**. There are no

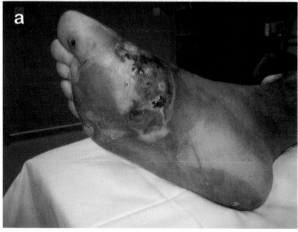
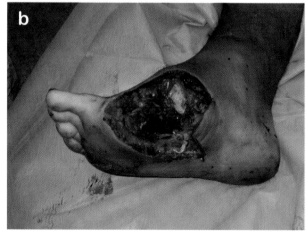

Figure 3. a) Severe acute diabetic foot infection. Note the entry point for infection - the chronic ulcer on the plantar surface of the hallux. b) This patient required urgent and extensive debridement.

important differences in outcome but improved cover against *Pseudomonas aeruginosa* or MRSA may be a clinical advantage where they are endemic in the vascular unit, or if they are invasive pathogens rather than colonists **(Ib/A)**.

Local wound toilet should be performed expeditiously, with de-roofing of ulcers and removal of dead skin and nails. Debridement of an infected foot may need to be extensive, but is likely to heal in patients with a palpable foot pulse (Figure 3). Simultanous or staged revascularisation may be needed to heal foot necrosis in diabetics with vascular disease. Dressings should be as simple as possible. Sloughy wounds can be cleaned with saline-soaked dressings changed frequently. For the medium term, a Cochrane review has recommended hydrogel dressings, which are widely available [15] **(Ia/A)**. Larval therapy has been the subject of only one clinical trial with mildly positive results [16] **(Ib/A)**.

Large open wounds may be left after debridement, which take many weeks to heal. Vacuum-assisted closure (VAC therapy) is currently a popular adjunct. It is useful to prepare wounds for split skin grafting by de-sloughing, reducing exudate, raising the ulcer floor and stimulating granulation tissue. In vascular practice it appears to be effective in reducing the area of open fasciotomy wounds and following digital or transmetatarsal amputation. There are, however, only small-scale trials of VAC therapy, probably due to the heterogeneous nature of the patient population; only one randomised trial describes positive results [17] **(IIa/B)**.

A similar situation pertains to hyperbaric oxygen treatment. The literature is full of small uncontrolled reports and short series, with only one tiny good quality trial in favour [18] **(Ia/A)**. The practicalities of attending 20-30 sessions, along with claustrophobia, seem to mitigate against the treatment.

Various small-scale studies have evaluated other adjuvant treatments, including recombinant epithelial growth factors, endothelial stimulation, ultrasound-delivered saline mist and other interventions, with encouraging results [19-21]. The cost and impracticality of such treatments, combined with relatively good results from simple debridement and dressings mean that they are unlikely to be introduced.

Revascularisation

The principles of restoration of blood flow to the ischaemic diabetic foot are exactly the same as for the ischaemic leg, except that more distal angioplasty and bypass are often required (Chapter 8). The results of bypass grafting are similar between diabetic and non-diabetic populations [22] **(IIb/B)**. Bypass procedures in diabetics are often long and complex, and benefit from discussion among a multidisciplinary team (Figure 4). Sometimes revascularisation attempts are futile and a primary amputation may be preferred, depending on the extent of the necrosis and patient factors such as immobility, the presence of suitable vein and infection with MRSA.

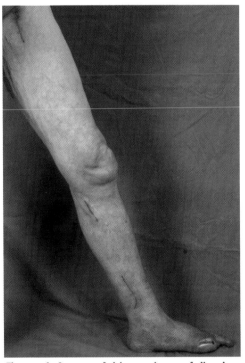

Figure 4. Successful leg salvage following *in situ* **femorotibial vein grafting with amputation of a gangrenous hallux.**

The surgery should be aimed at restoring a foot pulse to the affected leg. The first-line treatment is by subintimal angioplasty, which avoids the need for anaesthesia. Subintimal and tibial angioplasty is considered in Chapter 7. There are, as yet, no good studies comparing diabetic and non-diabetic patients.

Very distal bypass from popliteal to pedal artery is often required in diabetics, and has been considered in a meta-analysis. The five-year pooled estimate of primary patency was 63.1%, 70.7% for secondary patency, and 77.7% for foot preservation. There was a trend favouring reversed vein grafts and tibial bypasses for improved patency [23] **(IIb/B)**. The peroneal artery may, however, be the only target vessel available. Arm vein, contralateral long saphenous or short saphenous vein may be used, but there is seldom justification for the use of prosthetic material in this setting [23].

Amputation

Expeditious removal of infected and necrotic tissue is the mainstay of surgical management. Good clinical judgement and experience are essential to determine the extent of the resection and its relationship to any revascularisation procedure. In patients with ischaemia, blood flow continues to improve for six weeks after angioplasty, so it is prudent to delay minor amputation for a week or so, if possible.

Digital gangrene is treated by local amputation which should include the metatarsal head so that the web space can adduct. Wounds should not be closed with sutures. Web space infection should be treated by ray amputation with the same principles.

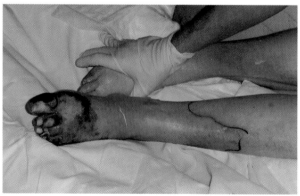

Figure 5. Severe, unsalvageable diabetic foot infection. Urgent major amputation may be life saving.

Transmetatarsal amputation, however, can preserve ankle function, and is an extremely valuable (occasional) option in the younger patient with extensive digital gangrene and a palpable foot pulse.

In fulminating infection a major amputation may be life saving (Figure 5). Emergency guillotine amputation can be done expeditiously, with the definitive procedure delayed until the patient's condition has improved and all signs of active sepsis have subsided.

The skew flap transtibial amputation is useful, particularly if there are anteromedial wounds from previous attempts at bypass grafting. A pneumatic orthopaedic tourniquet can safely be used in the diabetic patient to reduce blood loss during major amputation, and may be associated with a decreased revision rate [24] **(IIb/B)**.

Conclusions

As in many areas of surgery, multidisciplinary team working leads to improved outcome in the management of the diabetic foot [25] and can save money as well as legs **(Ib/A)** [26]. This may, paradoxically, be more difficult to achieve in isolated specialised vascular units than in district hospitals. Prevention is better than cure and a number of well-evidenced programmes are now available for the early diagnosis of the at-risk foot, with intervention such as education, regular monitoring and advice about foot wear to minimise the risk of deterioration [27, 28] **(Ia/A)**.

In managing the diabtetic foot, vascular specialists should have free access to expertise in surgical, radiological, diabetic, renal and elderly medicine, as well as physiotherapy, occupational therapy and a rehabilitation team. The diabetic patient with a septic foot and a palpable foot pulse has a good prognosis, and just needs effective debridement for infection that does not resolve with antibiotic treatment. The diabetic with critical ischaemia needs the full weight of vascular, medical and anaesthetic expertise to have a chance of limb salvage. The amputation rate is high in this group.

Key points	Evidence level

- ♦ Close collaboration between primary and secondary care improves the outcome for diabetic patients. — Ib/A
- ♦ X-ray contrast-related renal failure is reduced by hydration and sodium bicarbonate. — Ib/A
- ♦ Hydrogel dressings are optimal for diabetic foot ulcers. — Ia/A
- ♦ Larval therapy is effective. — Ib/A
- ♦ The results of distal bypass grafting are similar in diabetic and non-diabetic patients. — IIb/B

References

1. Nathan DM. Long-term complications of diabetes mellitus. *N Engl J Med* 1993; 328: 1676-85.
2. Glasgow RE, Nutting PA, King DK, *et al.* A practical randomized trial to improve diabetes care. *J Gen Intern Med* 2004; 19: 1167-74.
3. De Berardis G, Pellegrini F, Franciosi M, *et al.* QuED Study. Quality of care and outcomes in type 2 diabetic patients: a comparison between general practice and diabetes clinics. *Diabetes Care* 2004; 27: 398-406.
4. Tooke JE. Possible pathophysiological mechanisms for diabetic angiopathy in type 2 diabetes. *J Diabetes Complications* 2000; 14: 197-200.
5. Veves A, Akbari CM, Primavera J, *et al.* Endothelial dysfunction and the expression of endothelial nitric oxide synthetase in diabetic neuropathy, vascular disease and foot ulceration. *Diabetes* 1997; 47: 457-63.
6. Ackbari CM, Saouaf R, Barnhill DF, *et al.* Endothelial-dependent vasodilation is impaired in both micro and macrocirculation during acute hyperglycaemia. *J Vasc Surg* 1998; 28: 687-94.
7. Goldin A, Beckman JA, Schmidt AM, Creager MA. Advanced glycation end products: sparking the development of diabetic vascular injury. *Circulation* 2006; 114: 597-605.
8. Abbott CA, Carrington AL, Ashe H, *et al.* The North-West Diabetes Foot Care Study: incidence of, and risk factors for new diabetic foot ulceration in a community-based patient cohort. *Diabet Med* 2002; 19: 377-84.
9. Akbari CM, LoGerfo FW. Peripheral vascular disease in the person with diabetes. In: *Ellenberg and Rifkin's Diabetes Mellitus*, 6th Edition. Porte D, Sherwin RS, Baron AD, Eds. New York: McGraw Hill, 2003: 845-57.
10. Silvestro A, Diehm N, Savolainen H, *et al.* Falsely high ankle-brachial index predicts major amputation in critical limb ischemia. *Vasc Med* 2006; 11: 69-74.
11. Merten GJ, Burgess WP, Gray LV, *et al.* Prevention of contrast-induced nephropathy with sodium bicarbonate: a randomized controlled trial. *JAMA* 2004; 291: 2328-34.
12. Harkless L, Boghossian J, Pollak R, *et al.* An open-label, randomized study comparing efficacy and safety of intravenous piperacillin/tazobactam and ampicillin/sulbactam for infected diabetic foot ulcers. *Surg Infect* 2005; 6: 27-40.
13. Lipsky BA, Itani K, Norden C, *et al.* Linezolid Diabetic Foot Infections Study Group. Treating foot infections in diabetic patients: a randomized, multicenter, open-label trial of linezolid versus ampicillin-sulbactam/amoxicillin-clavulanate. *Clin Infect Dis* 2004; 38: 17-24.
14. Lipsky BA, Armstrong DG, Citron DM, *et al.* Ertapenem versus piperacillin/tazobactam for diabetic foot infections (SIDESTEP): prospective randomised controlled, double blinded multicenter trial. *Lancet* 2005; 366: 1695-703.
15. Smith J. Debridement of diabetic foot ulcers. *Cochrane Database Syst Rev* 2002; 4: CD003556.
16. Sherman RA. Maggot therapy for treating diabetic foot ulcers unresponsive to conventional therapy. *Diabetes Care* 2003; 26: 446-51.
17. Armstrong DG, Lavery LA, for the Diabetic Foot Study Consortium. Negative pressure wound therapy after partial diabetic foot amputation: a multicentre, randomised controlled trial. *Lancet* 2005; 366: 1704-10.
18. Abidia A, Laden G, Kuhan G, *et al.* The role of hyperbaric oxygen therapy in ischaemic diabetic lower extremity ulcers: a double-blind randomised-controlled trial. *Eur J Vasc Endovasc Surg* 2003; 25: 513-8.
19. Driver VR, Hanft J, Fylling CP, *et al*, for the Diabetic Foot Ulcer Study Group A prospective, randomized, controlled trial of autologous platelet-rich plasma gel for the treatment of diabetic foot ulcers. *Ostomy Wound Manage* 2006; 52: 68-70.
20. Hong JP, Jung HD, Kim YW. Recombinant human epidermal growth factor (EGF) to enhance healing for diabetic foot ulcers. *Ann Plast Surg* 2006; 56: 394-8.
21. Wolfle KD, Bruijnen H, Loeprecht H, *et al.* Graft patency and clinical outcome of femorodistal arterial reconstruction in diabetic and non-diabetic patients: results of a multicentre comparative analysis. *Eur J Vasc Endovasc Surg* 2003; 25: 229-34.

22. Albers M, Romiti M, Brochado-Neto FC, *et al*. Meta-analysis of popliteal-to-distal vein bypass grafts for critical ischemia. *J Vasc Surg* 2006; 43: 498-503.

23. Pomposelli FB Jr, Kansal M, Hamdan AB, *et al*. A decade of experience with dorsalis pedis artery bypasses. Analysis of outcome in more than 1000 cases. *J Vasc Surg* 2003; 37: 307-15.

24. Wolthuis AM, Whitehead E, Ridler BMF, *et al*. Use of a pneumatic tourniquet improves outcome following trans-tibial amputation. *Eur J Vasc Endovasc Surg* 2006; 31: 642-5.

25. A Trautner C, Haastert B, Giani G, Berger M. Amputations and diabetes: a case-control study. *Diabet Med* 2002; 19: 35-40.

26. Horswell RL, Birke JA, Patout CA, Jr. A staged management diabetes foot program versus standard care: a 1-year cost and utilization comparison in a state public hospital system. *Arch Phys Med Rehabil* 2003; 84: 1743-6.

27. Reiber GE, Smith DG, Wallace C, *et al*. Effect of therapeutic footwear on foot reulceration in patients with diabetes. *JAMA* 2002; 287: 2552-8.

28. Valk GD, Kreigsman DM, Assendelft WJ. Patient education for preventing diabetic foot ulceration. *Cochrane Database Syst Rev* 2005; 25: CD001488.

Chapter 12

Lower limb amputation in peripheral arterial disease

Kenneth R Woodburn MD FRCSG (Gen), Consultant Vascular Surgeon, Honorary Clinical Lecturer, Peninsula Medical School, and the Vascular Unit, Royal Cornwall Hospitals Trust, Truro, Cornwall, UK

Introduction

Major limb amputation is a constant presence in the practice of vascular surgery. Historical studies suggest that around 7% of patients with symptomatic arterial disease will undergo amputation within five years of diagnosis [1], an observation borne out by more recent work showing a 1.6% annual incidence of major limb amputation in patients with intermittent claudication [2]. Major limb amputation has been needed for many centuries as a result of mankind's preoccupation with armed conflict. While the techniques of limb amputation and anaesthetic and postoperative care have improved upon historical descriptions [3], there is little hard evidence as to its merits over alternative treatments. Outwith the field of trauma and orthopaedic surgery, major limb amputation is generally employed for acute and chronic critical limb ischaemia in the absence of any further realistic revascularisation option, or the presence of extensive lower limb tissue loss and/or sepsis in the diabetic (frequently neuropathic) foot.

This chapter summarises the evidence as it pertains to peripheral vascular and diabetic disease, which have become the commonest reasons for major limb amputation in the developed world.

Amputation and its alternatives

Many patients present with a clear need for major limb amputation and alternative strategies are not relevant: the presence of extensive established gangrene, extensive spreading foot sepsis in the diabetic neuropathic leg (Figure 1), intractable rest pain in the patient with a history of multiple failed revascularisation procedures over several years. These are all clinical presentations that mandate leg amputation, although hard scientific evidence in support of this course of action has not been documented.

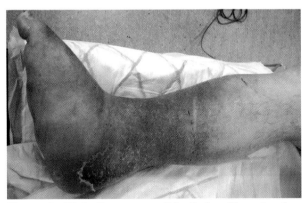

Figure 1. Diabetic neuropathic limb with extensive sepsis extending into the calf.

The patient who presents with advanced critical ischaemia without major tissue necrosis poses a more complex management problem. Many such patients could have an attempt at operative or percutaneous revascularisation surgery, or a primary major limb amputation. While some advocate an aggressive policy of reconstruction over amputation on the basis of improved operative mortality [4, 5], economic [6], or quality of life [7] considerations, the evidence is far from overwhelming. It is clear, however, that the patient with critical leg ischaemia has a limited survival, and treatments should be considered palliative rather than curative.

No reliable prospective comparative studies of primary amputation versus revascularisation exist. The evidence suggests a lower peri-operative mortality for revascularisation surgery over amputation [4, 5] **(III/B)**, although there is a clear selection bias in such studies, which reserved amputation for those with poor function and multiple comorbidities. Long-term survival is between 50% and 70% two years following leg amputation [8], and less than 50% five years after limb salvage surgery [9], confirming that measures other than crude survival data are required to evaluate the options for a patient with limb-threatening ischaemia.

Quality of life and functional outcome are thus often used to assess the outcomes of surgery for critical leg ischaemia but, as with mortality, there are no randomised studies, and the inevitable selection bias makes it difficult to interpret the findings; quality of life assessed by a variety of methods is generally reported to be better after limb salvage [7, 10] **(III/B)**, but this appears to be mainly a consequence of the restricted mobility following amputation [11]; around 50% of major limb amputees cannot walk within 18 months of surgery. In comparison, it is reported in at least one series that 97% of patients undergoing infra-inguinal bypass for limb salvage are able to walk [9]. Restricted mobility after amputation is, however, entirely compatible with continued independent living [12], and the desired outcome for individual patients with critical leg ischaemia should be to maintain an independent existence. In certain situations this may be best served by major limb amputation in preference to revascularisation.

Alternatives to surgical intervention for limb-threatening ischaemia are few: spinal cord stimulation is effective in reducing pain but does not prevent amputation; intravenous infusion of the prostacyclin analogue, Iloprost, has never established itself as a realistic alternative to amputation; and other pharmacological therapies for critical leg ischaemia have fared even worse (see Chapter 10). The decision remains one to be made between attempted limb salvage and primary amputation, depending on patient circumstances.

Leg amputation techniques

Despite some early claims for the superiority of a skewflap below-knee amputation (BKA) [13] over the traditional Burgess long posterior flap [14] (Figure 2), this was not supported in the only randomised controlled trial in patients with peripheral arterial disease reported in the literature to date [14]. Similarly, no benefit was demonstrated for a technique employing equal medial and lateral sagittal musculocutaneous flaps, when compared with the Burgess technique [15]. A recent Cochrane review concluded that the choice of technique for below-knee amputation had no effect on the outcome of the procedure [16] and it remains a question of surgeon preference **(Ib/A)**.

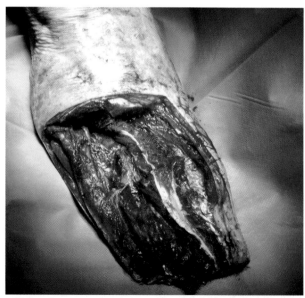

Figure 2. Below-knee amputation utilising the long posterior flap technique.

Table 1. Reported revision rates following major limb amputation.					
Study	Number of patients (legs)	AK:BK ratio	AK revisions	BK revisions	BK converted to AK
Termansen [15] (1977)	88 (88)	0:88	--	22 (25%)	17 (19%)
Keagy [29] (1986)	729 (971)	345:626	32 (9%)	118 (19%)	n/s
Harris [30] (1988)	189 (189)	63:126	6 (10%)	34 (27%)	23 (18%)
McCollum [31] (1988)	n/s (100)	19:81	--	n/s	6 (7%)
Ruckley [13] (1991)	191 (191)	0:191	--	31 (16%)	17 (9%)
Dormandy [32] (1994)	713 (n/s)	0:713	--	n/s	n/s (19%)
Nehler [12] (2003)	154 (172)	78:94	16 (20%)	23 (24%)	18 (19%)
Yip [19] (2006)	47 (51)	0:51	--	9 (18%)	9 (18%)
n/s - these data were not specified clearly in the article.					

Above-knee amputation (AKA) has been subject to even less scientific scrutiny than BKA, although it is believed that postoperative mobility is assisted by maintaining the maximum feasible femoral length and by carrying out a myoplasty to improve stump function [17]. In the presence of wet gangrene, patients undergoing leg amputation (above or below-knee) derive no significant benefit from a two-stage procedure (guillotine amputation followed by later definitive stump formation), over a one-stage procedure (definitive amputation with delayed closure of skin and subcutaneous tissue) [18] **(III/B)**. In the absence of any evidence to the contrary, it seems reasonable to conclude that definitive amputation at both the BK and AK levels should be carried out as a single procedure using the operative technique that the surgeon considers most appropriate.

Selection of level of amputation

A good amputation will leave the patient with enough leg to mobilise with a prosthesis, while ensuring primary healing without the need for revision to a higher level. Retrospective studies report that between 15-20% of cases will require revision following major leg amputation (Table 1) and revision is more common following BKA [12]. While approximately 15% of BKAs require conversion to AKA for early non-healing, once healed, the below-knee amputee has only a 4% chance of requiring later ipsilateral AKA. The improved primary healing of AKA is, however, offset by the greatly reduced mobility and use of an artificial limb compared with BKA [12].

Although all these studies suffer from significant selection bias, with the less mobile patients with more advanced disease undergoing amputation at the higher level, the evidence favours a healed BKA over a healed AKA for independent mobility. Selection of the appropriate level of primary amputation in those patients likely to mobilise postoperatively is, therefore, paramount. Many techniques that assist in the clinical decision-making process to maximise the number of healed BKAs have been investigated [19]. Peripheral pulses are of value in determining amputation level selection, as failure following BKA is rare in legs with a palpable popliteal pulse [20, 21]. Although many BKAs will heal when a popliteal pulse is absent, few heal when there is no femoral pulse [22]. Doppler ankle pressure measurement has been shown to predict healing of BKA with an accuracy of up to 90% [23], but these findings are not universal [24]. Objective measurements of skin temperature at the amputation site are reported to have an accuracy of at least 90% in predicting amputation healing [24, 25], with a similar success reported using temperature ratios [26]. Although a valuable adjunct to clinical judgement, these techniques require specialised equipment and there remains considerable uncertainty regarding the absolute temperature value that can be used for accurate level selection.

Study	Site of tcO_2 measurement (level of amputation)	Authors' "cut off" value (mmHg)	Healed amputations with $tcO_2>$ "cut off"	Failed amputations with $tcO_2>$ "cut off"	Healed amputations with $tcO_2<$ "cut off"	Failed amputations with $tcO_2<$ "cut off"
Wagner [24] (1988)	Calf (BKA)	16	94%	50%	6%	50%
Kram [33] (1989)	Calf (BKA)	20	96%	50%	4%	50%
Bacharach [28] (1992)	Calf (BKA) Thigh (AKA) Foot (transmetatarsal)	20	100%	33%	0%	67%
Bacharach [28] (1992)	Calf (BK) Thigh (AK) Foot (transmetatarsal)	40	70%	5%	30%	95%
Misuri [34] (2000)	Foot (digit or transmetatarsal) Calf (BKA)	20	88%	15%	12%	85%

Table 2. Transcutaneous oxygen tension and lower limb amputation healing.

Skin perfusion pressure determined by both radioisotope washout and also by laser Doppler has been shown to predict wound healing in almost 100% of major leg amputations, although there is a lack of consistency in the skin perfusion pressure at which healing will definitely occur [20, 27]. Transcutaneous oxygen measurements ($tcPO_2$) have consistently been reported to predict amputation wound healing with an accuracy of 85-100% [21, 23, 24, 28]. Most studies have used rather heterogenous patient populations and usually include a variety of amputation levels, and a variety of definitions of success and failure of the procedure. As a result a range of values have been reported to be useful in selecting the level for amputation and at best it can be concluded that a $tcPO_2$ at the proposed amputation site of greater than 40mmHg accurately predicts healing, while a level of less than 20mmHg is almost universally associated with stump breakdown [29-32] **(III/B)**(Table 2).

Thus, while clinical judgement based on the examination findings remains the key to selection of the level of amputation, accuracy in selection may be improved by the use of one or more adjunctive investigations. Even with these additional assessments, however, the failure rate for BKA remains between 15-25% in most series.

Postoperative management

Over the years a number of studies have reported benefits for the application of a rigid stump dressing immediately following leg amputation, particularly BKA (Figure 3). The advantages claimed over soft dressings include reduced postoperative oedema,

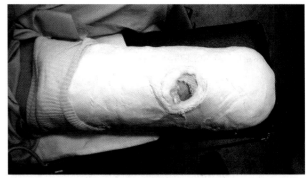

Figure 3. Rigid stump dressing applied to below-knee amputation at time of surgery. The window is cut over the patella to enable supervision of quadriceps exercises.

improved pain control, prevention of contractures, protection from injury and reduced length of hospitalisation [35, 36]. There is some evidence that the technique also reduces the time to first fitting with a prosthesis [37, 38]. However, much of the data are derived from non-vascular patients and, although the randomised trials of a rigid versus soft dressing in patients undergoing BKA for peripheral arterial disease have shown a clear trend towards earlier wound healing and limb fitting [39, 40], they have been statistically inconclusive. On balance, the evidence supports the use of a rigid or semi-rigid postoperative dressing to expedite wound healing and reduce stump volume [41] **(Ib/A)**, although larger multicentre trials remain essential if irrefutable evidence is to be obtained.

Management of phantom limb pain

Phantom pain is reported to occur in more than 75% of patients after leg amputation [42], although the incidence in patients undergoing amputation for peripheral arterial disease is not described specifically. While phantom pain decreases with time, its incidence is reported to be greatest in those patients with prolonged pre-operative leg pain [43] and efforts have been directed at reducing pain before surgery.

Trials of peri-operative epidural anaesthetic infusion were initially reported to show a reduction in phantom limb pain in those who had an epidural infusion for 24-72 hours before surgery [44, 45], but these trials were flawed in their small sample sizes, lack of randomisation and non-blinded nature of the trial designs. Both reported trials, however, suggested a colossal reduction in the rate of phantom pain one year postoperatively. More recently, a larger, randomised, double-blind Danish trial [46] **(Ib/A)** failed to show any reduction in phantom limb pain in patients who had a peri-operative epidural starting 18 hours before surgery; around 70% of patients in both groups reported phantom limb pain 12 months postoperatively. None of these trials clearly specified the indications for amputation in the study groups and the authors of the Danish trial acknowledged that a longer pre-operative epidural infusion may be of value, although the logistics of this probably make it impractical.

As an alternative, a perineural infusion of bupivacaine may reduce postoperative pain following major limb amputation [47], although the use of peri-operative epidural analgesia remains the method of choice since neither technique appears to have any significant effect on phantom limb pain [48]. Despite a clear advantage of epidural analgesia for postoperative pain control, there remains no good evidence of a beneficial effect on phantom limb pain.

Conclusions

Despite its long established place in the management of peripheral arterial disease, major leg amputation remains a surgical practice where clinical judgement and a holistic approach take some precedence over hard evidence. What evidence there is supports procedures that preserve the knee joint, but at a recognised cost of an increased number of revision operations. This must be tempered with the knowledge of the limited long-term survival of the vascular amputee. Adjunctive techniques may improve the accuracy of clinical judgement but have not gained widespread acceptance in routine vascular surgical practice, while the use of pre-operative epidural infusion to prevent phantom limb pain is not supported by the evidence. The role of postoperative dressing regimens in the ultimate outcome of leg amputation remains to be established through further study.

Key points	Evidence level

- ◆ There is no advantage of one surgical technique for below-knee amputation over any other. — Ia/A

- ◆ A rigid postoperative stump dressing appears to offer advantages over soft dressings after below-knee amputation. — Ib/A

- ◆ The use of peri-operative epidural analgesia reduces postoperative stump pain but not the rate of phantom limb pain. — Ib/A

- ◆ Selection of the most appropriate level of amputation is based on clinical judgement, but quantitative measures may assist in identifying patients who require above-knee amputation. — III/B

References

1. Bloor K. Natural history of arteriosclerosis of the lower extremities. *Ann R Coll Surg Eng* 1961; 28: 36-52.
2. Dormandy JA, Murray GD. The fate of the claudicant. *Eur J Vasc Surg* 1991; 5: 131-3.
3. Sachs M, Bojunga J, Encke A. Historical evolution of limb amputation. *World J Surg* 1999; 23: 1088-93.
4. Hobson RW, Lynch TG, Zafor J, *et al*. Results of revascularisation and amputation in severe lower extremity ischaemia: a five-year experience. *J Vasc Surg* 1985; 2: 174.
5. Taylor LM Jr, Hamre D, Dalman RL, Porter JM. Limb salvage vs amputation for critical ischaemia. The role of vascular surgery. *Arch Surg* 1991; 126: 1251-7.
6. Wolfe JHN, Tyrell MR. Justifying arterial reconstruction to crural vessels - even with a prosthetic graft. *Br J Surg* 1991; 78: 897-9.
7. Thompson MM, Sayers RD, Reid A, *et al*. Quality of life following infragenicular bypass and lower limb amputation. *Eur J Vasc Endovasc Surg* 1995; 9: 310-3.
8. Pell J, Stonebridge P. Association between age and survival following major amputation. The Scottish Vascular Audit Group. *Eur J Vasc Endovasc Surg* 1999; 17: 166-9.
9. Ahmed M, Abou-Zamzam AM, Lee RW, *et al*. Functional outcome after infrainguinal bypass for limb salvage. *J Vasc Surg* 1997; 25: 287-97.
10. Johnson BF, Singh S, Evans L, *et al*. A prospective study of the effect of limb-threatening ischaemia and its surgical treatment on the quality of life. *Eur J Vasc Endovasc Surg* 1997; 13: 306-14.
11. Pell JP, Donnan PT, Fowkes FGR, Ruckley CV. Quality of life following lower limb amputation for peripheral arterial disease. *Eur J Vasc Surg* 1993; 7: 448-51.
12. Nehler MR, Coll JR, Hiatt WR, *et al*. Functional outcome in a contemporary series of major lower extremity amputations. *J Vasc Surg* 2003; 38: 7-14.
13. Ruckley CV, Stonebridge PA, Prescott RJ. Skewflap versus long posterior flap in below-knee amputations: Multicenter trial. *J Vasc Surg* 1991; 13: 423-7.
14. Burgess EM, Romano RL, Zettl JH, Schrock RD Jr. Amputations of the leg for peripheral vascular insufficiency. *J Bone Joint Surg* 1971; 53: 874-90.
15. Termansen NB. Below-knee amputation for ischaemic gangrene. Prospective, randomized comparison of a transverse and a sagittal operative technique. *Acta Orthop Scand* 1977; 48: 311-6.
16. Tisi PV, Callam MJ. Type of incision for below-knee amputation. *The Cochrane Database Syst Rev* 2004; Issue 1: CD003749.pub2. DOI:10.1002/14651858. CD003749. pub2.
17. Woodburn KR, Ruckley CV. Lower extremity amputation: technique and perioperative care. In: *Vascular Surgery*. 6th Edition. Rutherford, Ed. New York: Elsevier Science, 2005; ch 172: 2460-73.
18. Fisher DF, Clagett GP, Fry RE, *et al*. One-stage versus two-stage amputation for wet gangrene of the lower extremity: a randomized study. *J Vasc Surg* 1988; 8: 428-33.
19. Yip VS, Teo NB, Johnstone R, *et al*. An analysis of risk factors associated with failure of below-knee amputations. *World J Surg* 2006; 30: 1081-87.
20. Dwars BJ, van den Brock TA, Rauwerda JA, Bakker FC. Criteria for reliable selection of the lowest level of amputation in peripheral vascular disease. *J Vasc Surg* 1992; 15: 536-42.
21. Ballard JL, Eke CC, Bunt TJ, Killeen JD. A prospective evaluation of transcutaneous oxygen measurements in the management of diabetic foot problems. *J Vasc Surg* 1995; 22: 485-92.
22. O'Dwyer KJ, Edwards MH. The association between lowest palpable pulse and wound healing in below-knee amputations. *Ann R Coll Surg Eng* 1985; 67: 232-4.
23. DeFrang RD, Taylor LM, Porter JM. Basic data related to amputations. *Ann Vasc Surg* 1991; 5: 202-7.

24. Wagner WH, Keagy BA, Kotb MM, *et al.* Noninvasive determination of healing of major lower extremity amputation: the continued role of clinical judgement. *J Vasc Surg* 1988; 8: 703-10.

25. Spence VA, Walker WF, Troup IM, Murdoch G. Amputation of the ischaemic limb: selection of the optimum site by thermography. *Angiology* 1981; 32: 155-69.

26. Stoner HB, Taylor L, Marcuson R. The value of skin temperature measurements in forecasting the healing of a below-knee amputation for end-stage ischaemia of the leg in peripheral arterial disease. *Eur J Vasc Surg* 1989; 3: 355-61.

27. Adera HM, James K, Castronuovo JJ, *et al.* Prediction of amputation wound healing with skin perfusion pressure. *J Vasc Surg* 1995; 21: 823-9.

28. Bacharach JM, Rooke TW, Osmundson PJ, Gloviczki P. Predictive value of transcutaneous oxygen pressure and amputation success by use of supine and elevation measurements. *J Vasc Surg* 1992; 15: 558-63.

29. Keagy BA, Schwartz JA, Koth M, *et al.* Lower extremity amputation: the control series. *J Vasc Surg* 1986; 4: 321-6.

30. Harris JP, Page S, Englund R, May J. Is the outlook for the vascular amputee improved by striving to preserve the knee? *J Cardiovasc Surg* 1988; 29: 741-5.

31. McCollum PT, Spence VA, Walker WF. Amputation for peripheral vascular disease: the case for level selection. *Br J Surg* 1988; 75: 1193-5.

32. Dormandy J, Belcher G, Broost P, *et al.* Prospective study of 713 below-knee amputations for ischaemia and the effect of a prostacyclin analogue on healing. *Br J Surg* 1994; 81: 33-7.

33. Kram HB, Appel PL, Shoemaker WC. Multisensor transcutaneous oximetric mapping to predict below-knee amputation wound healing: use of a critical PO_2. *J Vasc Surg* 1989; 9: 796-800.

34. Misuri A, Lucertini G, Nanni A, *et al.* Predictive value of transcutaneous oximetry for selection of the amputation level. *J Cardiovasc Surg* (Torino) 2000; 41: 83-7.

35. Burgess EM, Romano RL, Zettl CP. Amputation management utilising immediate postsurgical prosthetic fitting. *Prosthet Int* 1969; 3: 28-37.

36. Osterman H. The process of amputation and rehabilitation. *Clinics in podiatric medicine and surgery* 1997; 14: 585-602.

37. Mooney V, Harvey JP, McBride E, Snelson R. Comparison of post-operative stump management: plaster vs soft dressing. *J Bone Joint Surg* 1971; 53-A: 241-9.

38. McLean N, Fick GH. The effects of semirigid dressings on below-knee amputations. *Phys Ther* 1994; 74: 668-73.

39. Woodburn KR, Sockalingham S, Gilmore H, *et al.* On behalf of the Scottish Vascular Audit Group (SVAG) and Scottish Physiotherapy Amputee Research Group (SPARG). A randomised trial of rigid stump dressing following transtibial amputation for peripheral arterial insufficiency. *Prosthet Orthot Int* 2004; 28: 22-7.

40. Deutsch A, English RD, Vermeer TC, *et al.* Removeable rigid dressings versus soft dressings: a randomised controlled study with dysvascular transtibial amputees. *Prosthet Orthot Int* 2005; 29: 193-200.

41. Nawijn SE, van der Linde H, Emmelot CH, Hofstad CJ. Stump management after transtibial amputation: a systematic review. *Prosthet Orthot Int* 2005; 29: 13-26.

42. Ephraim PL, Wegener ST, MacKenzie EJ, *et al.* Phantom pain, residual limb pain, and back pain in amputees: results of a national survey. *Arch Phys Med Rehab* 2005; 86: 1910-9.

43. Jensen TS, Krebs B, Nielsen J, Rasmussen P. Immediate and long-term phantom limb pain in amputees: incidence, clinical characteristics and relationship to pre-amputation limb pain. *Pain* 1985; 21: 267-78.

44. Bach S, Noreng MF, Tjeliden NU. Phantom limb pain in amputees during the first 12 months following limb amputation, after pre-operative lumbar epidural blockade. *Pain* 1988; 33: 297-301.

45. Jahangiri H, Jayatunga AP, Bradley JW, Dark CH. Prevention of phantom pain after major lower limb amputation by epidural infusion of diamorphine, clonidine, and bupivacaine. *Ann R Coll Surg Eng* 1994; 76: 324-6.

46. Nikolajsen L, Ilkjaer S, Christensen JH, *et al.* Randomised trial of epidural bupivacaine and morphine in prevention of stump and phantom pain in lower-limb amputation. *Lancet* 1997; 350: 1353-7.

47. Pinzur MS, Garla PGN, Pluth T, Vrbos L. Continuous postoperative infusion of a regional anaesthetic after an amputation of the lower extremity. A randomized clinical trial. *J Bone Joint Surg* 1996; 78: 1501-5.

48. Lambert AW, Dashfield AK, Cosgrove C, *et al.* Randomized prospective study comparing preoperative epidural and intraoperative perineural analgesia for the prevention of postoperative stump and phantom limb pain following major amputation. *Reg Anesth Pain Med* 2001; 26: 316-21.

Chapter 13

Treatment of acute leg ischaemia

John F Thompson MS FRCSEd FRCS, Consultant Surgeon
Exeter Vascular Service, Royal Devon and Exeter Hospitals, Exeter, UK
Peninsula Medical School, Exeter, UK

Introduction

Acute leg ischaemia is a surgical and/or radiological emergency, caused by embolic occlusion or *in situ* thrombosis of either a native vessel, or pre-existing bypass graft. Rarely, thrombophilia, a hypercoagulable state, drugs, trauma or radiation may cause thrombosis. Thrombosis may also be a pre-morbid event, which in part explains the high mortality rate found in most series.

Emboli associated with valvular or ischaemic heart disease lodge at the common femoral artery bifurcation or popliteal trifurcation. In the absence of collateral vessels the ensuing ischaemia is profound, resulting in the classical presentation of a pale, paralyzed, pulseless, paraesthetic and perishing cold limb (Figure 1). Ischaemia caused by thrombosis is more insidious.

Over the last 20 years there has been a change in the spectrum of disease. Pure emboli are rarer, due to a fall in the incidence of rheumatic heart disease and an increase in the use of oral anticoagulation for the treatment of atrial fibrillation. Thrombosis, on the other hand, is more common in an ageing population with peripheral vascular disease, diabetes and previous vascular reconstructions [1]. There is a general acceptance that the incidence of profound lower limb ischaemia is declining, possibly due to more liberal prescription of statins.

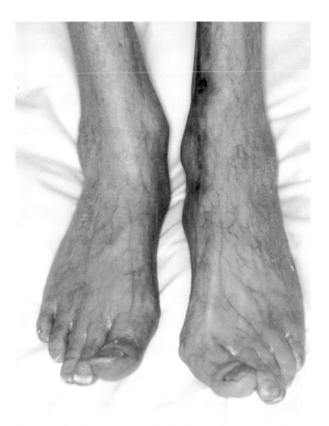

Figure 1. **Severe acute ischaemia caused by proximal embolus. Acute white leg, paralysed and paraesthetic.**

Historical perspective

In 1963, Thomas Fogarty described the balloon embolectomy catheter, which was a revolution as before this the only way to remove clot from an artery was by direct surgery. There was some disappointment that, despite its obvious efficacy, death (10-20%) and amputation rates (20-40%) remained high, due to the severity of the condition [2]. In 1997, the Swedish national vascular registry reported 1054 episodes of acute leg ischaemia; 44% were treated by thrombo-embolectomy, 31% by intra-arterial thrombolysis (at least initially), 7% by vascular reconstruction and the rest by graft revision. Thirty-day re-occlusion and mortality rates in the series were 9% and 15% for emboli and 24% and 14% for thromboses [3]. It has long been appreciated that mortality rates are higher following acute leg ischaemia caused by embolism, and amputation rates are higher after thrombosis.

In 1978, in recognition of the high fatality rate after acute leg ischaemia, Blaisdell proposed early heparinisation to prevent further clot propagation with delayed intervention by either surgical revascularisation or amputation. He suggested that this might save lives at the expense of a higher rate of amputation [4]. Aspirin decreases the incidence of secondary vascular events in patients with arterial disease [5]; heparin and aspirin are now universally accepted as the mandatory minimum treatment for acute leg ischaemia, but additional intervention is often required **(Ia/A)**.

The role of embolectomy

Balloon embolectomy under local anaesthetic is the standard treatment for the pure embolus. This situation is now relatively uncommon. Ideal candidates should have a good source for putative emboli (atrial fibrillation or recent myocardial infarction), a short history of ischaemia, and relatively normal vessels, suggested by palpable pulses or clear biphasic Doppler signals in the contralateral limb [6]. In this situation the following principles ensure the best possible outcome after embolectomy:

◆ operation under local anaesthetic (with sedation, as required) minimises cardiac morbidity, particularly if a myocardial infarction was the underlying problem;
◆ full anaesthetic monitoring, with an experienced anaesthetist present to administer sedation, fluids and oxygen, and treat any arrhythmias;
◆ the whole leg should be prepared for surgery, so that popliteal exploration or bypass are possible;
◆ if the result is disappointing, on-table angiography, on-table lysis or angioscopy may be employed;
◆ the operation should be done by a surgeon competent to perform a full range of interventional procedures.

Unfortunately, this scenario is rare and many patients have pre-existing vascular disease and associated cardiac, renal and pulmonary dysfunction. An experienced initial assessment by a vascular specialist is vital to plan a strategy, which will often involve angiography, percutaneous thrombolysis, angioplasty or reconstructive surgery. Extra-anatomic bypass or distal grafting may also be required. It is clear that the patient with acute leg ischaemia is best managed by a specialist [7] **(IIa/B)**.

The severity of ischaemia - what can wait?

In practice, very few legs need immediate intervention, but it takes experience to judge which patients admitted as an emergency can wait overnight to see a vascular specialist. The urgency of treatment can be planned according to the severity of the initial ischaemia. The Society for Vascular Surgery/ International Society of Cardiovascular Surgery (SVS/ISCVS) grading system is universally accepted [8] (Table 1).

Table 1. The Society for Vascular Surgery/ International Society of Cardiovascular Surgery (SVS/ISCVS) grading system.	
Class I (viable leg)	No sensory or motor function impairment and audible ankle Doppler signals
Class IIa (marginally threatened)	Symptoms limited to a mild sensory loss (usually in the toes). A delay of about six hours would be acceptable before treatment
Class IIb (immediately at risk)	Significant sensory loss, mild to moderate motor loss, but audible ankle Doppler signals. Delay is unacceptable and treatment should be prompt (Figure 2)
Class III (irreversible)	No audible ankle Doppler flow, muscle paralysis, total sensory loss and irreversible tissue damage with fixed skin mottling. Attempts to restore circulation may cause hyperkalaemia, myoglobinuria and death

Table 2. Algorithm for the treatment of acute leg ischaemia.

Ischaemic Class	Heparin	Treatment	Angiogram	Additional intervention
I	+	None	Elective	None
IIa	+	Low-dose thrombolysis or surgery	In X-Ray	If causative lesion identified
IIb	+	Embolectomy, reconstruction or accelerated thrombolysis	On table	If causative lesion identified
III	+	Delayed amputation	–	–

Treatment strategies should be based on the grading system as indicated in Table 2.

The role of thrombolysis

The development of *in situ* clot dissolution with thrombolytic agents such as streptokinase revolutionised the treatment of myocardial infarction. Vascular surgeons had high hopes that it would have a similar role in the management of peripheral ischaemia, the aim being to clear small vessels that the embolectomy catheter and surgery could not reach. After mixed initial success with intravenous thrombolytic therapy, which had a high complication rate and low efficacy, locally directed intra-arterial infusion of more fibrin-specific agents, such as tissue plasminogen activator (tPA) and urokinase, was introduced. The potential advantages of thrombolysis over surgery are that it is less invasive, less likely to dislodge atheromatous plaques, or rupture vessels and is capable of clearing smaller run-off vessels to improve patency [9].

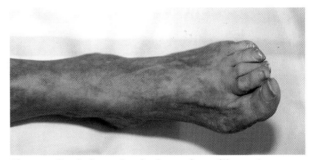

Figure 2. Subacute ischaemia with cutaneous mottling, and partial sensory loss. When mottling ceases to blanche on digital pressure (fixed staining) the limb is no longer viable.

The cause of the acute occlusion has a significant effect on management. Whereas pure emboli can be treated using lysis as sole therapy, treatment of an *in situ* thrombosis often unmasks the lesion underlying the occlusion, such as a high-grade atherosclerotic stenosis. These lesions require further treatment to prevent early rethrombosis after successful initial lysis; angioplasty or stenting are effective for short stenoses, but longer ones may be more appropriately treated by surgical bypass. As a result of this many would consider lysis to be pharmacological procrastination. After early enthusiasm there has been a fall in the number of patients treated by lysis, even by enthusiasts, but there remains a small number of patients with acute ischaemia for whom there is no obvious surgical alternative [10].

The Working Party on Thrombolysis made 30 recommendations regarding the objectives, indications, type of agent, monitoring and complications to help guide thrombolytic treatment of acute leg ischaemia [11] **(IV/C)**. The primary endpoint for intervention is amputation-free survival of the patient, but several surrogate endpoints were described, including the initial success rate of the intervention (complete/partial/no lysis).

A number of thrombolytic agents and dose regimens have been investigated. Streptokinase was the first drug used clinically and it was effective enough to become routine treatment for acute myocardial infarction and the standard for low-dose intra-arterial therapy of acute leg ischaemia (5,000u/h). A product of the bacteria streptococcus, it produced allergic reactions in many patients and could only be used once due to the generation of streptococcal antibodies. Newer, more fibrin-specific agents that act directly on the fibrin clot, such as urokinase and tPA, have become established as more effective agents with fewer side effects. Research continues into newer agents, but the ideal of an effective fibrin-specific agent with no systemic effects has not yet been achieved [12]. There are two main delivery methods for acute leg ischaemia: low-dose infusion and accelerated thrombolysis.

Low-dose thrombolysis

The common doses used are: tPA 0.5-1.0mg/h, urokinase 240,000IU/h for four hours then 120,000IU/h, streptokinase 5,000u/h. This technique is delivered using an end-hole catheter with the tip lodged in the occlusion. The patient is returned to the vascular ward and monitored closely whilst the infusion continues. If standard protocols for the safe management of lysis are not available then the patient is best treated on a high dependency or intensive care unit. Treatment often takes 18-24 hours and overnight infusion is common.

Accelerated thrombolysis

Alternative techniques include pulse-spray thrombolysis using a catheter with multiple side holes and a dedicated infusion pump [13], or accelerated thrombolysis with tPA (three 5mg boluses over 30 minutes, followed by 3.5mg/h for four hours, then 1mg/h as necessary) [14]. Both these techniques have been shown to speed up thrombolysis, often to less than eight hours. Direct comparison of accelerated and low-dose techniques have confirmed that the former is quicker, but that the overall results are similar [15] **(Ib/A)**. Accelerated lysis is specifically indicated in patients with Class IIb ischaemia, where there is a neurosensory deficit in the foot.

Contraindications to thrombolysis

The main risks from thrombolysis are catheter-related haemorrhage or stroke. These risks mitigate against treatment of any patient with acute leg ischaemia whose leg is not immediately threatened (e.g. acute onset claudication). To minimise the risks, a number of contraindications have been defined (Table 3).

Table 3. Contraindications to thrombolysis.

Absolute
Established cerebrovascular event within 2 months
Active bleeding diathesis
Recent gastrointestinal bleeding
Neurosurgery within 3 months
Intracranial trauma within 3 months

Relative major
Cardiopulmonary resuscitation within 10 days
Major surgery or trauma in the last 10 days
Uncontrolled hypertension
Puncture of uncontrollable vessel
Intracranial tumour
Recent eye surgery

Minor
Hepatic failure
Endocarditis
Pregnancy
Diabetic haemorrhagic retinopathy

Results of thrombolysis

There is remarkable consistency of results reported in the literature, regardless of the agent or dose. The UK Thrombolysis Study Group described the results of over 1100 episodes of thrombolysis (NATALI Database) [16]. A complete or partial lysis rate of 73% was recorded, with a limb salvage rate of 75%; 12.5% of patients needed amputation and 12.5% died. Complication rates are also consistent, the most important being stroke. The rate was from 1.2-2.1% in the randomised clinical trials (see below) and 2.3% in the NATALI database. Clearly, this is an effective but dangerous treatment.

Other indications

Several small studies have shown lysis to be effective in the treatment of thrombosed popliteal aneurysms, where it can be used to clear *in situ* thrombosis of the run-off vessels in preparation for aneurysm ligation and bypass. It should not be used to open the aneurysm itself, since this runs the risk of massive distal embolisation which often results in amputation [17]. Many surgeons now prefer intra-operative lysis for these patients [18]. Thrombolysis is also valuable for radiologists if there is a complication of endovascular intervention such as distal embolisation or thrombosis at an angioplasty site. The literature suggests that thrombolysis has a limited role in the resurrection of failed bypass grafts unless the thrombotic occlusion is fresh (less than two weeks old) [19]. Secondary patency rates of grafts successfully lysed are disappointing and revision surgery is usually required to deal with the underlying defect [20]. Antibiotic prophylaxis is essential to prevent graft infection during lysis. Surgical thrombectomy or replacement of the graft, if required on clinical grounds, is recommended. Table 4 is a guide to the ease and success rate of thrombolysis for graft thrombosis.

Acute limb ischaemia: surgery or thrombolysis

Lysis may be attempted in patients with SVS/ISCVS grade IIa ischaemia, if there is time. In clinical practice the guidewire traversal test is used. If a guidewire passes easily through the occlusion, or at least part of it, soft thrombus is present and lysis is worth trying. Case selection is important and complications are more common, especially when the patients are female and over 80 years of age [21].

There have been several randomised trials that compared surgery and thrombolysis for acute leg ischaemia. The first trial, from New York reported a higher mortality in patients who had initial surgery, although no difference in the rate of limb salvage [22] **(IIa/B)**. There were no differences in mortality and amputation between the lysis and surgical patients in the 392 patients included in the STILE (Surgery versus Thrombolysis for Ischaemia of the Lower Extremity) study, but this contained large numbers of

Table 4. A guide to the ease and success rate of thrombolysis for graft thrombosis.				
	Ease of access	Underlying defects	Risk of bleeding	Success rate
Femoropopliteal vein graft	difficult	+++	+	+
Femorodistal prosthetic graft	easy	+	+	++
Aorto-iliac/femoral Dacron graft	easy	++	+++	++
Extra-anatomic graft	easy	++	+	++

patients who presented late, and the radiologists were relatively inexperienced at thrombolysis [23] **(Ib/A)**. Post hoc analysis of surrogate endpoints, such as death and amputation, haemorrhage and peri-operative complications, favoured surgery, since recurrent ischaemia was more common in the lysis group. When recent occlusions (<14 days) were considered separately, however, fewer amputations were reported in the patients treated with thrombolysis.

The TOPAS (Thrombolysis or Peripheral Arterial Surgery) study was designed taking into account all the previous research and was supposed to provide the definitive answer; yet, amputation and mortality rates were similar at discharge and at one year follow-up after both initial surgery and thrombolysis in a large cohort of patients [24] **(Ib/A)**. Although both STILE and TOPAS studies claimed improved results for graft, compared to native vessel occlusions, adjuvant procedures were usually required to maintain patency.

Anticoagulation

There is a significant risk of rethrombosis after successful treatment of acute leg ischaemia by either surgery or thrombolysis. In addition, embolic occlusion has a high risk of further embolisation. Although there are no data to support the use of long-term anticoagulation after treatment of acute ischaemia, it seems logical and is used by most surgeons, especially if atrial fibrillation was implicated. In a study by the Vascular Surgical Society, anticoagulation appeared to confer long-term benefit [25]. The late mortality rate after acute leg ischaemia is very high due to the high incidence of other atherosclerotic complications and it should not be forgotten to offer these patients best medical therapy (see Chapter 5), whatever the outcome from their treatment.

Acute leg ischaemia as an end of life condition

There remains a high mortality rate, despite best management of acute leg ischaemia. It has become recognised that some elderly patients with comorbid diseases are reaching the end of their lives and that

intervention is hopeless. Patients who develop acute ischaemia while in hospital for another condition are a particular example [21]. Identification of these patients and formal palliative care, after discussion with relatives, may be the kindest treatment [26].

New techniques

High speed removal of thrombus without the bleeding risks of thrombolysis and the need for general anaesthesia is an attractive option. It can be quick and, if successful, the circulation is restored immediately. Thrombectomy can be achieved using adaptation of existing infusion catheters (aspiration embolectomy), but a large number of devices have been designed specifically for the purpose (mechanical thrombectomy).

Aspiration embolectomy

Any vascular interventionist has access to the equipment to perform percutaneous aspiration embolectomy. A simple 7F endhole catheter can be adapted for use by removing the taper at the end. The catheter is inserted into the occluding thrombus and a 50ml syringe is aspirated while the catheter is withdrawn through the occlusion. It is often possible to remove small quantities of clot this way and interventionists have used the technique for years when accidental distal embolisation has occurred during a radiological procedure.

Mechanical thrombectomy

Removal of larger amounts of thrombus requires more sophisticated equipment. The ideal thrombectomy device should have the following characteristics:

- remove all the thrombus;
- cause no endothelial injury;
- replace the need for a thrombolytic agent;
- cause no embolisation;
- cause minimal blood loss;
- easy to use;
- safe to use in arteries, veins and prosthetic grafts;
- cheap.

There are two main types of thrombectomy devices: those that macerate the thrombus but do not remove it and those that aspirate and remove the occluding material.

The macerating devices use high-speed rotating drills, or baskets, that convert solid material into microparticles that can be dissolved within the vessels without causing further harm (e.g. Amplatz thrombectomy device, Cragg brush). Particles from 1-3mm are generated that are easily dispersed. The advantage is that they do not remove blood or fluid, so transfusion is not required. They may be used as an adjunct to intra-arterial thrombolysis.

The aspiration devices use the venturi effect to create a vortex at the tip of the device that sucks in and macerates the thrombus material (e.g. Angiojet, Oasis device, Hydrolyser). The clot is then removed through an exhaust catheter; this does result in significant blood loss and transfusion of colloid and occasionally blood is sometimes required. Another hazard that affects both types of device is that significant haemolysis can occur if use is prolonged.

Clinicians have used percutaneous thrombectomy devices for treatment of occlusion of virtually every artery, vein and bypass graft. This has given an extensive but fragmented literature. Mostly reports concern acute arterial ischaemia, iliofemoral venous thrombosis and dialysis graft occlusion. Unlike thrombolysis, which works best for fresh thrombus, the mechanical devices can also deal with the more chronic occlusions, up to several months old. In acute arterial ischaemia, success rates vary from 12-95%, but on average seem little different from reports of patients treated using thrombolysis [27, 28]. There remains a problem from groin haematoma due to large catheter sizes, particularly when systemic heparinisation or thrombolysis are also needed.

Thrombectomy devices definitely work in selected patients, though it seems many require additional thrombolytic therapy. The principal problem is price; the devices are expensive and would have to produce significant savings to be cost-effective. If their results were equivalent to surgery, then they would have to avoid the expense of thrombolysis or shorten hospital stay. The cost and number of different devices and, therefore, the expense of organising a randomised trial hamper scientific study.

Conclusions

Successful management of acute lower leg ischaemia depends on accurate initial assessment; stratification is based on the severity of the ischaemia and selection of the appropriate treatment. This may be medical, surgical, or radiological and often involves a multidisciplinary approach. Hopefully, the future organisation of vascular services will continue to reflect this approach.

Key points	Evidence level

- All patients with acute limb ischaemia should receive aspirin and intravenous heparin (and probably oxygen and intravenous rehydration). — Ib/A
- The main cause of death in this group of patients is myocardial infarction. Appropriate medical and anaesthetic precautions are mandatory. — III/B
- Patients should be stratified according to the severity of their ischaemia. — IIa/B
- Randomised trials have not shown any advantage for surgery or thrombolysis in patients suitable for both; therefore, individual management decisions should be made by surgeons and radiologists working together. — Ia/A
- Local anaesthetic balloon embolectomy is a safe and effective treatment for recent arterial emboli. — IIb/B
- Thrombolysis is useful to unmask the causative lesion but further intervention is almost always required. — IIb/B

References

1. Earnshaw JJ. Demography and etiology of acute leg ischaemia. *Semin Vasc Surg* 2001; 14: 86-92.
2. Ericsson I, Holmberg JT Analysis of factors affecting limb salvage and mortality after arterial embolectomy. *Acta Chir Scand* 1977; 143: 237-40.
3. Jivegard L, Wingren U. Management of acute limb ischaemia over two decades: the Swedish experience. *Eur J Vasc Endovasc Surg* 1999; 18: 93-5.
4. Blaisdell FW, Steele M, Allen RF. Management of acute lower extremity ischaemia due to embolism and thrombosis. *Surgery* 1978; 84: 822-34.
5. Antiplatelet trialists' collaboration: collaborative overview of randomised trials of antiplatelet treatment. Part 1: Prevention of death, myocardial infarction and stroke by prolonged antiplatelet therapy in various categories of patients *Br Med J* 1994; 308: 81-106.
6. Whitman B, Parkin D, Earnshaw JJ. Management of acute leg ischaemia. In: *Pathways of care in vascular surgery.* Beard JD, Murray S, Eds. Shropshire: tfm publishing Ltd, 2002; 12: 99-106.
7. Campbell WB, Ridler BMF, Szymanska TH. Current management of acute leg ischaemia: results of an audit by the Vascular Surgical Society of Great Britain and Ireland. *Br J Surg* 1998; 85: 1498-503.
8. Rutherford RB, Baker JD, Ernst C, *et al.* Recommended standards for reports dealing with lower extremity ischaemia: revised version. *J Vasc Surg* 1997; 26: 517-38.
9. Marder VJ. The use of thrombolytic agents: choice of patient, drug administration, laboratory monitoring. *Ann Internal Med* 1979; 90: 802-12.
10. Richards T, Pittathankal AA, Magee TR, *et al.* The current role of intra-arterial thrombolysis. *Eur J Vasc Endovasc Surg* 2003; 26: 166-9.
11. Working party on thrombolysis in the management of lower limb ischaemia: thrombolysis in the management of lower limb peripheral arterial occlusion - a consensus document. *Am J Cardiol* 1998; 81: 207-18.
12. Ouriel K. Current status of thrombolysis for peripheral arterial occlusive disease. *Ann Vasc Surg* 2002; 16: 797-804.
13. Yusuf SW, Whitaker SC, Gregson RH, *et al.* Prospective randomized comparative study of pulse spray and conventional local thrombolysis. *Eur J Vasc Endovasc Surg* 1995; 10: 136-41.
14. Braithwaite BD, Buckenham TM, Galland RB, *et al.* Prospective randomised trial of high dose bolus versus low dose tissue plasminogen activator infusion in the management of acute limb ischaemia. *Br J Surg* 1997; 84: 646-50.
15. Plate G, Jansson I, Forssell C, *et al.* Thrombolysis for acute lower limb ischaemia - a prospective, randomised multicentre study comparing two strategies. *Eur J Vasc Endovasc Surg* 2006; 31: 651-60.
16. Whitman B, Foy C, Earnshaw JJ, on behalf of the Thrombolysis Study Group. National Audit of Thrombolysis for Acute Leg Ischemia (NATALI): clinical factors associated with early outcome. *J Vasc Surg* 2004; 39: 1018-25.
17. Galland RB, Earnshaw JJ, Baird RN, *et al.* Acute limb deterioration during intra-arterial thrombolysis. *Br J Surg* 1993; 80: 1118-20.
18. Thompson JF, Beard J, Scott DJA, *et al.* Intraoperative thrombolysis in the management of thrombosed popliteal aneurysms. *Br J Surg* 1993; 80:858-9.
19. Lacroix H, Suy R, Nevelsteen A, *et al.* Local thrombolysis for occluded arterial grafts: is the yield worth the effort? *J Cardiovasc Surg* 1994; 35:187-191.
20. Galland RB, Magee TR, Whitman B, *et al.* Patency following successful thrombolysis of occluded vascular grafts. *Eur J Vasc Endovasc Surg* 2001; 22: 157-60.

21. Braithwaite BD, Davies B, Birch PA, *et al.* Management of acute leg ischaemia in the elderly. *Br J Surg* 1998; 85: 217-20.

22. Ouriel K, Shortell CK, DeWeese JA, *et al.* A comparison of thrombolytic therapy with operative revascularisation in the treatment of acute peripheral arterial ischaemia. *J Vasc Surg* 1994; 19: 1021-30.

23. The STILE investigators. Results of a prospective randomised trial; evaluating surgery versus thrombolysis for ischaemia of the lower extremity. The STILE trial. *Ann Surg* 1994; 220: 251-68.

24. Ouriel K, Veith F, Sasahara AA, for the TOPAS investigators. A comparison of recombinant urokinase with vascular surgery as initial treatment for acute arterial occlusion of the legs. *N Engl J Med* 1998; 338: 1105-11.

25. Campbell WB, Ridler BM, Szymanska TH. Two-year follow-up after acute thromboembolic limb ischaemia: the importance of anticoagulation. *Eur J Vasc Endovasc Surg* 2000; 19: 169-73.

26. Campbell WB. Non-intervention and palliative care in vascular patients. *Br J Surg* 2000; 87: 1601-2.

27. Haskal ZH. Mechanical thrombectomy devices for the treatment of peripheral arterial occlusions. *Rev Cardiovasc Med* 2002; 3, suppl 2: S45-52.

28. Schmittling ZC, Hodgson KJ. Thrombolysis and mechanical thrombectomy for arterial disease. *Surg Clin North Am* 2004; 84: 1237-66.

Chapter 14

Haemodialysis access

Christopher P Gibbons MA DPhil MCh FRCS, Consultant Vascular Surgeon
Morriston Hospital, Swansea, UK

Introduction

Renal replacement therapy for end-stage renal failure requires an integrated approach including haemodialysis, peritoneal dialysis and renal transplantation to maximise life expectancy. The majority of patients will require haemodialysis at some stage.

Most patients present electively with deteriorating renal function, allowing the possibility for permanent access to be established in advance; about 30% present acutely and require emergency haemodialysis using a central venous catheter until permanent dialysis access has been established. The subsequent choice between haemodialysis and continuous ambulatory peritoneal dialysis (CAPD) depends on patient preference, lifestyle and ability to cope.

Principles of haemodialysis access

Effective haemodialysis requires blood to circulate through a dialyser at 300ml/min or greater for about four hours, three times per week. The arterial inflow and venous return must be sufficiently separate to avoid recirculation. Most patients undergo hospital haemodialysis as an outpatient, although some can be trained for home dialysis. Access to the circulation can be provided in three ways:

- a double-lumen central venous line (CVC) in the superior vena cava can be used immediately, providing excellent blood flows. Recirculation is prevented by a 3cm gap between the luminal openings;
- an autogenous arteriovenous fistula (AVF) increases the flow within a superficial vein sufficiently for dialysis via one needle near the fistula, returning blood to the circulation through a more proximal needle. When only a short length of vein is available, a single needle may be used for alternating withdrawal and return of blood but dialysis times are prolonged. An AVF requires several weeks' maturation before use, to allow the fistula flow to increase as the vessels dilate [1] and the vein to arterialise for easier and safer needling;
- when there is no suitable vein a prosthetic graft (e.g. polytetrafluoroethylene - PTFE) run superficially between a deep artery and vein can be needled directly for dialysis. Prosthetic AV grafts can be used as soon as the wounds are healed.

Temporary or emergency haemodialysis access

The Scribner shunt

The first haemodialysis access device was the Scribner shunt described in 1960. However, repeated thrombosis and infection, poor patency and patient discomfort led to its replacement by CVCs for emergency and AVFs for permanent access.

Temporary central venous lines

The internal jugular vein is the best site for a CVC [2, 3]. Subclavian lines have an increased risk of pneumothorax or haemothorax on insertion and have a higher incidence of central vein thrombosis and stenosis, leading to the loss of upper limb access sites [2]. Femoral lines have a greater incidence of infection, may cause recirculation and carry a small risk of retroperitoneal haematoma or femoral, iliac or inferior vena cava thrombosis [2, 3]. They are uncomfortable for longer-term use and are usually reinserted for each dialysis.

Patients may be allowed home with a temporary CVC while awaiting permanent access. However, the waiting time for lines should be minimised because of the ever-present risk of septicaemia and central venous thrombosis [4]. The USA National Kidney Foundation Dialysis Outcomes Quality Initiative (NKF-DOQI) guidelines recommend that less than 10% of patients should be dialysed on lines beyond three months [4]. CVCs are associated with a higher mortality compared with autologous AVFs or grafts [5-7] **(IIa/B)**. Moreover, previous use of temporary access seems to compromise the patency of subsequent AVFs [8] **(IIa/B)**. In the Dialysis Outcomes and Practice Patterns Study (DOPPS) more than 50% of UK patients started dialysis with a CVC in contrast to a European average of 33% [9, 10]; in the 2005 UK Renal Registry Report [11], 68% started dialysis with a CVC, reflecting the under-provision of access surgery in the NHS.

Insertion of central venous catheters

Catheters are usually inserted under local anaesthesia using ultrasound control, which minimises complications [2, 12] **(Ia/A)**. Complications of insertion are infrequent but include pneumothorax, haemorrhage from inadvertent arterial puncture, chylothorax from thoracic duct puncture, brachial plexus trauma and air embolism [2]. The internal jugular approach on the right is easier and has fewer complications [3].

Long-term complications of central venous catheters

Long-term complications of central venous catheters are as follows:

♦ infection is the cause of death in 16-36% of dialysis patients and is access-related in 50-70% [13]. Bacteraemia is most frequent with central lines, with an incidence of 1-6.5 episodes per 1000 catheter days, and is most commonly due to *Staphylococcus aureus* [13]. This may lead to metastatic infections such as bacterial endocarditis, mycotic aneurysms, osteomyelitis or septic arthritis. It is minimised by careful aseptic technique for inserting, changing or using lines, cleaning with chlorhexidine, which is superior to povidone iodine [14] **(Ib/A)**, and the early establishment of permanent access. Established infection requires systemic antibiotic therapy and temporary catheter removal [3, 4, 13]. Antibiotic prophylaxis is not recommended [3] **(Ib/A)**;

♦ catheter thrombosis is prevented by heparin instillation after use [15] **(Ia/A)**. Heparin also reduces microbial adherence [15]. Urokinase may clear a clotted catheter and obviate its replacement [16];

♦ a fibrin cuff may occlude the tip of the line. Patency may be restored by catheter replacement, local thrombolysis or by 'stripping' under angiographic control using a percutaneously introduced snare [16];

♦ central venous thrombosis and subclavian stenosis may preclude further access in the arms. Percutaneous angioplasty is often effective but one-year patencies are usually less than 40% [17]. Primary stenting may give better patencies but restenosis occurs within one to two years in the majority [17]. Others have reserved stents for recurrent or resistant stenoses. Covered stents and brachytherapy have no advantage [17]. Venous bypass (e.g. internal jugular turndown or right atrium-subclavian bypass) may be used and reported patencies are 80-90% at one year but the surgery is a major undertaking [18]. Finally, the arm may need to be abandoned in favour of a lower limb AVF;

- displacement or malposition usually requires repositioning of the line [3].

Permanent central venous catheters

When other options have been exhausted, a permanent double-lumen catheter (e.g. PermCath or Vascath) may be used. These have a Dacron cuff within a subcutaneous tunnel for sutureless fixation and as a barrier to infection. They have a relatively short life, requiring removal or replacement within 18 months [19], although secondary patency varies greatly between centres [16]. The risks of infection, central venous thrombosis and death are less than with uncuffed catheters, but much greater than for AVFs [13]. The relative risk of infection for tunnelled compared with non-tunnelled catheters was 0.61 in a meta-analysis [20] **(Ia/A)**. In one study the relative risk of infection relative to AVFs was as high as 13.6 for tunnelled catheters and 32.6 for temporary catheters [6]. In other studies the relative risk for CVCs compared with AVFs was somewhat less at 1.5 and was higher in men than women [5, 7]. A tunnelled CVC is recommended for temporary access longer than three weeks [4] **(IV/C)**.

Permanent vascular access

Vascular access planning

The veins on the back of the hand should be used preferentially for intravenous infusions and venepuncture to preserve the cephalic veins for dialysis [4]. Permanent access is best provided by an arteriovenous fistula (AVF), although in the absence of adequate superficial veins a prosthetic AV graft may be used [4]. Access should make maximum use of available sites, starting as distally as possible. The non-dominant arm is used preferentially to allow use of the dominant arm during dialysis and self-needling if home dialysis is anticipated. When access sites on the non-dominant arm are unavailable, the dominant arm and, finally, the leg can be used. The arterial inflow must be good, but considerable adaptation may occur so that even small vessels such as the distal radial artery may be used. In diabetes and long-standing renal failure, arterial calcification may prevent adaptation and necessitate a more proximal fistula. Any haemodynamically significant (>70%) upstream arterial stenosis will impair inflow and may cause thrombosis or failure of maturation. The vein must be superficial, of adequate size (>2mm) and without stenosis [21] **(IIa/B)**. In obese patients forearm veins may be difficult to locate and this sometimes requires a more proximal fistula or graft.

Pre-operative investigation

Routine pre-operative arterial and venous duplex imaging has been suggested to increase the rate of autogenous fistula formation and improve overall fistula patency rates [21] **(IIa/B)**. It is especially useful before secondary or tertiary access and in patients such as the obese in whom veins are poorly visible [22]. It is probably unnecessary for primary access in patients with a good radial pulse and visible forearm veins [23] **(IIa/B)**.

Before constructing a radiocephalic AVF, it is standard advice to perform an Allen test [4] (observation of digital perfusion with the radial artery occluded - blanching indicates an inadequate ulnar artery), but there is no evidence that it is necessary in practice. Venography of the axillary and subclavian veins has been advocated in all patients with subclavian lines and is mandatory in patients with signs of venous engorgement, oedema or venous collaterals around the shoulder [4].

Techniques

Techniques involve the following:

- aspirin (75-300mg daily) with, or without, dipyridamole (100mg t.d.s.) is given pre-operatively for at least 24 hours and continued postoperatively to reduce the risk of thrombosis [24, 25] **(Ib/A)**;
- most procedures can be performed under local anaesthetic and about half are suitable for day-case surgery. General anaesthesia may be preferable for brachio-axillary grafts, basilic vein transpositions and lower limb fistulae;
- some surgeons prefer axillary block, believing that the resulting vasodilatation improves fistula flow, but a qualified anaesthetist is usually required;
- postoperatively, the arm is warmed in a gamgee sleeve to promote vasodilatation. A glyceryl trinitrate patch is sometimes placed over the vein near the fistula in an attempt to improve patency as this is known to reduce thrombosis after intravenous catheter insertion and has been shown to increase flow in AV fistulae [26].

Possible fistula sites

The radiocephalic (Breschia-Cimino) AVF

The radiocephalic (Breschia-Cimino) AVF (Figure 1) at the wrist was first described in 1966 and remains the gold standard for primary access [4, 27]. Originally a side-to-side configuration was described but an end-to-side (vein to artery) fistula is preferred to reduce the incidence of distal venous hypertension. Retrograde flow from the distal radial artery represents 30% of the total fistula flow, leading some to advocate an end-to-end configuration with distal arterial and venous ligation to minimise digital ischaemia [27], but steal is relatively uncommon in practice. A primary radiocephalic fistula is possible in over 60% of patients and becomes usable in 80% within six weeks, with reasonable long-term primary patency (63% at one year) [27, 28] **(Ia/A)**. If it fails, further radiocephalic fistulae are often possible in the forearm provided the arterial inflow is satisfactory (Figure 2) [27].

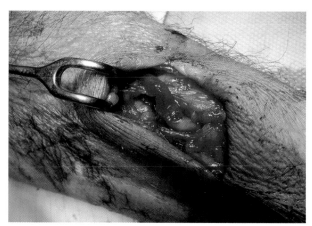

Figure 1. The wrist radiocephalic AV fistula.

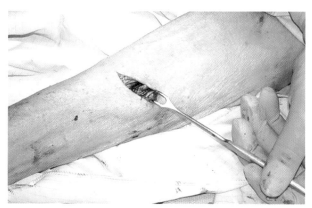

Figure 2. A radiocephalic AV fistula in the mid forearm.

The snuffbox AVF

The snuffbox AVF (Figure 3), a more distal radiocephalic fistula in the anatomical snuffbox, is possible in 50% of patients who need primary access and is preferred by the author [29]. Patency is similar to the standard radiocephalic fistula, which, in the event of failure, can still be constructed in 45% [27, 29].

The brachiocephalic AVF

If forearm veins are inadequate, the cephalic vein or one of its tributaries in the antecubital fossa can be anastomosed to the brachial artery to produce an excellent high-flow fistula (Figure 4). Needles are placed in the upper arm cephalic vein for dialysis [27, 30].

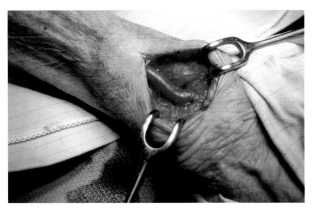

Figure 3. The snuffbox AV fistula.

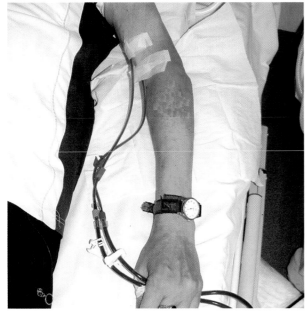

Figure 4. Dialysis on a brachiocephalic AV fistula.

Brachiocephalic or brachiobasilic forearm loops

When the veins are adequate but the arteries poor in the forearm, the distal cephalic or basilic vein can be looped to create a brachiocephalic fistula (Figure 5), leaving options open for a standard brachiocephalic AVF in the event of failure. Other options include transposition of the basilic vein to the radial artery or the cephalic vein to the ulnar artery in the forearm [30].

The ulnobasilic AVF

The basilic vein is less accessible and rarely used for intravenous infusions leaving it available for a fistula to the ulnar artery at the wrist, although needling can be more difficult. A previously failed radiocephalic or brachiocephalic AVF does not preclude it, even if the radial artery is occluded, as the interosseous artery provides a good collateral supply to the hand [27, 31].

The basilic vein transposition

A brachiobasilic AVF in the antecubital fossa only permits single needle dialysis as the median basilic vein dives deeply after 2-3cm. However, rerouting the basilic vein in a subcutaneous tunnel in the upper arm renders it available for needling (Figure 6) [30, 32]. This can be done in a single stage, but some prefer to perform a brachiobasilic anastomosis first, with transposition and re-anastomosis of the basilic vein to

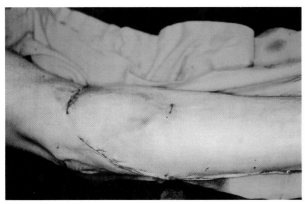

Figure 5. A brachiobasilic forearm loop.

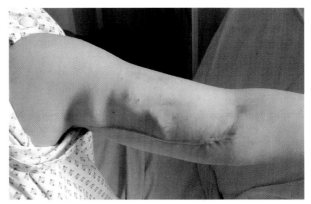

Figure 6. A basilic vein transposition AV fistula.

the brachial artery at a second stage after a period of maturation. Patency may be superior to upper arm prosthetic grafts [32] **(IIb/B)**.

Vein grafts

Long saphenous vein can be used as an AV graft either *in situ* or transposed to the arm, but is more difficult to needle and patency is poor [30, 33]. Femoral vein is better, providing a high flow but the incidence of steal is high [33].

Prosthetic AV grafts

Prosthetic AV grafts may be used in the absence of suitable superficial veins. The usual configurations are brachial AV forearm loops, straight radiobasilic grafts or brachio-axillary grafts. If access is impossible in the arms a femoro-femoral AV loop may be constructed in the thigh (Figure 7) but infection rates are higher [33]. Usually 6mm PTFE is used. Grafts that are tapered or stepped at the arterial end have been advocated to reduce steal, but seem to have no advantage in practice [34] **(Ib/A)**. An externally supported central section or internal support throughout prevents kinking of looped grafts. Wider grafts [35] and the addition of a vein cuff [36] or an expanded distal end of a PTFE graft (Venaflo) [37] at the venous anastomosis improves patency **(Ib/A)**. Prosthetic grafts such as PTFE are easy to needle and can be used within two to three weeks. However, they require long periods of compression following removal of dialysis needles, have poorer patency [19] (58% vs 72% at six months

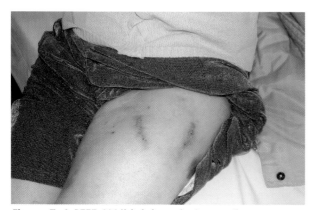

Figure 7. A PTFE AV thigh loop between the common femoral artery and vein.

and 33% vs 51% at 18 months in a recent meta-analysis) [38] **(Ia/A)**, require more frequent revisions [19], and have higher rates of infection (9% vs. 1% per annum) [5, 19] **(Ia/A)**.

The mortality risk relative to autologous AVFs has been estimated to be 1.2 and 2.2 in different reports [6, 7] and in another study was greater in diabetics (1.54) than non-diabetics (1.08) [11] **(IIa/B)**. Despite their drawbacks, prosthetic grafts have been popular in the USA, even for primary access, with a graft usage of 76% in the DOPPS, which is probably representative of the majority of US dialysis units [39]. NKF-DOQI recommended that more than 50% of primary access procedures should be autologous fistulae, which would be regarded as unnecessarily low in Europe, where prosthetic graft usage (<30%) is much less than in the USA [39]. In Swansea prosthetic grafts were used in only 63 / 1748 (3.5%) access procedures and only 3 / 1037 (0.3%) primary procedures over the last 21 years.

Biological grafts

Biological grafts, such as cryopreserved cadaveric femoral vein, bovine mesenteric vein and bovine ureter have the theoretical advantage of increased resistance to infection in comparison with artificial grafts but most have been prone to aneurysmal dilatation and thrombosis [33].

Organisation of services

Dedicated operating lists for vascular access are essential and it has been recommended that one such weekly list should be available for every 120 patients on dialysis [17]. Access nurses and co-ordinators can identify problems, prioritise patients and organise operating lists to shorten the patient pathway and reduce waiting times, which have been hitherto unacceptably high in the UK [9-11]. Some units have specific clinics for assessment, investigation and postoperative follow-up, but an experienced access nurse can perform pre-operative assessment, directly listing most patients for surgery and identifying the small number of patients who require more detailed consideration by the surgeon before admission.

Complications

Thrombosis

Thrombosis is the most common cause of access failure. This may result from an inadequate inflow due to upstream arterial stenosis, but more commonly from a stenosis in the venous outflow following previous intravenous infusions, or scarring after traumatic dialysis needle placement. Intimal hyperplasia is particularly common beyond the venous anastomosis in prosthetic grafts. Thrombosis may also result from dehydration or hypercoagulability during intercurrent illness.

Failure is more common with small vessels; in one study all fistulae with arterial or venous diameters of less than 1.6mm thrombosed [2] **(IIa/B)**. A minimum diameter of 2mm is now generally recommended for the successful creation of an AVF [21]. Flow velocity, measured by duplex imaging, of more than 300cm/sec at 5-10cm from the anastomosis the day after surgery is a strong predictor of fistula patency [21] **(IIa/B)**. In most studies, fistula thrombosis is more common in women [27] **(IIb/B)**. Prosthetic grafts have poorer patency [38] **(IIa/B)**. Anastomosis with non-penetrating vascular clips improved patency in randomised trials but they cannot be used in diseased or calcified vessels [40] **(Ib/B)**. Whereas diabetes has often been implicated as an adverse factor, the evidence is conflicting [27]. Smoking reduces access patency [41] **(IIb/B)**. Lipoprotein abnormalities seem to be an adverse factor only in patients of African origin [42] **(IIa/B)**.

Dialysis patients are generally anaemic and have reduced platelet stickiness, which may improve fistula patency. Fears that erythropoietin therapy to increase haemoglobin might also reduce fistula patency have not been realised in practice [27], and even improved patency of grafts in one study [43] **(IIa/B)**. Hypercoagulable states, hyperfibrinogenaemia and vasculitis are risk factors for access thromboses [44, 45] **(IIa/B)**. Antiplatelet agents such as aspirin and dipyridamole prolong fistula patency and are used routinely [24, 25] **(Ib/A)**. Anticoagulation with warfarin reduces AVF thrombosis in patients with a hypercoagulable state [44] but more widespread use is unwise in view of the risk of haemorrhagic complications [46] and warfarin was even associated with poorer patency in the DOPPS study [47] **(IIa/B)**. The combination of aspirin and clopidogrel increased haemorrhagic complications without influencing patency in prosthetic AV grafts [48], although the results of a larger randomised trial are awaited. Fish oil reduced access thrombosis in one randomised trial [49] **(Ib/A)**. In the DOPPS study, fistula patency was better in patients on calcium channel blockers and ACE inhibitors [47], but others have failed to confirm any effect of ACE inhibitors [50]. Patency can be restored by thrombolysis with streptokinase or tPA and percutaneous angioplasty (PTA) under angiographic control or by surgical thrombectomy and revision. The choice may depend on local expertise but there is some evidence that the subsequent patency of AV grafts is better after surgery [51] **(IIb/B)**.

Steal

Distal to a high-flow fistula the arterial pressure is reduced, resulting in impairment or reversal of blood flow. If the collateral supply is inadequate, distal ischaemia with rest pain, paraesthesiae or even digital gangrene results. Steal may also result from a significant upstream arterial stenosis. Steal occurs in 1-8% of haemodialysis access procedures and is more common in brachial fistulae or grafts than distal fistulae [52, 53]. It is also said to be more frequent in diabetics and the elderly [52]. The diagnosis is confirmed by the absence of a radial pulse and by measuring the arterial pressure at the wrist using continuous-wave Doppler [54], or in the fingers by photoplethysmography [52]. By analogy with lower limb ischaemia, a wrist pressure of <50mmHg or a finger pressure of <40mmHg may indicate critical ischaemia. Occlusion of the fistula restores the radial pulse and distal perfusion pressure to normal.

Fistula ligation is curative but loses the access. Reduction of fistula flow by banding or interposition of a narrowed segment of graft is unreliable [55]. For wrist or snuffbox fistulae, simple ligation of the radial artery distal to the AVF prevents distal reversed flow and relieves symptoms by improving perfusion to the thumb [53]. For brachial AVFs, distal ligation of the artery beyond the AVF, together with revascularisation by a saphenous vein graft from the proximal brachial

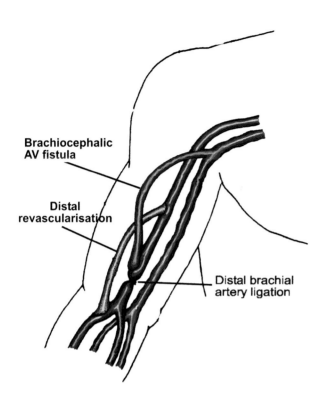

Brachiocephalic AV fistula

Distal revascularisation

Distal brachial artery ligation

Figure 8. Diagram of the DRIL procedure.

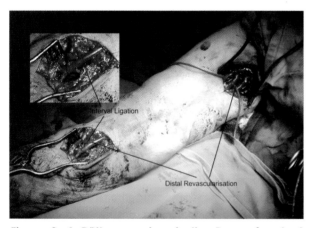

Interval Ligation

Distal Revascularisation

Figure 9. A DRIL procedure in the R arm for steal following a brachial AV fistula.

artery to the brachial artery beyond the fistula (the DRIL procedure) is often successful [52] **(IIb/B)** (Figures 8 and 9). An alternative is to detach the vein from the brachial artery and extend it to the proximal

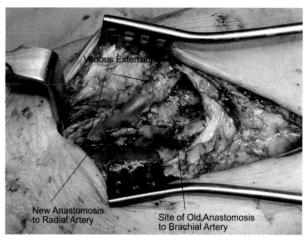

Venous Extension

New Anastomosis to Radial Artery

Site of Old Anastomosis to Brachial Artery

Figure 10. The extension procedure for steal following a brachiocephalic AV fistula.

radial artery (the extension procedure) [56] (Figure 10). When distal pressure measurements confirm the adequacy of collaterals, simple distal brachial artery ligation may occasionally be effective [57] **(III/B)**.

Ischaemic monomelic neuropathy

Disabling neuropathic pain occasionally occurs after AV fistula placement. It usually accompanies steal and may persist after successful revascularisation. It can be confirmed by electrophysiology but treatment is difficult [58].

Infection

Bacteraemia is frequent in patients undergoing haemodialysis and may respond to systemic antibiotics. Local infection is more common in prosthetic grafts than autologous fistulae [5, 13]. In early postoperative graft infection the whole prosthesis is usually involved and should be excised. Later, localised infection at needle sites may be treated by partial graft excision and bypass through a clean area, but total excision often eventually becomes necessary [33]. Infection in autologous fistulae usually responds to antibiotics but grossly purulent needle sites may result in uncontrollable haemorrhage requiring fistula ligation.

Haemorrhage

Haemorrhage can result from repeated needling at the same site. It is more common in prosthetic grafts, which often require prolonged compression after removing needles. Haematoma formation (the blown fistula), results in scarring, stenosis and fistula failure, and should be avoided. Self-sealing grafts may reduce leakage but have poorer patency [59] **(IIa/B)**.

Aneurysm

The venous dilatation proximal to an AVF sometimes becomes excessive. This is rarely a problem but pain, thrombosis or impending rupture may necessitate fistula ligation with creation of a more proximal AVF.

Venous hypertension

Distal venous flow in a side-to side AVF occasionally causes swelling of the radial aspect of the hand or even ulceration of the thumb. Ligation of the distal venous outflow is usually curative. It is rare after end-to-side (vein to artery) fistulae. Subclavian vein thrombosis or stenosis may cause gross arm swelling and can be treated by angioplasty with, or without a stent, but if this fails fistula ligation may be required.

Cardiac failure

High output cardiac failure may occur with proximal fistulae or bridge grafts, where flow often exceeds one litre per minute. Digital occlusion of the fistula may cause a reduction in pulse rate (Branham's sign). Treatment is either by fistula ligation or by interposing a narrow segment of prosthetic graft.

Needle placement

A new AV fistula is usually allowed to mature for one to three months before use [4], although there was no evidence that early cannulation was detrimental in the DOPPS [60] **(IIa/B)**. Cannulation is performed aseptically by one of three methods [61] (Figure 11):

 ◆ rope ladder: systematic evenly spaced cannulation along the length of the vein draining

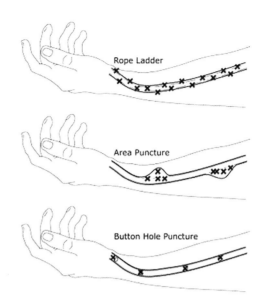

Figure 11. Strategies for needling AV fistulae. Crosses represent needle sites.

the fistula causes mild and well-distributed dilatation throughout an autologous AVF and is also recommended for prosthetic grafts;

 ◆ area puncture: repeated cannulation over short segments of the vein, may encourage localised dilatation in a new fistula but may lead to interspersed stenoses and is inadvisable for long-term use;

 ◆ buttonhole: repeated puncture through the same needle site causes little dilatation and reduces the pain of cannulation but is not recommended for prosthetic grafts as it tends to cause false aneurysms.

Vascular access surveillance

In some patients, a reduction in the palpable thrill or in dialysis flow rates, or an increase in venous pressure on dialysis may herald fistula failure. In others, thrombosis occurs suddenly for no apparent reason. Many such fistulae have asymptomatic stenoses, which, with timely detection, could be treated prophylactically by angioplasty or surgery. Surveillance by duplex imaging, static and dynamic pressure measurements within the fistula, or measurement of access blood flow have all been advocated [62]. Deterioration in fistula flow or an increase in venous pressure is more predictive of a significant stenosis than a single value [62]. There is evidence from randomised [63, 64] and non-randomised [62] studies that patency is prolonged by surveillance of both autologous fistulae and prosthetic AV grafts **(Ib/A)**, although other studies have failed to show any benefit [65]. Comparisons between different surveillance methods have also been contradictory [62].

Once stenoses have been identified, balloon angioplasty may obviate the need for surgery and prevent occlusion. There is some evidence that SMART stents improve patency [66] and cutting balloons are showing some promise [67]. The results of a trial of brachytherapy to reduce recurrent intimal hyperplasia are awaited.

Vascular access in children

Children present particularly difficult access problems. Transplantation is ideal and achieves optimal growth and development. While CAPD is the next best option, haemodialysis is often required. Distal autologous fistulae are more difficult to create, requiring microsurgical skills, but several European units have shown that they are preferable [68] **(IIb/B)**. Many other units rely on permanent central venous lines or prosthetic grafts, risking the loss of available access sites.

Conclusions

The dialysis population is increasing at about 8% per year throughout the world because of the increasing incidence of diabetes and the aging population [69]. Vascular access is now accepted as a major part of vascular surgery in may countries, including the UK, and is one of the areas of expansion within the vascular field. Appropriate organisation of services with dedicated access operating lists and enthusiastic interventional radiology is essential to improve and maintain standards. Haemodialysis access surgery should become an essential part of vascular surgical training to ensure adequate expertise and the maintenance of high standards for the future.

Key points	Evidence level
◆ Early AV fistula construction minimises the use of central venous catheters, reduces infection, hospitalisation and mortality.	Ia/A
◆ An autogenous AV fistula is the optimum access, having the lowest incidence of infection and thrombosis, and the lowest mortality.	Ia/A
◆ When suitable veins are unavailable for an autogenous AVF, a prosthetic AV graft is the next best option as most biological grafts are prone to thrombosis and aneurysm formation.	III/B
◆ Pre-operative duplex imaging improves fistula patency but is probably unnecessary for primary access in patients with good vessels on clinical examination. For a successful AV fistula, vessels should be greater than 2mm in diameter.	IIa/B
◆ Aspirin with, or without, dipyridamole prolongs fistula patency and is recommended routinely.	Ib/A
◆ Surveillance of AVFs or AV grafts by flow measurement, duplex imaging or pressure measurement remains controversial but the available evidence suggests that fistula patency may be prolonged and the number of surgical procedures reduced.	Ib/A

References

1. Wong V, Ward R, Taylor J, *et al.* Factors associated with early failure of arteriovenous fistulae for haemodialysis access. *Eur J Vasc Endovasc Surg* 1996; 12: 207-13.
2. Farrell J, Abraham KA, Walshe JJ. Acute vascular access. In: *Haemodialysis Vascular Access: Practice and Problems.* Conlon PJ, Schwab SJ, Nicholson ML, Eds. Oxford: Oxford University Press, 2000: 3-22.
3. Frankel A. Temporary access and central venous catheters. *Eur J Vasc Endovasc Surg* 2006; 31: 417-22.
4. NKF-K/DOQI Clinical Practice Guidelines for Vascular Access: Update 2000. *Am J Kidney Dis* 2001; 37 Suppl 1: S137-81.
5. Dhingra RK, Young EW, Hulbert-Shearon TE, *et al.* Type of vascular access and mortality in U.S. hemodialysis patients. *Kidney Int* 2001; 60: 1443-51.
6. Stevenson KB, Hannah EL, Lowder CA, *et al.* Epidemiology of hemodialysis vascular access infections from longitudinal infection surveillance data: predicting the impact of NKF-DOQI clinical practice guidelines for vascular access. *Am J Kidney Dis* 2002; 39: 549-55.
7. Astor BC, Eustace JA, Powe NR, *et al;* CHOICE Study. I. Type of vascular access and survival among incident hemodialysis patients: the Choices for Healthy Outcomes in Caring for ESRD (CHOICE) Study. *J Am Soc Nephrol* 2005; 16: 1449-55.
8. Rayner HC, Pisoni RL, Gillespie BW, *et al.* Dialysis Outcomes and Practice Patterns Study creation, cannulation and survival of arteriovenous fistulae: data from the Dialysis Outcomes and Practice Patterns Study. *Kidney Int* 2003; 63: 323-30.
9. Goodkin DA, Mapes DL, Held PJ. The Dialysis Outcomes and Practice Patterns Study (DOPPS): how can we improve the care of hemodialysis patients? *Semin Dial* 2001; 14: 157-9.
10. The Kidney Alliance. End Stage Renal Failure - A Framework for Planning and Service Delivery. Munro and Forster. London, 2001.
11. UK Renal Registry Report 2005. UK Renal Registry, Bristol, UK. Ansell D, Feest T, Williams AJ, Winearls C, Eds. Chapter 6; The National Dialysis Access Survey - preliminary results: 87-102. (http://www.renalreg.com/Report%202005/Cover_Frame 2.htm).
12. Randolph AG, Cook D, Gonzales CA, Brun-Buisson Cl. Ultrasound guidance for placement of central venous catheters: a meta-analysis of the literature. *Crit Care Med* 1996; 24: 2053-8.
13. Kirkland KB, Sexton DJ. Dialysis-access infection. In: *Haemodialysis Vascular Access: Practice and Problems.* Conlon PJ, Schwab SJ, Nicholson ML, Eds. Oxford: Oxford University Press, 2000: 84-100.
14. Maki DG, Ringer M, Alvardo CJ. Prospective randomised trial of povidone-iodine, alcohol, and chlorhexidine for prevention of infection associated with central venous and arterial catheters. *Lancet* 1991; 338: 339-43.
15. Randolph AG, Cook DJ, Gonzales CA, Andrew M. Benefit of heparin in peripheral venous and pulmonary artery catheters: a meta-analysis of randomised controlled trials. *Chest* 1998; 113: 165-71.
16. Blankenstijn PJ. Cuffed tunnelled catheters for long-term vascular access. In: *Haemodialysis Vascular Access: Practice and Problems.* Conlon PJ, Schwab SJ, Nicholson ML, Eds. Oxford: Oxford University Press, 2000: 67-84.
17. Mickley V. Central vein obstruction in vascular access. *Eur J Vasc Surg* 2006; 32: 439-44.
18. Dammers R, de Haan MW, Planken NR, *et al.* Central vein obstruction in hemodialysis patients: results of radiological and surgical intervention. *Eur J Vasc Endovasc Surg* 2003; 26: 317-21.
19. Hodges TC, Fillinger MF, Zwolak RM, *et al.* Longitudinal comparison of dialysis access methods: factors for failure. *J Vasc Surg* 1997; 26: 1009-19.
20. Randolph AG, Cook DJ, Gonzales CA, Brun-Buisson C. Tunneling short-term central venous catheters to prevent catheter-related infection: a meta-analysis of randomized, controlled trials. *Crit Care Med* 1998; 26: 1315-6.
21. Brown PW. Preoperative radiological assessment for vascular access. *Eur J Vasc Endovasc Surg* 2006; 31: 64-9.
22. Vassalotti JA, Falk A, Cohl ED, *et al.* Obese and non-obese hemodialysis patients have a similar prevalence of functioning arteriovenous fistula using pre-operative vein mapping. *Clin Nephrol* 2002; 58: 211-4.
23. Wells AC, Fernando B, Butler A, *et al.* Selective use of ultrasonographic vascular mapping in the assessment of patients before haemodialysis access surgery. *Br J Surg* 2005; 92: 1439-43.
24. Andrassy K, Malluche H, Bornfeld H, *et al.* Prevention of PO clotting of AV Cimino fistulae with acetylsalicyl acid: results of a prospective double blind study. *Klin Wochenschr* 1974; 52: 348-9.
25. Sreedhara R, Himmelfarb J, Lazarus JM, Hakim RM. Antiplatelet therapy in graft thrombosis: results of a prospective randomised double blind study. *Kidney Int* 1994; 45: 1477-83.
26. Akin EB, Topcu O, Ozcan H, *et al.* Haemodynamic effect of transdermal glyceryl trinitrate on newly constructed arteriovenous fistula. *World J Surg* 2002; 26: 1256-9.
27. Gibbons CP. Primary vascular access. *Eur J Vasc Endovasc Surg* 2006; 31: 523-9.
28. Rooijens PP, Tordoir JH, Stijnen T, *et al.* Radiocephalic wrist arteriovenous fistula for hemodialysis: meta-analysis indicates a high primary failure rate. *Eur J Vasc Endovasc Surg* 2004; 28: 583-9.
29. Wolowczyk L, Williams AJ, Gibbons CP. The snuffbox arteriovenous fistula for vascular access. *Eur J Vasc Endovasc Surg* 2000; 19: 70-76.
30. Tordoir JH, Keuter X, Planken N, *et al.* Autogenous options in secondary and tertiary access for haemodialysis. *Eur J Vasc Endovasc Surg* 2006; 31: 661-6.
31. Salgado OJ, Chacon RE, Henriquez C. Ulnar-basilic fistula: indications, surgical aspects, puncture technique, and results. *Artif Organs* 2004; 28: 634-8.
32. Dix FP, Khan Y, Al-Khaffaf H. The brachial artery-basilic vein arterio-venous fistula in vascular access for haemodialysis - a review paper. *Eur J Vasc Endovasc Surg* 2006; 31: 70-9.
33. Berardinelli L. Grafts and graft materials as vascular substitutes for haemodialysis access construction. *Eur J Vasc Endovasc Surg* 2006; Epub ahead of print. http://dx.doi.org/10.1016/j.ejvs.2006.01.001.
34. Dammers R, Planken RN, Pouls KP, *et al.* Evaluation of 4-mm to 7-mm versus 6-mm prosthetic brachial-antecubital forearm loop access for hemodialysis: results of a randomized multicenter clinical trial. *J Vasc Surg* 2003; 37: 143-8.
35. Garcia-Pajares R, Polo JR, Flores A, *et al.* Upper arm polytetrafluoroethylene grafts for dialysis access. Analysis of

two different graft sizes: 6mm and 6-8mm. *Vasc Endovascular Surg* 2003; 37: 335-43.

36. Lemson MS, Tordoir JH, van Det RJ, *et al.* Effects of a venous cuff at the venous anastomosis of polytetrafluoroethylene grafts for hemodialysis vascular access. *J Vasc Surg* 2000; 32: 1155-63.

37. Sorom AJ, Hughes CB, McCarthy JT, *et al.* Prospective, randomized evaluation of a cuffed expanded polytetrafluoroethylene graft for haemodialysis vascular access. *Surgery* 2002; 132: 135-40.

38. Huber TS, Carter JW, Carter RL, *et al.* Patency of autogenous and polytetrafluoroethylene upper extremity arteriovenous hemodialysis accesses: a systematic review. *J Vasc Surg* 2003; 38: 1005-11.

39. Pisoni RL, Young EW, Dykstra DM, *et al.* Vascular access use in Europe and the United States: results from the DOPPS. *Kidney Int* 2002; 61: 305-16.

40. Shenoy S, Miller A, Petersen F, *et al.* A multicentre study of permanent hemodialysis access patency: beneficial effect of clipped vascular anastomotic technique. *J Vasc Surg* 2003; 38: 229-35.

41. Wetzig GA, Gough IR, Furnival CM. One hundred cases of arteriovenous fistula for haemodialysis access: the effect of cigarette smoking on patency. *ANZ J Surg* 1985; 55: 551-4.

42. Astor BC, Eustace JA, Klag MJ, *et al*; CHOICE Study. Race-specific association of lipoprotein(a) with vascular access interventions in hemodialysis patients: the CHOICE Study. *Kidney Int* 2002; 61: 1115-23.

43. Martino MA, Vogel KM, O'Brien SP, Kerstein MD. Erythropoietin therapy improves graft patency with no increased incidence of thrombosis or thrombophlebitis. *J Am Coll Surg* 1998; 187: 616-9.

44. LeSar CJ, Merrick HW, Smith MR. Thrombotic complications resulting from hypercoagulable states in chronic haemodialysis vascular access. *J Am Coll Surg* 1999; 189: 73-9.

45. Baumann M, Niebel W, Kribben A, *et al.* Primary failure of arteriovenous fistulae in auto-immune disease. *Kidney Blood Press Res* 2003; 26: 362-7.

46. Biggers JA, Remmers AR Jr, Glassford DM, *et al.* The risk of anticoagulation in haemodialysis patients. *Nephron* 1977; 18: 109-13.

47. Saran R, Dykstra DM, Wolfe RA, *et al.* Dialysis Outcomes and Practice Patterns Study Association between vascular access failure and the use of specific drugs: the Dialysis Outcomes and Practice Patterns Study (DOPPS). *Am J Kidney Dis* 2002; 40: 1255-63.

48. Kaufman JS, O'Connor TZ, Zhang JH, *et al.* Randomized controlled trial of clopidogrel plus aspirin to prevent hemodialysis access graft thrombosis. *J Am Soc Nephrol* 2003; 14: 2313-21.

49. Schmitz PG, McCloud LK, Reikes ST, *et al.* Prophylaxis of hemodialysis graft thrombosis with fish oil: double-blind, randomized, prospective trial. *J Am Soc Nephrol* 2002; 13: 184-90.

50. Heine GH, Ulrich C, Kohler H, *et al.* Is AV fistula patency associated with angiotensin-converting enzyme (ACE) polymorphism and ACE inhibitor intake? *Am J Nephrol* 2004; 24: 461-8.

51. Marston WA, Criado E, Jaques PF, *et al.* Prospective randomised comparison of surgical versus endovascular management of thrombosed dialysis access grafts. *J Vasc Surg* 1997; 26: 373-81.

52. Wixon CL, Mills JL. Haemodynamic basis for the diagnosis and treatment of angioaccess-induced steal syndrome. *Adv Vasc Surg* 2000; 8: 147-59.

53. Duncan H, Ferguson L, Faris I. Incidence of the radial steal syndrome in patients with Brescia fistula for haemodialysis: its clinical significance. *J Vasc Surg* 1986; 4: 144-7.

54. Bakran A, Singh UP, Ahmed A, How TV. Wrist/brachial pressure index - a simple method for assessing steal syndrome after proximal arm AV fistulae. Angioaccess for Haemodialysis. Proceedings of the 2nd International Multidisciplinary Symposium, Tours, 1999: 223.

55. DeCaprio JD, Valentine RJ, *et al.* Steal syndrome complicating hemodialysis access. *Cardiovascular Surgery* 1997; 5: 648-53.

56. Ehsan O, Bhattacharya D, Darwish A, Al-khaffaf H. 'Extension technique': a modified technique for brachio-cephalic fistula to prevent dialysis access-associated steal syndrome. *Eur J Vasc Endovasc Surg* 2005; 29: 324-7.

57. Balaji S, Evans JM, Roberts DE, Gibbons CP. Treatment of steal syndrome complicating a proximal arteriovenous bridge graft fistula by simple distal arterial ligation without revascularisation using intraoperative pressure measurements. *Ann Vasc Surg* 2003; 17: 320-2.

58. Hye RJ, Wolf YG. Ischemic monomelic neuropathy: an under-recognised complication of hemodialysis access. *Ann Vasc Surg* 1994; 8: 578-82.

59. Coyne DW, Lowell JA, Windus *et al.* Comparison of survival of an expanded polytetrafluoroethylene graft designed for early cannulation to standard wall polytetrafluoroethylene grafts. *J Am Coll Surg* 1996; 183: 401-5.

60. Saran R, Dykstra DM, Pisoni RL, *et al.* Timing of first cannulation and vascular access failure in haemodialysis: an analysis of practice patterns at dialysis facilities in the DOPPS. *Nephrol Dial Transplant* 2004; 19: 2334-40.

61. Andrew J, Gibbons CP. Vascular access for haemodialysis. In: *Pathways of care in vascular surgery.* Beard JD, Murray S, Eds. Shrewsbury, UK: tfm Publishing Ltd., 2002: 241-54.

62. Henry ML. Routine surveillance in vascular access for haemodialysis. *Eur J Vasc Endovasc Surg* 2006; in press.

63. Tessitore N, Lipari G, Poli A, *et al.* Can blood flow surveillance and pre-emptive repair of subclinical stenosis prolong the useful life of arteriovenous fistulae? A randomized controlled study. *Nephrol Dial Transplant* 2004; 19: 2325-33.

64. Malik J, Slavikova M, Svobodova J, Tuka V. Regular ultrasonographic screening significantly prolongs patency of PTFE grafts. *Kidney Int* 2005; 67: 1554-8.

65. Dember LM, Holmberg EF, Kaufman JS. Randomized controlled trial of prophylactic repair of hemodialysis arteriovenous graft stenosis. *Kidney Int* 2004; 66: 390-8.

66. Vogel PM, Parise C. Comparison of SMART stent placement for arteriovenous graft salvage versus successful graft PTA. *J Vasc Interv Radiol* 2005; 16: 1619-26.

67. Singer-Jordan J, Papura S. Cutting balloon angioplasty for primary treatment of hemodialysis fistula venous stenoses: preliminary results. *J Vasc Interv Radiol* 2005; 16: 25-9.

68. Bourquelot P. Vascular access in children: the importance of microsurgery for creation of autologous arteriovenous fistulae. *Eur J Vasc Surg* 2006; Epub ahead of print. http://dx.doi.org/10.1016/j.ejvs.2006.04.010.

69. Donovan K. Population requirements for vascular access surgery. *Eur J Vasc Endovasc Surg* 2006; 31: 176-80.

Chapter 15

Screening for abdominal aortic aneurysm

Brian P Heather MS FRCS, Consultant Vascular Surgeon
Gloucestershire Royal Hospital, Gloucester, UK

Introduction

Ruptured abdominal aortic aneurysm (AAA) accounts for approximately 10,000 deaths annually in the UK [1] **(IV/C)** and there is evidence of an increasing incidence of the condition [2, 3] **(III/B)**. While some of the recorded deaths occur in the extremely elderly, many are seen in patients in the sixth and seventh decades of life, where such a premature death represents loss of considerable potential years of life.

Mortality rates for elective, open aneurysm repair are generally regarded as being between 5% and 8%, with a figure of 6.8% reported for all non-ruptured aneurysm surgery in the Vascular Society's own voluntary audit for the years 2001 - 2004 [4] **(III/B)**. Many centres are able to claim better figures than this for conventional open surgery [5, 6] **(III/B)** and recent randomised trials have confirmed early expectations that operative mortality for elective endovascular aneurysm repair (EVAR) would be lower still [7, 8] **(Ib/A)**.

In contrast, there is little evidence of any significant improvement in the outcome of surgery for ruptured aneurysms, where the overall community mortality remains in excess of 80%. Improvements in surgical, anaesthetic and postoperative techniques do not seem to have realised the same benefits for ruptured aneurysms as they have for elective procedures [9-12]

(III/B). The reported variations in mortality after surgery for ruptured AAA probably owe more to differences in referral patterns and case selection than to different treatment techniques.

The huge difference in outcome between elective and emergency aneurysm surgery clearly suggests that the overall mortality from the condition would be reduced by an increase in the number of elective operations performed. The wider use of diagnostic ultrasound, CT and MR imaging and, to a lesser extent, increased public and professional awareness of the condition, have probably resulted in a small increase in incidental discovery of AAA and subsequent elective repair. However, large numbers of aortic aneurysms still remain asymptomatic, unsuspected and undiagnosed until they rupture; logically, the only way in which this situation can be improved is by a deliberate policy of widespread screening of the at-risk population.

The evidence

Despite the fact that the benefits of a population screening programme have appeared self-evident to many vascular surgeons for over 20 years, the only scientific evidence available to support this view when this book was first published in 1999 came from a single, small randomised study carried out in the

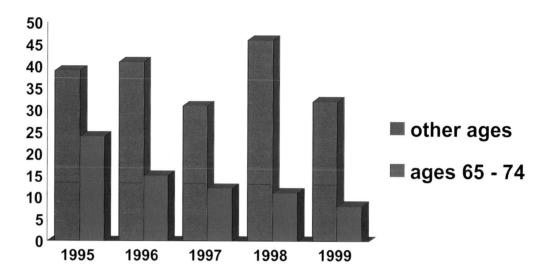

Figure 1. Total aneurysm-related deaths in Gloucestershire men 1995-1999.

Chichester area [13] **(Ib/A)** and from reports of a significant reduction in overall population deaths from aortic aneurysm in the non-randomised Gloucestershire screening programme [14] **(III/B)**, shown in Figure 1.

The situation has now changed dramatically and level I evidence is now available from two large randomised controlled trials of the efficacy of population screening for aortic aneurysms in men.

The Multicentre Aneurysm Screening Study (MASS) [15] **(Ib/A)**, which reported in 2002, randomised 67,800 men to screening or observation and, based on intention to treat, reported a 42% reduction in overall mortality from aneurysm disease in the screening group. Mortality reduction was, obviously, considerably better than this in those who actually attended for ultrasound examination after allocation to the screening group.

A smaller Danish study, published in 2005 [16] **(Ib/A)**, randomised 12,639 men and achieved a somewhat better reduction in aneurysm-related mortality of 66% based, again, on intention to treat.

It is, in fact, likely that both studies have under-estimated the full potential of a population screening

programme to reduce deaths from aneurysms for two important reasons:

- follow-up in both trials was limited to four years, whereas the full benefits of early detection of a small, asymptomatic aortic aneurysm would continue to accrue for as long as 10 to 15 years - for as long as patients with such aneurysms remained suitable candidates for elective aneurysm surgery [17] **(III/B)**;
- recruitment in both trials included men with a range of ages (65 to 74 years in MASS, 65 to 77 years in the Danish study) and it is inevitable that some deaths from ruptured AAA would already have occurred in such a cohort. Significantly greater benefit would eventually result from screening men only at the age of 65, as would almost certainly be the case in any national screening programme, albeit that such benefits would take some time to be realised fully.

Many of those with an interest in aneurysm screening will recall the BMJ sub-editor's unfortunate headline "Screening for AAA does not reduce overall death rates", when reporting in 2004 the results of a randomised trial carried out in Western Australia [18] **(Ib/A)**. This was an unusual study in a number of ways: recruitment included men up to the age of 83, many of whom could not possibly be expected to benefit from screening and there was often a significant time delay between randomisation to the screening group and the actual performance of the test, during which a number of men randomised to screening died from rupture of an undetected AAA. Despite this inherent bias against a positive result, the trial still showed a trend towards an advantage in screening, although this did not reach statistical significance. The authors of the paper have since pointed out that their study was not intended as a trial of aneurysm screening *per se* but as a study of any possible additional advantage of screening in a population in whom incidental AAA detection was already high.

Population screening

It is now widely accepted that the clinical advantages of screening men for AAA are proven; such a policy would result in a very significant reduction in premature deaths from aneurysm rupture.

The actual costs of implementing large-scale aneurysm screening are less well understood and various published estimates of the overall cost-effectiveness have varied from extremely favourable to unaffordable. The MASS study included a robust analysis of costs both for the four years of the trial itself and for a future projection extending over ten years [19] **(IIb/B)**. Calculated costs per quality adjusted life-year (QALY) gained by screening were £36,000 during the trial, estimated to fall to £8,000 per QALY gained in a programme running over ten years. This latter figure certainly falls well within what is recognised as an acceptable cost / benefit ratio for health-related expenditure within the NHS.

As a result of the additional supportive evidence gained over the last five years, the centre of debate has gradually switched from whether there should be a national screening programme for AAA in the UK to when such a programme can be introduced and how it would be organised. This change in emphasis is exemplified by the letter from Sir Muir Gray, Programme Director of the UK National Screening Committee to Directors of Public Health in June 2006: "The NSC has

advised that screening men aged 65 for AAA can be recommended in principle subject to two critical issues of reconfiguring treatment services and providing information and support to enable men to make an informed choice. A working group has been set up to consider these issues and the NHS protocols that should be in place if an aneurysm is found."

The optimistic view is that NHS screening for AAA in men could begin to be implemented in England during 2007 and would be widespread by 2010. Similarly, the equivalent committee in the US has recommended reimbursement for aneurysm screening, based on the results of the randomised trials [20] **(Ia/A)**. In this prevailing climate the current questions for debate now include:

◆ organising favourable publicity for a screening programme, looking at ways of obtaining maximum attendance and providing suitable information for invited men to make an informed decision about whether to attend for an ultrasound scan;

◆ deciding at what age screening should be offered, what aortic diameter requires follow-up surveillance and whether re-screening, after a suitable interval, of patients with an initial normal aortic diameter has any value;

◆ deciding the optimal venues and methods for offering screening and arranging suitable training for those who will carry out the ultrasound tests, together with robust quality control arrangements to ensure accurate aortic diameter measurements;

◆ organising the participation of vascular surgeons and vascular surgery units, which will almost certainly involve a re-organisation into screening units covering a population of approximately 1,000,000 and will, almost inevitably involve audit of the outcomes of such units, if not of individual surgeons.

Publicity, attendance and information

The Gloucestershire screening programme for AAA has consistently achieved attendance rates of 86% for screening 65-year-old men since its introduction in 1990 [21] **(III/B)**. This is largely attributable to invitations coming from patients' own GPs, holding screening sessions in the relatively non-threatening environment of the GP surgery and providing clear, accurate information on the purpose of screening.

An attendance rate of at least 80% would be desirable in a national programme if there is to be a significant and worthwhile reduction in emergency aneurysm surgery and mortality in the population as a whole. This will only be achieved by expert publicity and good public relations management of the programme, clarifying both the benefits and the limitations of screening.

The National Screening Committee has made it clear that it regards attendance for a screening test as an issue of informed consent. Information must, therefore, be made available in a variety of formats (leaflets, verbal advice, websites etc.) and possibly in a variety of languages. Very basic research is required at this stage into the best ways in which such information can be provided and, for example,

into how many 65-year-old men have easy internet access.

It will, for example, be quite challenging to explain the differences between overall benefits on population mortality (which AAA screening undoubtedly provides) and the variety of possible outcomes from screening for individuals, some of which are actually harmful.

What age to screen, what size to follow-up

As shown in Figure 2, the questions of what age to screen, what size of aorta to monitor and whether a second round of screening is cost-effective are all interlinked.

Most trials of AAA screening have, with good effect, used the age of 65 years as a starting point. The disadvantage is that between 5% and 10% of

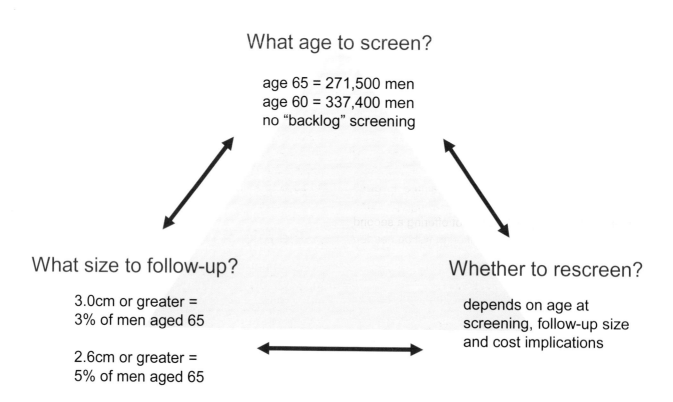

What age to screen?

age 65 = 271,500 men
age 60 = 337,400 men
no "backlog" screening

What size to follow-up?

3.0cm or greater =
3% of men aged 65

2.6cm or greater =
5% of men aged 65

Whether to rescreen?

depends on age at screening, follow-up size and cost implications

Figure 2. Interlinking factors in screening for AAA.

AAA ruptures occur before this age and are therefore missed. The resource implication of reducing the age of screening to 60 years, in an attempt to identify a larger proportion of AAAs before they rupture, is an increase in the number of men in the UK eligible for screening from approximately 271,500 to approximately 337,400 - a potential increase in screening activity of nearly 25%.

The choice of what aortic diameter to follow-up by serial ultrasound surveillance lies between accepting the arbitrary definition of an AAA as 3cm or greater in diameter (resulting in approximately 3% of 65-year-old men requiring follow-up) or adopting a slighter safer threshold of 2.6cm or greater (involving approximately 5% of screened men). The cost implications of adopting the lower size threshold are significant and may not be justified by the small, but definite number of 65-year-old men with an aortic diameter between 2.6cm and 2.9cm who subsequently develop a clinically significant AAA while they are at an age where elective repair might be considered.

The re-screening, after a number of years, of men who have a 'normal' aortic diameter when first examined has been shown to have a relatively small chance of identifying new AAAs [22] (III/B). The costs of such a second round of screening would be high.

An ideal programme, ignoring costs, would probably involve initial screening of men at 60 years of age, follow-up of all aortas with a diameter of 2.6cm or greater and a second round of screening at age 70 years. In practice, cost-benefit considerations are likely to mean that a national programme involves screening of men at age 65, following-up aortic diameters of 3cm or greater and not offering a second round of screening. Careful monitoring will be needed to see whether this policy results in a secondary rise in AAA rupture in men of 75 years and above after the first ten years of a national programme.

It is generally accepted that, for resource reasons, there will be no attempt to screen a backlog of men who are older than 65 years when national screening begins and that screening will not routinely be offered to women. Both these perfectly reasonable decisions will present a challenge to those involved in the public relations aspect of a national screening programme.

Where to screen and who to train

The Gloucestershire policy of performing the great majority of ultrasound scans in a room provided by individual GP surgeries has worked extremely well in that particular environment. It is, however, recognised that such a policy may not be applicable in either very sparsely populated regions or in deprived inner city areas. It is likely that the first phase of national screening will include a number of trials of offering screening in local hospitals, village halls or in mobile units, as used successfully for breast cancer screening.

It is estimated that approximately 250,000 new ultrasound scans of 65-year-old men would be required in a national programme, rising to a need for 375,000 annual scans after ten years with the follow-up of enlarged aortas discovered on screening. Performance of the ultrasound scans themselves will require the equivalent of an estimated 100 full-time personnel.

Fully trained ultrasonographers are in short supply and their full range of skills is not required for the relatively straightforward task of measuring aortic diameter. The MASS trial showed that it is possible to train suitable individuals without previous ultrasound experience to perform accurate aortic diameter measurement within a relatively short time. Work is currently in hand to develop suitable training courses to provide both the necessary ultrasound techniques and the basic understanding of dealing with patients, data recording and confidentiality that would be needed to fulfil the role of an aneurysm screener.

The role of vascular surgeons

It is likely that patients with an enlarged aorta would be followed-up within a national programme until their aortic diameter reached 5.5cm, at which time they would be referred to a vascular surgeon for discussion of elective aneurysm repair.

The long-term credibility and effectiveness of a national screening programme are very largely dependent on the availability of consistent, high quality advice from vascular surgeons who can provide elective surgical repair of aneurysms with the lowest possible morbidity and mortality. It is, therefore, inevitable that vascular surgeons who wish to take part in a national screening programme should be willing to submit their data for audit and be willing to work in co-operative groups large enough to allow meaningful, multidisciplinary discussion and management of individual patients. Although it is not necessary for every participating surgeon individually to offer both open and endovascular aneurysm repair, the environment in which they work should enable patients to be offered the most appropriate form of surgery when this is required.

One of the most important roles of vascular surgeons participating in a programme that may involve offering a potentially life-threatening operation to asymptomatic patients is the assessment of peri-operative risk in patients who are likely to have comorbid conditions and the selection of those patients most likely to benefit from elective aneurysm surgery. Too high a threshold for offering surgery may benefit the surgeon's personal mortality figures at the expense of denying surgery to patients who may benefit from aneurysm repair; too low a threshold may result in operations that are not beneficial, and in avoidable peri-operative deaths. There would appear to be other advantages for surgeons, since the peri-operative mortality rate is lower in patients having surgery for a screen-detected AAA compared to those discovered incidentally [23] **(III/B)**.

Although very considerable, detailed work still needs to be done on all of the above, all the necessary criteria to begin screening are entirely achievable within the next year or two. It would, therefore, be reasonable now to look forward another ten or 15 years to a time when ruptured AAA and emergency AAA repair are limited to:

- women, for whom no screening programme is proposed, since the cost / benefit ratio would be approximately ten times less favourable than a screening programme for men;
- men whose aneurysms rupture before the age of 65 (approximately 5% of all ruptured AAA in men);

- men who do not accept their invitation for a screening ultrasound test. Hopefully, good quality publicity and information would reduce this to less than 15% of those invited;
- a very small number of men whose aneurysms rupture during surveillance;
- the difficult group of men found to have an aneurysm, who have significant comorbidity that renders elective surgery either out of the question or, at least, very high risk. This group represents a significant challenge to the clinical acumen of vascular surgeons involved in a screening programme.

Conclusions

Overall, the case for widespread screening of men for AAA can be regarded as proven. If a national screening programme is established successfully along the lines suggested and emergency surgery becomes limited to the categories described above, the effects on population mortality from AAA, on the provision of emergency vascular surgery and on the quality of life of vascular surgeons would be immense. Vascular surgeons could then spend more of their off-duty time on more appropriate activities (Figure 3).

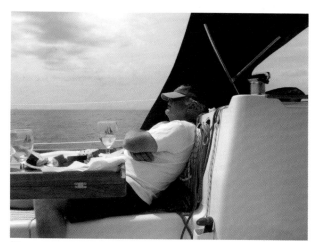

Figure 3. The author enjoying leisure time resulting from a screening programme.

Key points	Evidence level

- The clinical benefits of screening 65-year-old men for AAA are proven beyond reasonable doubt. — Ia/A

- The costs and benefits of AAA screening compare favourably to other health care expenditure. — Ia/A

- A national screening programme for AAA in men is entirely feasible and is likely to commence in England within two or three years. — IV/C

- Additional work is required to determine such issues as the best ways to maximise attendance, the information available to men offered screening, the exact way in which screening tests will be offered and carried out, and how the quality of the programme will be monitored. — IV/C

- Very significant improvements in mortality from AAA and very significant reductions in the numbers of emergency operations should be achieved within ten years of the introduction of a national screening programme. — Ia/A

References

1. Office of Population Censuses and Surveys. Mortality Statistics, England and Wales. London: HMSO, 1989.

2. Fowkes FGC, MacIntyre CCA, Ruckley CV. Increasing incidence of aortic aneurysms in England and Wales. *Br Med J* 1989; 298: 33-5.

3. Melton LJ, Bickerstaff LK, Hollier LH, *et al.* Changing incidence of abdominal aortic aneurysms. A population-based study. *Am J Epidemiol* 1984; 120: 379-86.

4. Vascular Society of Great Britain and Ireland. Fourth National Database Report 2004. Henley on Thames: Dendrite Clinical Systems, 2005.

5. Veith FJ, Goldsmith J, Leather RP, *et al.* The need for quality assurance in vascular surgery. *J Vasc Surg* 1991; 13: 523-6.

6. Akkersdijk GJ, van de Graaf Y, Van Bockel JH, *et al.* Mortality rates associated with operative treatment of infrarenal abdominal aortic aneurysms in the Netherlands. *Br J Surg* 1994; 81: 706-9.

7. EVAR trial participants. Endovascular aneurysm repair versus open repair in patients with abdominal aortic aneurysm (EVAR trial 1): randomised controlled trial. *Lancet* 2005; 365: 2179-86.

8. Prinssen M, Verhoeven ELG, Buth J, *et al.* A randomized trial comparing conventional and endovascular repair of abdominal aortic aneurysms. *N Engl J Med* 2004; 351: 1607-18.

9. Bengtsson H, Bergqvist D. Ruptured abdominal aortic aneurysm: a population-based study. *J Vasc Surg* 1993; 18: 74-80.

10. Mealy K, Salman A. The true incidence of ruptured abdominal aortic aneurysms. *Eur J Vasc Surg* 1988; 2: 405-8.

11. Johansson G, Swedenborg J. Ruptured abdominal aortic aneurysms: a study of incidence and mortality. *Br J Surg* 1986; 73: 101-3.

12. Katz DJ, Stanley JC, Zeienock GB. Operative mortality rates for intact and ruptured abdominal aortic aneurysms in Michigan: an 11-year statewide experience. *J Vasc Surg* 1994; 19: 804-15.

13. Scott RA, Wilson NM, Ashton HA, *et al.* Influence of screening on the incidence of ruptured abdominal aortic aneurysm: 5-year results of a randomized controlled study. *Br J Surg* 1995; 82: 1066-70.

14. Heather BP, Poskitt K, Earnshaw J, *et al.* Population screening reduces the mortality from aortic aneurysms in men. *Br J Surg* 2000; 87: 750-3.

15. Ashton HA, Buxton MJ, Day NE, *et al.* The Multicentre Aneurysm Screening Study (MASS) into the effect of abdominal aortic aneurysm screening on mortality in men: a randomised controlled trial. *Lancet* 2002; 360: 1531-9.

16. Lindholt J, Juul S, Fasting H, *et al.* Screening for abdominal aortic aneurysms: single-centre randomised controlled trial. *Br Med J* 2005; 330: 750-4.

17. Wilmink T, Claridge MWC, Fries A, *et al.* A comparison between the short-term and long-term benefits of screening for abdominal aortic aneurysms from the Huntingdon Aneurysm Screening Programme. *Eur J Vasc Endovasc Surg* 2006; 32: 16-20.

18. Norman PE, Jamrozik K, Lawrence Brown MM, *et al.* Population-based randomised controlled trial on impact of screening on mortality from abdominal aortic aneurysm. *Br Med J* 2004; 329: 1259-62.

19. Multicentre Aneurysm Screening Study Group. Multicentre aneurysm screening study (MASS): cost-effectiveness analysis of screening for abdominal aortic aneurysms based

on four-year results from randomised controlled trial. *Br Med J* 2002; 325: 1135-41.

20. US Preventive Services Task Force. Screening for abdominal aortic aneurysm: recommendation statement. *Ann Int Med* 2005; 142: 198-202.

21. Gujral S, Shaw E, Earnshaw J, *et al*. Improving attendance rates for abdominal aortic aneurysm screening. *Ann R Coll Surg Engl* 1997; 79: 71-4.

22. Lederle F, Johnson G, Wilson S, *et al*. Yield of repeated screening for abdominal aortic aneurysm after a 4-year interval. *Arch Intern Med* 2000; 60: 1117-21.

23. Irvine CD, Shaw E, Poskitt KR, *et al*. A comparison of the mortality rate after elective repair of aortic aneurysms detected either by screening or incidentally. *Eur J Vasc Endovasc Surg* 2000; 20: 374-8.

Chapter 16

Indications for elective surgery for abdominal aortic aneurysm

Felicity J Meyer MA BM BCh FRCS, Consultant Vascular Surgeon
Department of General and Vascular Surgery, Norfolk and Norwich University Hospital, Norwich, UK

Introduction

The first successful abdominal aortic aneurysm (AAA) repairs were performed in the 1950s [1, 2]. The standard technique of endo-aneurysmorrhaphy was subsequently described in 1966 [3]. Since then, AAA repair has become one of the mainstays of vascular surgery, although until recently there was little level I evidence of its efficacy. Elective AAA repair is primarily a prophylactic operation with a definite risk of death or serious complication, so patient and procedure selection must be stringent.

Asymptomatic abdominal aortic aneurysm

The aim of elective repair of asymptomatic AAA is to prolong life by preventing premature death from rupture. Therefore, the risk of death or major morbidity from operation must be balanced against the probability of death from rupture. This may appear to be a relatively simple equation, but there are several variables to consider.

Operative risk

The reported operative risk for elective open AAA repair is variable, but may reach 10.6% [4] **(Ia/A)**. Publication of results from specialist single centres and selection bias, however, may give a false impression of much lower mortality rates. Consequently, the mortality rate in the surgical community as a whole is likely to be greater than it appears in the literature [5]. Case mix is a crucial determinant of outcome and better results may be obtained by denying operation to high-risk patients; published series seldom itemise those who are not offered surgery. The results of surgery in patients entered into multicentre trials are often worse than single-centre series, yet even these do not represent the generality, since trial protocols, and surgeon/patient selection processes reduce the likelihood of unfavourable outcomes. A modern vascular surgeon should be aware of their personal results, although these may only be meaningful when a large enough series of procedures has accrued, which may take many years in smaller units. In the UK, members of the Vascular Society of Great Britain and Ireland may contribute to a risk-adjusted database (National Vascular Database), where their outcomes are compared with colleagues. In the latest report, peri-operative mortality was 6.3% after elective AAA surgery [6].

Individual risk

There is some evidence that may assist the estimation of individual risk of death after elective operation for AAA **(IIb/B)** [7]. The established risk factors are increasing age, ischaemic heart disease, chronic obstructive pulmonary disease and renal impairment [7-9]. The presence of these factors is known to increase mortality rates, but the precise risk for an individual patient remains difficult to calculate. Scoring systems, such as the Physiological and Operative Severity Score for the enUmeration of Mortality and morbidity (POSSUM), or the Glasgow Aneurysm Score are helpful for groups of patients, but not individuals [10, 11]. Complex procedures such as AAA repair need their own POSSUM risk equation. Other studies have investigated the possibility of optimising unhealthy patients before surgery, particularly to reduce the risk of cardiac complications. So far, this has not been shown to be cost-effective [12, 13] **(III/B)**. It is prudent, however, to ensure that all patients have been appropriately medically managed prior to undergoing AAA repair. This may include treatment with beta blockers and statins [13-15].

Size

It is generally accepted that the major determinant for rupture is the maximum diameter of the aneurysm, but precise rupture rates for different sizes of aneurysms are not clearly defined. Large aneurysms (>6cm diameter) carry a high risk of rupture, of the order of 25% at one year [16] **(III/B)**. Small aneurysms (<5cm diameter) may rupture, but do so uncommonly and several uncontrolled series have shown that, given an elective operative mortality of 5-10%, expectant management is the safer option [16-18] **(III/B)**.

Until recently, many surgeons were uncertain about exact indications for surgery in patients with an AAA between 4-6cm. The argument for early surgery of smaller AAA is that operation is likely to be required eventually, so it is safer to intervene when the patient is younger and fitter. The counter argument is that it is unwise to risk death when operation could possibly be deferred for several years. Many patients with aneurysm die from other causes before the AAA reaches 6cm. Age and life expectancy must be considered in relation to aneurysm size and general fitness, and the options should be discussed fully with the patient and their relatives.

This controversy over management of small aneurysms, particularly in the size range 4.0-5.5cm, where surgeons had the most equipoise, led to three randomised trials of early surgery versus observation. The Canadian Small Aneurysm Treatment Trial commenced in 1991 but was abandoned due to poor recruitment. The enrolled patients are still being followed and some data may eventually become available. The UK Small Aneurysm Trial [19, 20] and the Aneurysm Detection and Management (ADAM) study [21], carried out in Veterans Administration hospitals in the US, produced definitive results.

The UK Small Aneurysm Trial

This study included 1090 patients, aged 60-76 years and fit for surgery, who had an asymptomatic AAA 4.0-5.5cm in diameter. They were randomised to early surgery or ultrasound surveillance until the aneurysm either reached 5.5cm, or became symptomatic, when operation was undertaken [19]. The first analysis was after a mean follow-up of 4.6 years when there was no difference in the mortality rate between the two groups on an intention-to-treat analysis **(Ib/A)** [19]. Cost analysis indicated that surveillance was the cheaper option [22]. At second analysis after eight years, the survival curves had crossed, and those who had early surgery had a lower mortality rate, although this did not reach statistical significance [20] (Figure 1). This difference was attributed to lifestyle changes adopted by the early surgery group. This study was well designed and conducted and the large numbers made it statistically robust. The conclusion that aneurysms of <5.5cm maximum diameter may safely be managed by ultrasound surveillance therefore appears clear-cut, and has been adopted by most vascular surgeons **(Ib/A)**. There are some details of the study that require further discussion.

The 30-day postoperative mortality rate for patients in the early surgery groups was 5.8% - higher than in many published single-centre series and almost three

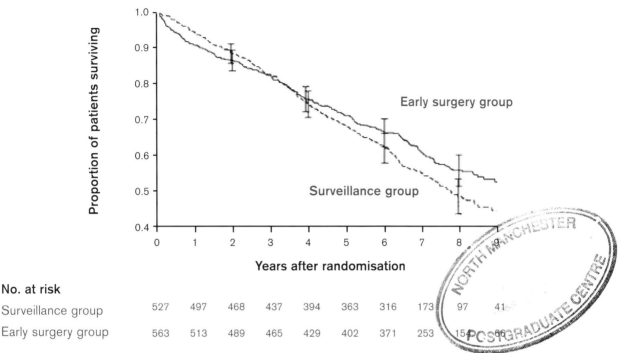

Figure 1. Comparison of survival after early surgery versus surveillance for aortic aneurysms 4-5.5cm in diameter after eight-year follow-up. Data from the UK Small Aneurysm Trial. *Reproduced with permission from the Massachusetts Medical Society. © 2002 Massachusetts Medical Society. All rights reserved* [20].

times the expected rate used in the power calculations for the study design. This mortality rate, however, was similar to that of other unselected multicentre studies [5]. Surgeons with mortality rates significantly lower than this may argue that early surgery in their hands could yet confer a long-term benefit.

The trial was not stratified for age and aneurysm size, but subgroup analysis indicated that younger patients (aged 60-66 years) and patients with larger aneurysms (4.9-5.5cm) may benefit from early surgery, although this did not reach statistical significance [23].

As with any randomised trial, the results cannot be extrapolated to patients who fall outside the inclusion criteria and the trial protocol (especially surveillance rates) must be followed to achieve similar results. For example, the findings cannot be applied to patients aged under 60 years, in whom there remains uncertainty about whether early repair might be advisable.

The ADAM Trial

In the ADAM trial, 1136 US veterans, aged between 50 and 79 years and fit for surgery, with AAA between 4.0 and 5.4cm diameter were randomised to receive either early elective surgery or six-monthly surveillance with ultrasound or CT [21]. The patients were stratified for age, sex and aneurysm size. The mean follow-up was 4.9 years and the primary outcome was death. The overall operative mortality was only 2.7%, and yet there was still no survival advantage demonstrated for early surgery. One reason for this is that the rupture rate in the surveillance group was only 0.6% per year. In addition, over 60% of the surveillance group had undergone operative repair by the end of the study. Another concern is that although 5038 patients with an AAA were considered for randomisation, fewer than a quarter of these were entered into the study. Nevertheless, ADAM provided further evidence that surveillance of AAA less than 5.5cm is safe in men, even when operative mortality is low **(Ib/A)**.

Although a clinician can present the evidence and offer advice, the final decision about surgery lies with the patient. The anxiety produced may be such that some patients prefer early surgery, even when it involves risk. There is evidence to support this from the UK Small Aneurysm Study where quality of life analysis showed that those undergoing early surgery had an improvement in health perception compared with those undergoing surveillance [22].

Sex

The UK Small Aneurysm Trial only included 188 women, but subgroup analysis showed no survival advantage after early operation in this group [18]. Analysis of all 2257 patients who were enrolled, but then excluded from the trial (464 women, 39 of whom ruptured their AAA), revealed that women were three times more likely to rupture their AAA than men, and that the mean diameter at rupture was 5cm, compared with 6cm in men [23] **(IIb/B)**. An observational study of 103 AAA also found rupture was three times more likely in women [24] **(III/B)**. Unfortunately, fewer than ten women were entered into the ADAM trial. There is sufficient evidence to support a more relaxed indication for AAA surgery in women and many surgeons offer elective repair once the aortic diameter reaches 5cm.

Expansion rate

The mean rate of expansion of an AAA is in the order of 3mm per year, rising with increased aneurysm diameter [25]. However, expansion rates are variable, both between patients and in the same patient over different time intervals. The risk of rupture is thought to be related to the rate of expansion [25] **(III/B)**. Aneurysms that expand rapidly (>5mm over six months) may be regarded as high risk and could be considered for early surgery.

Compliance and wall stress

The compliance of the distal aorta in normal subjects relates to its elastin content. Aneurysmal dilatation of the aorta is associated with loss of elastin fibres and an increase in collagen content. The aortic wall, therefore, becomes less compliant (stiffer) as the aneurysm increases in size. There is evidence that aneurysms which do not conform to this pattern and are more compliant than expected, or which do not become less compliant as they grow, are more likely to rupture [26] **(III/B)**. Now that compliance can be measured non-invasively with ultrasound equipment, there are likely to be further studies in this area. Wall stress can also be calculated, using three-dimensional CT and may be a useful predictor of rupture in small aneurysms [24].

Open versus endovascular repair

The two large randomised trials have defined intervention policy for AAA, yet both were done using open aneurysm repair. If the peri-operative mortality rates are lower with endovascular aneurysm repair (EVAR) the indications for elective repair may be different (see Chapters 17 and 18). This has led to the inception of the Comparison of Surveillance versus Aortic Endografting for Small Aneurysm Repair (CAESAR) trial. This European study aims to randomise patients with AAA of 4.0-5.4cm in size to receive either EVAR or surveillance. Its findings are awaited, but again, the problem of smaller aneurysms in women may not be addressed by this trial, since fewer women have an AAA anatomically suitable for EVAR.

Symptomatic aneurysm

AAA may cause symptoms either of pain or from distal embolisation. Pain is usually felt in the abdominal or lower lumbar region and is constant in nature. It may be referred to groin, genitalia or thigh. Painful or tender aneurysms should be repaired in patients fit for surgery, not only for pain relief but also because of the possibility of contained leak or the threat of impending rupture.

The first difficulty in a patient with pain and an aneurysm is to determine whether the aneurysm is the cause of the pain, rather than some other intra-abdominal pathology or musculoskeletal disorder. Second, many symptomatic aneurysms may have already had a small leak. The results of operation within four hours of admission are worse than for elective repair, even in non-ruptured AAA; surgery is safer when delayed for up to seven days [27] **(III/B)**. This does not necessarily imply, however, that surgery for the symptomatic aneurysm should always be delayed. Differences in outcome may simply reflect the less favourable circumstances under which urgent surgery may be undertaken and the more serious pathology in these patients. The decision whether it is safe to defer operation can be difficult and CT has not proved to be an entirely reliable arbiter [28]; if in doubt, clinical judgment should override CT findings.

Distal embolism from an AAA usually presents with multiple small necrotic patches on the legs and feet, commonly described as 'trash foot'. Occasionally, the aneurysm itself may thrombose, causing profound lower torso ischaemia. Aneurysm repair is indicated, regardless of AAA diameter, to prevent tissue loss. A lumbar sympathectomy can be performed at the same time. Very rarely, intact aneurysms can cause disseminated intravascular coagulation which can present as a bleeding disorder. Such patients should be stabilised on low-dose heparin before operation.

AAA and synchronous pathology

Iliac aneurysms

Aortic aneurysms are often associated with more distal iliac aneurysms (Figure 2), although isolated iliac aneurysms are rare. Iliac aneurysms should be repaired if they are causing compressive problems, such as ureteral obstruction or iliac vein thrombosis, but the size threshold for intervention in asymptomatic iliac aneurysms remains uncertain. There is not a clear relationship between size and rupture in iliac aneurysms [29], but mortality from iliac rupture is high [30]. Iliac aneurysms are usually repaired, therefore, if an associated AAA has reached the size threshold for repair or if the iliac aneurysm itself is over 3-4cm in diameter.

Coincidental occlusive and aneurysm disease

In patients undergoing aorto-iliac or renovascular reconstruction for occlusive disease it is usually

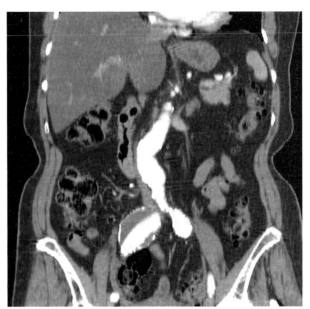

Figure 2. CT showing 4.5cm right common iliac aneurysm associated with a small AAA.

prudent to undertake repair of a coincidental aortic aneurysm, even when it is below the size that would normally be considered for repair.

Coincidental non-vascular intra-abdominal pathology

There remains debate about performing aneurysm repair concurrently with other intra-abdominal surgical procedures. The advantages of a joint procedure are that under a single anaesthetic the risk of aneurysm rupture is minimised and the risk or potential complications of the other pathology are reduced. The drawback may be an increased risk of the specific complications of AAA surgery such as graft infection and aorto-enteric fistula, together with the general complications associated with greater dissection and blood loss. There are several case series with adequate results to support the practice of concurrent renal and ureteric surgery [31] **(III/B)**, since this is limited to retroperitoneal dissection, provides easy access to the renal arteries and is usually sterile. AAA repair should not usually be undertaken if there is peritoneal contamination. There is little good evidence to provide optimal management protocols for other procedures, such as cholecystectomy or colectomy for cancer, but it may be appropriate to perform concurrent procedures if both conditions are life-threatening, or there would be a significant risk from a second anaesthetic. Staged procedures, EVAR or even delayed retroperitoneal AAA repair are alternative options.

Conclusions

Most vascular surgeons have now adopted the conclusions of the two randomised small aneurysm trials and follow most patients with an asymptomatic aneurysm of less than 5.5cm in maximum diameter by regular ultrasound surveillance **(Ia/A)**. Once the diameter reaches 5.5cm, elective repair is usually offered if the patient is fit. Variations from this protocol are considered if the aneurysm growth exceeds 5mm in any six-month interval, in young patients and in women. Symptomatic aneurysms should be considered for urgent repair, particularly if assessment suggests there is the possibility of a localised leak. In stable symptomatic aneurysms, better results may be achieved if repair is delayed until the next available routine operating list.

Key points	Evidence level
◆ Patients with an AAA >5.5cm and fit for surgery should be offered elective repair.	IIa/B
◆ Patients with AAA <5.5cm aged over 60 years should be offered ultrasound surveillance.	Ib/A
◆ There is a lack of evidence on when to offer surgery to men under 60 years of age with a small aneurysm, and to women of any age.	IV/C

References

1. Dubost C, Allory M, Oeconomos N. Resection of an aneurysm of the abdominal aorta: re-establishment of the continuity by a preserved arterial graft, with result after five months. *Arch Surg* 1952; 64: 405.
2. Schaffer PW, Hardin CW. The use of temporary and polythene shunts to permit occlusion, resection and frozen homologous artery graft replacement of vital vessel segments. *Surgery* 1952; 31: 186.
3. Creech O. Endo-aneurysmorrhaphy and treatment of aortic aneurysm. *Ann Surg* 1966; 154: 935-46.
4. Blankenstein JD. Mortality and morbidity rates after conventional abdominal aortic aneurysm repair. *Semin Interv Cardiol* 2000; 5: 7-13.
5. Michaels JA. Use of mortality rate after aortic surgery as a performance indicator. *Br J Surg* 2003; 90: 827-31.
6. Vascular Society of Great Britain and Ireland. National Vascular Database report 2004. Oxford: Dendrite Clinical Systems Ltd, 2004. ISBN 1-903968-12-7.
7. Johnston KW, Scobie TK. Multicenter prospective study of nonruptured abdominal aortic aneurysms. *J Vasc Surg* 1988; 7: 69-81.
8. Katz DJ, Stanley JC, Zelenock GB. Operative mortality rates for intact and ruptured aortic aneurysms in Michigan: an eleven-year statewide experience. *J Vasc Surg* 1994; 19: 804-15.
9. Steyerberg EW, Kievit J, de Mol Van Otterloo JC, *et al.* Perioperative mortality of elective aortic aneurysm surgery. A clinical prediction rule based on literature and individual patient data. *Arch Int Med* 1995; 155: 1998-2004.
10. Neary WD, Heather BP, Earnshaw JJ. The Physiological and Operative Severity Score for the enUmeration of Mortality and morbidity (POSSUM). *Br J Surg* 2003; 90: 157-65.
11. Biancari F, Leo E, Ylonen K *et al.* Value of the Glasgow Aneurysm Score in predicting the immediate and long-term outcome after elective open repair of infrarenal abdominal aortic aneurysm. *Br J Surg* 2003; 90: 838-44.
12. Bry JD, Belkin M, O'Donnell TF, *et al.* An assessment of the positive predictive value and cost-effectiveness of

dipyridamole myocardial scinitgraphy in patients undergoing vascular surgery. *J Vasc Surg* 1994; 19: 112-21.

13. McFalls EO, Ward HB, Moritz TE, *et al.* Coronary artery revascularisation before elective major vascular surgery. *N Engl J Med* 2004; 351: 2795-804.

14. POBBLE Trial Investigators. Perioperative beta blockade (POBBLE) for patients undergoing infrarenal vascular surgery: results of a randomized double blind controlled trial. *J Vasc Surg* 2005; 41: 602-9.

15. O'Neil-Callaghan K, Katsimalagis G, Tepper MR, *et al.* Statins decrease perioperative cardiac complications in patients undergoing non-cardiac vascular surgery: the Statins for Risk Reduction in Surgery (StaRRS) study. *J Am Coll Cardiol* 2005; 45: 336-342.

16. Johansson G, Nydahl S, Olofsson P, *et al.* Survival in patients with abdominal aortic aneurysms. Comparison between operative and non-operative management. *Eur J Vasc Surg* 1990; 4: 497-502.

17. Scott RA, Wilson NM, Ashton HA, *et al.* Is surgery necessary for abdominal aortic aneurysm less than 6cm in diameter? *Lancet* 1993; 342: 1395-6.

18. Brown PM, Pattenden R, Vernooy C, *et al.* Selective management of abdominal aortic aneurysms in a prospective measurement program. *J Vasc Surg* 1996; 23: 213-22.

19. The UK Small Aneurysm Study Participants. Mortality results for the randomised controlled trial of early elective surgery or ultrasonographic surveillance for small abdominal aortic aneurysms. *Lancet* 1999; 352: 1649-55.

20. The United Kingdom Small Aneurysm Trial Participants. Long-term outcomes of immediate repair compared with surveillance of small abdominal aortic aneurysms. *N Engl J Med* 2002; 346: 1445-52.

21. Lederle FA, Wilson SE, Johnson GR, *et al.* Immediate repair compared with surveillance of small abdominal aortic aneurysms. *N Engl J Med* 2002; 346: 1437-44.

22. The UK Small Aneurysm Study Participants. Health service costs and quality of life for early elective surgery or ultrasonic surveillance for small abdominal aortic aneurysms. *Lancet* 1998; 352: 1656-60.

23. Brown LC, Powell JT, on behalf of The UK Small Aneurysm Study Participants. Risk factors for aneurysm rupture in patients kept under ultrasound surveillance. *Ann Surg* 1999; 230: 289-97.

24. Fillinger MF, Marra SP, Raghaven ML, *et al.* Prediction of rupture risk in abdominal aortic aneurysm during observation: wall stress versus diameter. *J Vasc Surg* 2003; 37: 724-32.

25. Bengtsson H, Bergqvist D, Ekberg O, *et al.* Expansion pattern and risk of rupture of abdominal aortic aneurysms that were not operated on. *Eur J Surg* 1993; 159: 461-7.

26. Wilson K, Bradbury AW, Whyman MR, *et al.* Relationship between abdominal aortic aneurysm wall compliance and clinical outcome: a preliminary analysis. *Eur J Vasc Endovasc Surg* 1998; 15: 472-7.

27. Cambria RA, Gloviczki P, Stanson AW, *et al.* Symptomatic, non-ruptured abdominal aortic aneurysms: are emergent operations necessary? *Ann Vasc Surg* 1994; 8: 121-6.

28. Adam DJ, Bradbury AW, Stuart WP, *et al.* The value of computed tomography in the assessment of suspected ruptured abdominal aortic aneurysm. *J Vasc Surg* 1998; 27: 431-7.

29. Brin BJ, Busuttil RW. Isolated hypogastric artery aneurysms. *Arch Surg* 1982; 176: 1329-33.

30. Richardson JW, Greenfield LJ. Natural history and management of iliac aneurysms. *J Vasc Surg* 1988; 8: 165-71.

31. Hafez KS, El Fettouh HA, Novick AC, *et al.* Management of synchronous renal neoplasm and abdominal aortic aneurysm. *J Vasc Surg* 2000; 32: 1102-10.

Chapter 17

The evidence for endovascular aneurysm repair

Geoffrey Gilling-Smith MS FRCS, Consultant Vascular Surgeon
Royal Liverpool University Hospital, Liverpool, UK

Introduction

Since 1991, when Juan Parodi [1] and colleagues reported the successful isolation of an abdominal aortic aneurysm (AAA) by transfemoral endovascular placement of a simple home-made endograft, there has been huge interest in endovascular aneurysm repair (EVAR). Previously many patients with significant comorbidities were refused open repair (OR) because of the perceived risks of intervention. Parodi's less invasive endovascular approach offered the possibility of treating such patients (Figure 1).

Early enthusiasm for endovascular repair was soon tempered by reports of late failure. In a significant number of cases, migration of the endograft resulted in endoleak, late rupture and death. It also became apparent that the endografts themselves were structurally flawed. Distortion of the endograft, fracture of the supporting stents and tears in the graft fabric were all reported with increasing frequency, leading to the suggestion that endovascular repair was a 'failed experiment'.

Analysis of the causes of late failure led to refinement of the indications for endovascular repair, improved planning and technique, increased focus on

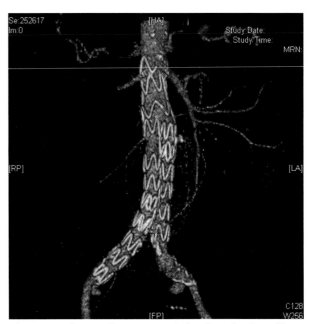

Figure 1. Infrarenal aneurysm following stent grafting.

surveillance and secondary intervention, as well as redesign of the endograft concept. Enthusiasts retained their optimism, but it is only recently that reliable evidence for the safety, efficacy and durability of contemporary EVAR has become available.

The evidence

For many years the only sources of data about endovascular repair were single-centre series and small cohort studies. More recently, data have become available from a number of large registries such as the British RETA Registry [2, 3] **(III/B)**, the European EUROSTAR Registry [4] **(III/B)** and the US-based LIFELINE Registry [5] **(III/B)**. This has in the last year or so been supplemented by data from three prospective randomised trials comparing EVAR with open repair in patients considered suitable for both treatments (the UK EVAR 1 [6, 7] **(Ib/A)** and the Dutch DREAM [8, 9] **(Ib/A)** trials) and comparing endovascular repair with best medical therapy in patients considered unfit for open repair (the UK EVAR 2 [10] **(Ib/A)** trial). The US-based OVER trial and the French ACE trial have yet to report.

Endovascular repair in patients fit for open surgical repair

In the UK EVAR 1 trial 1082 patients aged 60 years or more who were deemed fit for open surgical repair and who had an infrarenal aneurysm of at least 55mm diameter which was suitable for endovascular repair, were randomised to receive either open (n=539) or endovascular repair (n=543). The Dutch DREAM trial included 345 patients with aneurysms of at least 50mm diameter but was otherwise similar to EVAR 1.

Safety

Both trials reported similar early results. In EVAR 1, 30-day operative mortality was 1.7% after EVAR and 4.7% after OR (p<0.01). In DREAM, 30-day operative mortality was 1.2% after EVAR and 4.6% after OR. The trials therefore confirmed a clear advantage for EVAR consistent with previously reported comparisons between data from the RETA and EUROSTAR registries (1-2% operative mortality after EVAR) and data from trials comparing OR with surveillance in patients with small aneurysms (3-6% operative mortality after OR).

Efficacy

Endovascular and open repair are performed to prevent death from aneurysm rupture. The most reliable indicator of efficacy is therefore the incidence of aneurysm-related death (any death due to repair of the aneurysm or occurring as a consequence of late complications of aneurysm repair, or late rupture of the aneurysm). In DREAM, the cumulative rate of aneurysm-related death after two years was 2.1% after EVAR and 5.7% after OR. In EVAR 1, the cumulative incidence of aneurysm-related death at four years (by Kaplan-Meier estimate) was 4% after EVAR and 7% after OR (Figure 2). Neither trial demonstrated any difference in late all-cause mortality.

The most conservative conclusion that may be reached is that EVAR is at least as effective as OR at preventing late aneurysm-related death. Failure to demonstrate any difference in survival (freedom from late death of any cause) is neither an endorsement nor an indictment of either technique.

Durability

Endovascular repair relies on the intravascular deployment of a covered stent graft to isolate the aneurysm from the circulation and thus prevent rupture. The aneurysm is not in fact 'repaired'. It remains *in situ* and susceptible to rupture should it again be exposed to aortic pressure and/or flow. For the repair to be durable, the endograft must remain in place and continue effectively to isolate the aneurysm for the remainder of the patient's life.

It became apparent during the early years of endovascular grafting for AAA that the endograft did not always remain where it had been deployed and/or that it did not always continue to isolate the aneurysm from the circulation. In some cases, failure of attachment of the endograft to normal arterial wall above the aneurysm resulted in caudal migration and restoration of flow into the aneurysm sac. Migration could also result in distortion, fracture and disintegration of the stent graft or kinking and thrombosis of a graft limb.

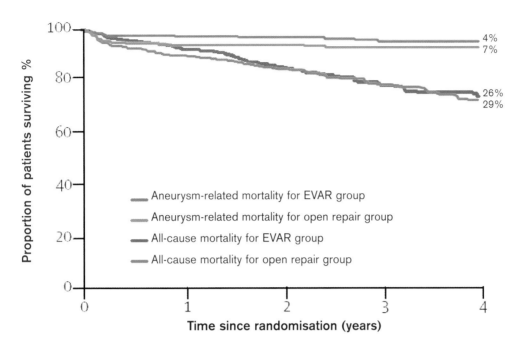

Figure 2. Kaplan-Meier curve of survival and survival free from aneurysm-related death in patients randomised to open or endovascular repair of aortic aneurysm (EVAR 1 trial). *Reproduced with permission from Elsevier* [7].

Another complication unique to endovascular repair and observed in significant numbers of patients was persistent or recurrent flow of blood within the aneurysm sac but outside the endograft (endoleak). A number of different types have been defined:

◆ Type I - failure of the seal between the stent graft and the arterial wall, either proximal or distal to the aneurysm;
◆ Type II - persistent reperfusion of the aneurysm sac via patent inferior mesenteric or lumbar arteries;
◆ Type III - disconnection of the component parts of a modular stent graft;
◆ Type IV - leak through the graft itself.

With increasing experience, the clinical significance of such complications and the indications for secondary intervention have become clearer. It is now recognised that migration and graft-related endoleak are associated with a significant risk of late aneurysm rupture and death. In most cases they should be treated by secondary intervention. It is also recognised that Type II endoleak is usually benign and can, in most cases, be left alone.

Both the RETA and EUROSTAR registries reported an overall incidence of late complications of between 10% and 15% per annum. The DREAM trial included both systemic and graft-related complications in its analysis. Overall, the freedom from severe complications at two years was 80.6% after OR and 83.1% for EVAR. Freedom from moderate or severe complications was 65.9% for OR and 65.6% for EVAR. It is probable that these figures masked a higher rate of systemic complications after OR and a higher rate of graft-related complications after EVAR, but the specific data are not available.

The EVAR 1 trial reported late complications in more detail. Overall, non-systemic graft-related complications were reported in 35% of patients after EVAR, but in only 8% of patients after OR. Secondary interventions were performed in 15% of patients after EVAR and in only 7% of patients after OR. It should be noted, however, that almost half of the complications reported after EVAR were of doubtful clinical significance (Type II endoleak), while almost a third of the secondary interventions were performed for indications that many would now question.

Cost and quality of life

The EVAR 1 trial included an analysis of both cost and quality of life. It found that EVAR was significantly more expensive than OR over a four-year interval. Unsurprisingly, the costs of hospital accommodation including ITU/HDU were higher after OR but this deficit was negated by the costs of the endografts, follow-up imaging and secondary intervention after EVAR. It also found no difference in quality of life after EVAR or OR. Quality of life was better after EVAR than OR between one and three months after operation but this difference was not maintained thereafter.

Critique of trial data

There has been much debate since the trial results were published with proponents and sceptics employing the same evidence to support arguments for and against endovascular repair in patients who are suitable for either procedure. Proponents of EVAR point out that operative and late aneurysm-related mortality are both significantly reduced and that, in the short term, quality of life is better. Sceptics argue that endovascular repair offers only marginal survival benefit, is more expensive and is associated with a higher rate of re-intervention. While true, these statements overlook a number of important points.

The survival benefit may be marginal to a statistician but it is not marginal to a patient whose chance of periprocedural death is three times greater after open than after endovascular repair. The cost of endovascular repair reflects not only the cost of endografts (which is likely to fall) but also the cost of follow-up imaging and secondary intervention. With increasing experience many centres are refining protocols to reduce the frequency of follow-up examination, and moving away from reliance on routine CT examination and employing cheaper imaging modalities to monitor the integrity of the stent graft repair. The incidence of late complications and

the need for secondary intervention is also reducing [11] and is likely to continue to reduce as stent graft design continues to improve. In addition, many complications of endografting are now known to be relatively benign, so that secondary intervention is indicated in fewer patients than during the early years of the trials.

The late results from the randomised trials are awaited, but it is clear that, in patients who are suitable for both treatments, EVAR is safer than open repair in the short term and at least as effective at preventing death from aneurysm rupture. In the author's opinion, patients who are suitable for both treatments should at least be offered the choice.

Endovascular repair in patients unfit for open surgery

Endovascular repair was initially developed to permit treatment of patients who were medically or surgically unfit for open surgery. It was thought that avoidance of laparotomy and aortic cross-clamp, reduced blood loss, avoidance of lower limb ischaemia and reperfusion injury, as well as the possibility of repair under local anaesthesia, would all result in lower physiological stress and therefore lower operative morbidity and mortality.

There is no doubt that endovascular repair is associated with lower physiological stress than open repair [12]. In patients who are medically unfit, however, this reduction in stress and associated reduction in the risk of both fatal and non-fatal systemic complications of intervention may not be sufficient to offset the risk of death from rupture of an untreated aneurysm. Perhaps more importantly, the risk of intervention is upfront, whereas the risk of death from rupture is spread over time. Thus, intervention can only be justified if patients are likely to live long enough to derive any benefit.

Evidence from registries

Buth et al [13] retrospectively compared outcomes after EVAR in 450 patients considered unfit for open surgery and/or general anaesthesia with those in

2525 patients who were considered fit. Patients who were unfit tended to be older, have less favourable aorto-iliac anatomy and underwent more complex procedures. Operative mortality in this group was 5.1% compared with 2% in patients who were fit. In addition, two-year survival in the unfit group was also lower. Based on these data, a mathematical model was constructed to calculate whether or not EVAR would be likely to offer a survival advantage in patients who were unfit for open surgery. This model assumed an annual rupture rate of 11% in untreated aneurysms. It confirmed that endovascular repair offered no survival advantage during the first year after operation (the risk of death from intervention outweighed the risk of death from rupture). Thereafter, however, EVAR conferred a significant survival advantage that increased with time.

Evidence from the EVAR 2 trial

The UK EVAR 2 trial compared endovascular repair with best medical therapy in patients who were anatomically suitable for endovascular repair but considered unfit for open surgical repair. A total of 338 patients aged 60 years or older with an aneurysm of at least 55mm diameter were randomised to receive endovascular repair (166) or no intervention (172).

Operative mortality in those who underwent EVAR repair was 9%. After mean follow-up of 3.3 years, estimated survival at four years was 64% (Kaplan-Meier). On an intention-to-treat analysis there was no difference in aneurysm-related or all-cause mortality between the two groups (Figure 3). In addition, the cost of EVAR, surveillance and secondary intervention was significantly higher in the endovascular group while there was no discernible improvement in quality of life.

Critique of trial data

The results of EVAR 2 have been widely interpreted as evidence that endovascular repair offers no benefit

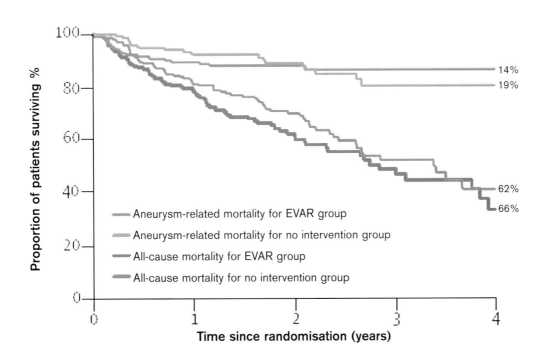

Figure 3. Kaplan-Meier curve of survival and survival free from aneurysm-related death in patients randomised to no intervention or endovascular repair of aortic aneurysm (EVAR 2 trial). *Reproduced with permission from Elsevier* [10].

to patients who are considered unfit for open surgical repair. In reality the conclusions are somewhat less definite.

On an intention-to-treat analysis there was no difference in the incidence of aneurysm-related death between those assigned to EVAR (20/166) and those assigned to best medical therapy (22/172). However, nine of the 20 aneurysm-related deaths in those assigned to EVAR were due to rupture before planned elective intervention. The median delay between randomisation and treatment in the endovascular group was 57 days (IQR 39 - 82) and the median delay between randomisation and rupture in those who ruptured before treatment was 98 days. It is highly likely that the number of aneurysm-related deaths in the endovascular group would have been less if intervention had been performed expeditiously. Almost three quarters of aneurysm-related deaths in the trial population occurred in patients who had not undergone elective endovascular repair. In addition, a significant number of patients randomised to best medical therapy within the trial (47/172: 27%) subsequently underwent endovascular (35) or open (12) repair when their aneurysms enlarged and/or became symptomatic, or when their fitness improved. One can only speculate as to the natural history of these aneurysms had they been left untreated but it is evident that a small reduction in the number of aneurysm-related deaths before intervention in those assigned to EVAR, combined with a small increase in the number of ruptures in those assigned to best medical therapy, would have altered the trial outcome significantly.

Operative mortality in those assigned to endovascular repair was perhaps higher than many expected at 9%. This may simply reflect the fact that the patients were unfit and that the physiological stress of endovascular repair is not negligible. It may, however, also reflect the fact that local or regional anaesthesia was employed in only 50% of patients and that measures to reduce operative risk (aspirin, statins and/or beta blockers) were employed in only a third. It is also interesting to note that operative mortality was only 2% in those assigned to best medical therapy who subsequently underwent endovascular or open repair. It is not known to what extent the fitness of these patients was improved before intervention.

One of the most striking findings of the trial was the significantly lower than expected rate of rupture of untreated aneurysms (nine per 100 person years). Was this because aneurysms that are anatomically suitable for endovascular repair are less likely to rupture than aneurysms with short or angulated necks, or was this because best medical therapy is more effective at preventing rupture than many believed? It is well known that aneurysm diameter alone is a relatively poor surrogate marker for risk of rupture and it is clear that further research is required to identify patients who are truly at high risk of rupture and in whom intervention can more readily be justified.

What is clear from EVAR 2 is that patients considered unfit for open surgery have a poor prognosis whether or not their aneurysm is treated, with only two thirds surviving four years. At the very least this underlines the need for careful patient selection. As with carotid intervention, prophylactic EVAR, with its associated morbidity and mortality cannot be justified unless the patient is likely to live long enough to benefit. On the other hand, the EVAR 2 trial should not be interpreted as justification to deny intervention to all who are considered unsuitable for open surgery. Patients who are medically very unfit, whose condition cannot readily be improved by medical intervention and who as a result have a limited life expectancy will probably not benefit from intervention, particularly if their aneurysm is relatively small. However, it is likely that endovascular repair does confer a survival advantage in patients whose fitness and life expectancy can be improved by medical therapy or intervention, in those in whom the contraindications to open repair are primarily surgical (the hostile abdomen) and in those with an aneurysm that is large and/or enlarging rapidly. Further subgroup analysis and late follow-up data are awaited.

Conclusions

Endovascular repair has been confirmed as a safe alternative to open surgery in patients who are medically and anatomically suitable for both treatments. Such patients should be informed of the advantages and disadvantages of each technique and offered the choice between endovascular and open repair.

The role of endovascular repair in patients who are not fit for open repair remains uncertain. Endovascular repair is clearly inappropriate in those who are very unfit and/or have a very limited life expectancy, but this should not be extrapolated to deny treatment to all who are deemed unfit. Those with larger aneurysms and those in whom fitness can be improved should probably be considered for endovascular repair but this should be delayed to enable optimisation of medical fitness.

Endovascular repair is more expensive than open repair but the cost of endogafts, the need for expensive follow-up imaging and the requirement for secondary intervention are all likely to reduce with further refinements in endograft design, patient selection and interventional techniques.

Key points	Evidence level
◆ In patients who are anatomically suitable and fit for both EVAR and open repair, EVAR offers a small but significant reduction in 30-day operative mortality and is at least as effective at preventing mid-term aneurysm-related death.	Ib/A
◆ EVAR is more expensive due to the cost of the endograft and follow-up and has a higher rate of secondary intervention.	Ia/A
◆ Quality of life is better after EVAR than open repair for the first three months after intervention; thereafter there is no difference.	Ib/A
◆ In patients who are considered unfit for open repair the incidence of aneurysm-related death is less in those who undergo elective EVAR than in those who are simply observed.	Ib/A

References

1. Parodi JC, Palmaz JC, Barone HD. Transfemoral intraluminal graft implantation for abdominal aortic aneurysms. *Ann Vasc Surg* 1991; 5: 491-9.
2. Thomas SM, Gaines PA, Beard JD. Short-term (30-day) outcome of endovascular treatment of abdominal aortic aneurysms: results from the prospective registry of endovascular treatment of abdominal aortic aneurysms (RETA). *Eur J Vasc Endovasc Surg* 2001; 21: 57-64.
3. Thomas SM, Beard JD, Ireland M, *et al*. Results from the prospective registry of endovascular treatment of abdominal aortic aneurysms (RETA): mid-term results to five years. *Eur J Vasc Endovasc Surg* 2005; 29: 563-70.
4. Harris PL, Vallabhaneni SR, Desgranges P, *et al*. Incidence and risk factors of late rupture, conversion, and death after endovascular repair of infrarenal aortic aneurysms: the EUROSTAR experience. *J Vasc Surg* 2000; 32: 739-49.
5. Lifeline Registry Publications Committee. Lifeline registry of endovascular aneurysm repair: long-term primary outcome measures. *J Vasc Surg* 2006; 43: 1-10.
6. The EVAR Trial Participants. Comparison of endovascular aneurysm repair with open repair in patients with abdominal aortic aneurysm (EVAR trial 1) - 30-day operative mortality: randomised controlled trial. *Lancet* 2004; 364: 843-8.
7. The EVAR Trial Participants. Endovascular aneurysm repair versus open repair in patients with abdominal aortic aneurysm (EVAR trial 1): randomised controlled trial. *Lancet* 2005; 365: 2179-86.
8. Prinssen M, Verhoeven EL, Buth J, *et al*. A randomized trial comparing conventional and endovascular repair of abdominal aortic aneurysm. *N Engl J Med* 2004; 351: 1607-18.

9. Blankensteijn JD, De Jong S, Prinssen M, *et al*. Two-year outcomes after conventional or endovascular repair of abdominal aortic aneurysms. *N Engl J Med* 2005; 352: 2398-405.

10. EVAR Trial Participants. Endovascular aneurysm repair and outcome in patients unfit for open repair of abdominal aortic aneurysm (EVAR trial 2): a randomised controlled trial. *Lancet* 2005; 365: 2187-92.

11. Torella F, on behalf of the EUROSTAR collaborators. Effect of improved endograft design on outcome of endovascular aneurysm repair. *J Vasc Surg* 2004; 40: 216-21.

12. Pearson S, Hassen T, Spark J, *et al*. Endovascular repair of abdominal aortic aneurysm reduces intraoperative cortisol and perioperative morbidity. *J Vasc Surg* 2005; 41: 919-25.

13. Buth J, Van Marrewijk CJ, Harris PL, *et al*. Outcome of abdominal aortic aneurysm repair in patients considered unfit for an open procedure: a report on the EUROSTAR experience. *J Vasc Surg* 2002; 35: 211-20.

Chapter 18

Endovascular aneurysm repair: state of the art 2006

Tim J Parkinson MB BS MRCS(Glasg), Vascular Research Fellow

John D Rose FRCP FRCR, Consultant Radiologist

Mike G Wyatt MSc MD FRCS, Consultant Vascular Surgeon

Northern Vascular Centre, Freeman Hospital, Newcastle upon Tyne, UK

Introduction

The endovascular repair (EVAR) of abdominal aortic aneurysms (AAAs) was first reported by Parodi et al in 1990 [1]. Over the last 16 years EVAR has evolved from the early home-made stent graft to commercially produced devices of the highest quality.

The devices are available in tubular (aorto-aortic), aorto-uni-iliac (AUI) or bifurcated configurations. They may be one piece or modular (several components requiring construction during deployment), and are attached to either the infrarenal or suprarenal abdominal aorta via an uncovered portion of stent. Recently, stent grafts have been manufactured individually with fenestrations corresponding to the visceral arteries for the treatment of juxtarenal aneurysms. The stent graft fabric consists either of polyester (Dacron) or polytetrafluoroethylene (PTFE) and can be either balloon-expanded or self-expanding.

Stent grafts are used to treat aneurysms of the abdominal and, more recently, thoracic aorta, as well as thoracic dissection, traumatic aortic transection, penetrating ulcers, pseudo-aneurysms, aortobronchial fistulae and mycotic aneurysms [2].

While stent graft technology continues to develop and gain acceptance as an alternative to open aneurysm repair, lack of long-term data regarding durability, the higher financial cost [3] and lack of randomised controlled trials have delayed widespread acceptance.

The evolution of EVAR

Tube grafts

The first tube grafts were constructed from Dacron with a Palmaz stent attached either proximally, or both proximally and distally. Unsuitable distal aortic neck and failure to effect an adequate distal seal led to post-procedure aneurysm rupture [4] and a high rate of conversion to open surgery [5] **(IIa/B)**.

May et al [6] from Australia reported their five-year experience of EVAR using a variety of stent grafts. There was no significant difference in the peri-operative mortality rate between the different graft configurations; however, the success rate of tube grafts was only 50% at 40 months, compared to 80% for the other types (aorto-iliac, bifurcated). Similarly, Faries et al reported on 65 tube grafts from various manufacturers [7]. They found no aortic ruptures, but proximal attachment failure in two patients, and distal failure in 12, with a mean interval to failure of 12.9 months. With several centres reporting similar results and late complications, and the acknowledgement that proximity to the aortic bifurcation meant that only 5% of AAAs were suitable for exclusion with a tube graft, these are seldom used [5] **(IIa/B)**.

Aorto-uni-iliac grafts

These were easier to develop than bifurcated grafts, and it was accepted that iliac fixation was needed to overcome the problems associated with distal seal using tube grafts. They involve a single tubular stent graft attached to both the infrarenal aorta and the more suitable iliac artery (no aneurysm, occlusion or tortuosity). The contralateral iliac artery is then occluded with an endovascular plug (Figure 1), and a femoro-femoral crossover graft performed. Parodi *et al* were one of the first groups to document the successful insertion of eight AUI grafts with encouraging early results [8].

Following this, Hopkinson *et al* described the use of a modified Gianturco stent, Dacron graft and Wallstent in 30 patients, with successful insertion in 25 (83.3%) and a 30-day overall operative mortality of two (6.6%) [9]. Bell *et al* complemented this with their tapered aorto-mono-iliac graft constructed from an 8mm thin-walled expanded PTFE tube graft, pre-dilated proximally to 35mm and tapered distally to 15mm, with the graft sutured proximally to a 5cm long predilated Palmaz stent. There was success in 52 (87%) of the 60 patients treated, with aneurysm exclusion in 49 (82%) and a peri-operative mortality rate of 3% [10, 11].

The recent EVT/Guidant trials compared AUI stent grafts for complex aorto-iliac aneurysms with bifurcated grafts, tube grafts and open repair [12]. Endpoints were operative morbidity and outcome at one year. Implantation was achieved in 94.2% of the AUI group (comparable to the other endovascular techniques) and there was no significant difference in operative mortality between the groups (4.2% AUI, 2.6% bifurcated, 0% tube, 2.7% open repair). The rates of Type 1 endoleak at one year were 2.4%,

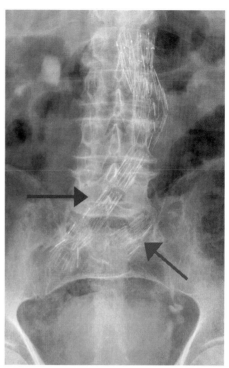

Figure 1. Plain radiograph showing an AUI stent graft, the red arrow indicating the ipsilateral long limb and the blue arrow the contralateral iliac plug. A femoro-femoral crossover is present but not visualised.

2.3% and 3.8% for the AUI, bifurcated and tube groups, respectively and there were no reported late aneurysm ruptures or cross-over graft thromboses. The authors concluded that AUI results were competitive with bifurcated and tube repair, and that all had lower mortality than open repair.

While sacrificing anatomical continuity, AUI stent grafts have a role, particularly in the presence of unilateral iliac artery occlusion; due to their rapid deployment, many advocate their use in the treatment of ruptured AAA **(IV/C)**. The associated femoral cross-over grafting is low risk; Hopkinson *et al* described 136 cases and, after a median follow-up of seven months, found two late graft infections and one graft thrombosis [13].

Bifurcated grafts

Non-modular (unipiece)

Chuter *et al* were the first to describe bifurcated endovascular grafts in 1994 [14, 15]. The devices comprised a standard bifurcated Dacron graft with Gianturco stents sutured at both the proximal and distal extremities. Fifty-two grafts were inserted over a three-year interval during which the device underwent modification, eventually resulting in professional production. Early results were promising: 92% successful deployment of the home-made devices and 100% for the ten commercial endografts. However, long-term success was only 64% in the home-made and 90% in the commercial group. Device failures were attributed to graft thrombosis secondary to kinking and proximal graft migration.

Endovascular technologies (EVT) developed the first commercially available bifurcated device, based on a graft designed and patented by Lazarus [16], with two identical limbs including self-expanding stents attached to the distal extremities [17]. Unipiece stent grafts have attracted criticism due to the relative difficulty in deployment of the contralateral limb (frequently requiring open surgical access), and the inflexibility of the devices due to equal dimensions of the limbs **(IV/C)**. The Endologix (Powerlink) is currently the only commercially available one-piece bifurcated stent graft and, in a multicentre trial in the USA, it had fewer adverse postoperative events than open repair [18].

Modular stent graft

Modular grafts consist of a main aortic body, plus a long and a short limb. The main body is inserted via one iliac system to attach to the aorta, while the long limb attaches to the iliac artery on the ipsilateral side. The short limb, which opens into the aneurysm sac, is catheterised from the contralateral groin, allowing deployment of the contralateral iliac limb and completion of the bifurcated graft (Figure 2). The graft components are self-expanding and adhere by radial force. They are thus adaptable to different anatomy.

The first commercially produced modular graft was the MinTec Stentor which was supported along its entire length by the stent; it eventually evolved into the Vanguard stent graft. Unfortunately, these early modular devices were prone to late failure with device migration, graft limb occlusion, ligature breakage, stent kinking and limb dislocation (Figure 3) **(III/B)**. Jacobs *et al* from the Mount Sinai Medical Center reported 60 patients with stent failure out of 686 procedures; 43 had metallic stent fractures and 14 had suture disruption [19]. The two most affected were the Vanguard (16/60 failures with nine body separations) and the Talent stent graft (24/60 with 23 metal stent fractures). Holtham *et al* described 55 Vanguards with median follow-up of 40 months; there

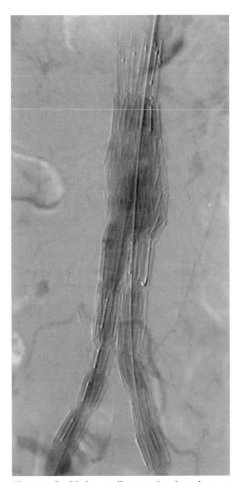

Figure 2. Plain radiograph showing a fully constructed bifurcated modular stent graft. Both limbs have been extended to the common iliac artery bifurcations.

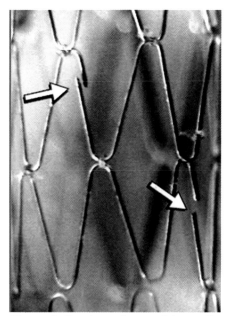

Figure 3. Fractures (arrows) in aortic stent.

were three device migrations, 12 occluded limbs and nine Type 3 endoleaks [20].

The Vanguard and Guidant Ancure/EVT were subsequently withdrawn due to structural failure. Developments resulted in higher quality stents and design to reduce these worrying complications. The currently available devices are shown in Table 1. Despite concerns regarding the long-term durability of these grafts, an analysis of the 6787 patients in the EUROSTAR database found the Excluder, Talent and Zenith stent grafts were associated with a lower risk of migration, kinking, occlusion and need for secondary intervention compared to the Vanguard [21].

Suprarenal versus infrarenal fixation

Some of the first-generation stent grafts with infrarenal fixation were prone to late proximal attachment failure [22], often resulting in stent graft

Table 1. Currently available aortic and thoracic endografts (2006).

Aortic endografts

Device name (manufacturer)	Device configuration	Suprarenal component	Aortic diameters available (mm)	
Endologix (Powerlink)	Unipiece	Optional	25 or 28	
Zenith (Cook)	Modular +/- fenestrated	Yes	22-36	
Talent (Medtronic)	Modular	Yes	24-34	
Anaconda (Terumo)	Modular	No	19.5-34	
Excluder (Gore)	Modular	No	23 or 26 or 28.5	

Thoracic endografts

Device name (manufacturer)	Device configuration	Framework	Thoracic diameters available (mm)	Lengths available (mm)
Zenith TX2 (Cook)	Unipiece/modular + extensions, uncovered distally	Stainless steel	28-42	108-216
Relay (Bolton)	Unipiece + extensions, uncovered proximally	Nitinol	22-46	90-200
Valian (Medtronic)	Unipiece + extensions, covered/uncovered proximally	Nitinol	24-46	110-215
TAG (Gore)	Unipiece + extensions, covered proximally & distally	Nitinol	26-40	100-200

migration, failure of aneurysm exclusion and continued risk of rupture **(III/B)** [20]. Several companies took advantage of the relative sparing of the suprarenal aorta to develop stent grafts with an uncovered section of proximal stent that crosses the renal artery ostia and attaches to the suprarenal aorta with barbs or hooks (Figure 4).

Tonnessen *et al* compared the mid to long-term migration rates for 235 patients who had either an infrarenal (Medtronic AneuRx) or suprarenal (Cook Zenith) stent graft [23]. Freedom from migration for each of the first four years was 96.1%, 89.5%, 78.0% and 72.0%, respectively, for the AneuRx, compared to 100%, 97.6%, 97.6% and 97.6% for the Zenith (p=0.01). Despite initial concerns that the renal arteries could be occluded by the metal struts, several short to mid-term studies failed to show any significant difference in renal function after suprarenal compared with infrarenal fixation [24, 25] **(IIa/B)**.

Fenestrated/branched stent grafts

For aortic aneurysms with a short proximal neck (<10mm), EVAR remained limited until the development of fenestrated grafts in 1999. A Dacron-covered suprarenal stent was accurately cut to size with fenestrations according to pre-imaging studies and successfully deployed in a canine model [26]. These grafts can be employed in the perirenal or suprarenal aorta by including fenestrations in the proximal graft fabric, allowing blood flow to the viscera. The stent grafts are based on the Zenith (Cook) platform and each is manufactured individually, based on the visceral arteries to be included.

There are three types of fenestration, dependent on their position relative to the graft fabric. The most proximal is a U-shaped gap (scallop) in the leading edge of the graft fabric (Figure 5). This may incorporate a single renal artery into the stent graft or the superior mesenteric artery in combination with distal fenestrations for the renal arteries. The remaining two types of fenestration are situated away from the leading edge in the body of the graft fabric.

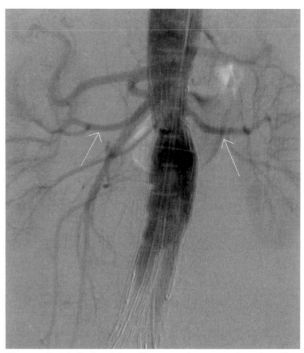

Figure 4. Digital subtraction angiogram showing the uncovered suprarenal portion of a stent graft in relation to the renal arteries (shown by the arrows).

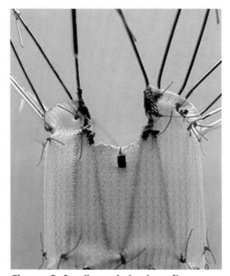

Figure 5. Scalloped stent graft.

They are either large fenestrations (stent struts crossing them), or small (lying between the stent struts and requiring secondary stenting to prevent occlusion).

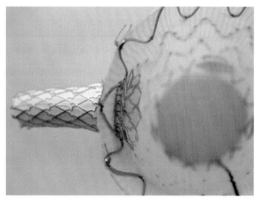

Figure 6. Branched stent graft.

Branched grafts are a further development of fenestrated grafts. These use covered renal stent grafts at the level of the fenestrations, creating a fully sealed system and allowing the treatment of aneurysms with no infrarenal neck (Figure 6).

Thoracic stent grafts

Volodos *et al* first described the use of endovascular prostheses to exclude thoracic aneurysms [27]. They documented the treatment of a post-traumatic aneurysm of the descending thoracic aorta that remained successful after five years, the treatment of an anastomotic aneurysm following reconstruction for coarctation and the treatment of a Type 3 dissecting thoracic aneurysm. Subsequently, endografts have been used for thoracic aneurysms, Type B thoracic dissections, penetrating ulcers and pseudo-aneurysms of the thoracic aorta [2, 28].

Like early abdominal aortic endografts, the first home-made stent grafts consisted of a graft with stents attached proximally and distally for fixation, the main body of the graft being unsupported. Loss of fixation led to device migration, kinking due to lack of support and failure to exclude the aneurysm. The first generation of commercially produced stent grafts (Gore Excluder and Medtronic Talent) had longitudinal support struts to avoid this. However, fracture of these struts [19] led to their modification and re-design, and there are now four commercially produced devices (Table 1). Disadvantages at present include large

delivery systems, frequently requiring formal surgical access, and the slow development of fenestrated stent grafts for more complex aortic arch aneurysms.

Patient selection for EVAR

Abdominal aortic aneurysm

Up to 66% of AAAs may be suitable for EVAR, depending on the morphological characteristics of the aneurysm [29]. Factors include long infrarenal aneurysm neck, no angulation and, absence of thrombus or conical shape. Also, the size, tortuosity and presence of any aneurysm in the iliac vessels are important (Table 2) **(III/B)**.

Table 2. Selection criteria for endovascular repair.
Aortic endografts
Aneurysm diameter >55mm or symptomatic
Neck length >15mm
Neck angulation <60 degrees
Iliac vessels >7mm diameter
Minimal tortuosity/calcification of iliacs
Thoracic endografts
Descending thoracic aortic diameter >65mm (60mm in Marfan's syndrome) or symptomatic
Iliac vessels suitability as for aortic endografts
20mm proximal and distal landing zone required

For infrarenal AAA, ideally the neck length should be at least 15mm for EVAR. Stanley *et al* reported data from their database of 238 patients with a Cook Zenith graft [30]. Over a median follow-up of 13.4 months, the endoleak rate for infrarenal necks less than or equal to 10mm was 57%; endoleak was also significantly associated with both a contour change of 3mm along the neck and a neck length <20mm. They concluded that neck contour, length and diameter are the most important factors in predicting endoleak. Sampaio *et al* similarly found that patients with short and heavily calcified aortic necks were at increased risk of Type 1 endoleaks [31].

As well as no calcification, the angle between the main axis of the aneurysm and the neck should ideally be less than 60°. Sternbergh *et al* described a series of 81 procedures [32]. The risk of an adverse postoperative event (death, conversion to open repair and Type 1 endoleak) was 70%, 54.5% and 16.6% in patients with severe (≥60°), moderate (40-59°) and mild (<40°) angulation, respectively. The authors recommended caution in patients with neck angulation >40°.

In addition, the iliac arteries should be at least 7mm in diameter to accommodate the large delivery systems of EVAR. Tortuosity of the iliac arteries precludes device delivery and accounts for up to 15% of exclusions from EVAR [33]. Iliac artery pre-dilation or stenting can be used to overcome iliac stenoses. The use of a guidewire passed retrogradely from brachial to femoral artery and held under tension can also aid delivery of the stent graft. If all else fails, formal surgical access of the iliac artery can be achieved through a small retroperitoneal incision.

Thoracic endografts

It is accepted that aneurysm repair is indicated once the ascending thoracic aorta reaches 5.5cm and the descending thoracic aorta reaches 6.5cm in diameter. These should be reduced to 5.0cm and 6.0cm, respectively, for those with Marfan's disease and repair should be considered for symptomatic aneurysms, regardless of size [34].

The suitability of patients for endovascular repair of thoracic aneurysms depends on three factors, the first of which is an adequate iliac system for device introduction. This follows the same specifications as for infrarenal AAA repair. Chuter *et al* have described the carotid artery as an alternative introduction vessel, although formal carotid access was required anyway for adjuvant procedures in a complex case [35]. The remaining factors are the proximal and distal landing zones, each of which ideally requires 2cm of normal aortic tissue to effect an adequate seal.

Proximal landing zone

At the proximal landing zone in the distal aortic arch, the stent graft must counter the concavity of the arch and accommodate the aortic branches supplying the head, neck and arms. To effect an adequate seal, the origin of the left subclavian artery (LSA) must be covered in up to 17% of procedures [36], causing concern for upper limb ischaemia. Rehders *et al* reported 171 thoracic EVAR procedures, 22 (13%) of which occluded the LSA [37]. Despite lower systolic blood pressure in the left arm, only seven of the 22 (32%) suffered arm symptoms, none requiring intervention. Transposition of the LSA is not usually required before intentional stent graft occlusion in the presence of intact vertebral and carotid arteries.

The more proximal the aneurysm in the aortic arch, the greater the likelihood that the left carotid artery will also need to be covered. Carotid-carotid bypass or carotid-subclavian bypass or transposition can be done before or simultaneously with EVAR. These hybrid procedures will be considered later.

At the distal landing zone, the need for 2cm of aorta to effect an adequate seal may impede on the origins of the visceral and renal arteries. Fenestrated and branched grafts have been used to solve this, as have hybrid procedures to revascularise the visceral and renal arteries [38] (Chapter 19).

Current status of EVAR

Since its introduction 15 years ago, much research has been undertaken and EVAR has now become an evidence-based intervention. There has been a huge number of open trials of EVAR, two randomised trials, and two large databases - RETA and EUROSTAR (Chapter 17).

Abdominal aortic aneurysm

The EVAR 1 trial [3, 39] compared open vs. endovascular repair of AAA in a multicentre randomised controlled trial. The endpoints were mortality (aneurysm-related and overall), durability, cost and health-related quality of life. In total, 1082 patients were randomised. The 30-day mortality for EVAR was 1.7% vs. 4.7% for open repair; although after four years follow-up overall mortality was similar in both groups, the aneurysm-related mortality was still lower after EVAR (4% vs. 7%) **(Ib/A)**. Quality of life scores were similar between the two procedures within six months, after an initial advantage for EVAR. The cost of EVAR was significantly higher over the four years. This was due to the cost of the stent grafts and the high re-intervention rate during follow-up. It is hoped that, as EVAR becomes more commonplace, the cost will reduce.

It was expected that the ideal role of EVAR would be in patients at high risk from open AAA repair. The EVAR 2 trial [40] compared EVAR vs. best medical treatment in patients deemed unfit for open AAA repair. Ultimately, following per-protocol analysis, there was no benefit in favour of EVAR **(Ib/A)**.

Endoleak

Failure to exclude the aneurysm from the circulation continues to be of concern following EVAR, as the patient remains liable to rupture.

A recent systematic review of all the published data on the safety and efficacy of EVAR included 61 studies describing 19,804 procedures [41]. Endoleak rates were as follows: Type 1 (6.8%), Type 2 (10.3%) and Type 3 (4.2%). Regular routine follow-up is important and may need to be life-long.

The greatest concern with endoleak is continued aneurysm sac expansion and possible rupture. Peppelenbosch et al reviewed the 4392 cases from the EUROSTAR Registry and at four years found a freedom from rupture rate of 90%, 98% and 98% for aneurysms with pre-operative dimensions of >6.5cm, 5.5-6.4cm, and 4.0-5.4cm, respectively [42].

Although continued aneurysm sac expansion usually means an endoleak is present, it can still occur in the absence of radiological confirmation. This is commonly considered to be due to endotension. The cause is not clear, although it has been theorised that direct pressure transmission by thrombus or adjacent aortic lumen, undetected low-flow endoleak and porosity of the stent graft to serous fluid may be to blame.

Fenestrated/branched stent grafts

While there are no randomised controlled trials, in the setting of short aortic neck or juxtarenal aneurysm there are promising early results from small series of procedures in specialist centres **(III/B)**. Anderson et al from Australia reported 13 patients with an unsuitable infrarenal aortic neck who had 100% successful deployment, no 30-day mortality and no endoleak during 3-24 months' follow-up [43]. Verhoeven et al described similar results in 18 patients [44].

A Cleveland Clinic report included 32 patients (22 with a short aortic neck and ten with angulation or thrombus compromising neck quality) [45]. All devices were successfully deployed and 83 visceral vessels were incorporated (renal arteries and superior mesenteric artery). One patient died within 30 days from pneumonia. The endoleak rate at 30 days was 6.5%; there was one case of persistent Type 2 endoleak and continued aneurysm sac growth. Mean follow-up was 9.2 months, during which six patients had transient or permanent elevation of serum creatinine (one requiring haemodialysis). Of the 83 incorporated vessels, three had late stenoses (all successfully treated) and two renal occlusions were detected.

In a second series of 72 patients, the focus was on renal function following fenestrated EVAR. Twenty-four patients had deterioration in renal function during follow-up (mean six months, range 1-24), and 17 patients experienced 19 renal events (ten renal artery stenoses, five renal artery occlusions and four patients required haemodialysis). Renal events and death were more common in the group of 23 patients with pre-operative renal dysfunction [46]. The authors concluded that fenestrated EVAR is associated with a significant risk of adverse renal outcome (16% in patients with normal renal function and 39% in those with pre-existing renal dysfunction).

Thoracic EVAR

Although there are no controlled trials of thoracic EVAR, there have been over 40 case series reported in the last decade, covering both elective and emergency procedures. A recent review of the available literature up to 2004 described 1518 procedures [2] **(III/B)**. There was a primary technical success rate of 97%, a 30-day mortality of 5.5%, a hospital mortality rate of 6%, a paraparesis rate of 0.7%, paraplegia in 1.3%, an endoleak rate of 7.7%, graft kinking in 0.1% and graft infection in 0.7%. A more recently published series in 2006 [47] seems only to continue these promising results, which contrast strongly with the results of open surgery.

EVAR for ruptured AAA

To date, the use of EVAR for the treatment of AAA rupture has involved only small series **(III/B)**. Against a background of 50% mortality for open repair of ruptured AAA, the potential for EVAR has excited considerable controversy. It has been suggested by some that only 20% of ruptured AAAs are suitable for EVAR [48], based on adverse anatomical neck features. In contrast, Reichart et al stated this figure could be as high as 42% [49]. The patient must be haemodynamically stable to enable pre-procedure computed tomography, so it remains unclear how many aneurysms would be eligible for EVAR.

A recent review reported that peri-operative mortality for EVAR of ruptured AAA ranged from 9-45% [50]. After 91 procedures, there were seven peri-operative endoleaks (two Type 1 and five Type 2), 15 patients developed renal failure and hospital stay ranged from 2-70 days. The results were comparable to those of open repair. Peppelenbosch et al described an international multicentre study of the Talent AUI stent graft [51]. Of the 49 treated patients, operative blood loss, duration of ICU admission and mechanical ventilation were all significantly shorter than for open repair. The 30-day mortality rate was 35% compared to 39% after open repair, with similar three-month all-cause mortality rates, 40% and 42%, respectively.

There is still no consensus about which stent graft should be used for EVAR of ruptured AAA; many advocate the use of an AUI device, as this only requires cannulation of one iliac system **(IV/C)**. Femoral crossover grafting is done once haemodynamic stability is restored. The occasional difficulty in cannulating and attaching the short limb of a modular stent graft can prolong surgery and increase the rate of haemorrhage. The logistical requirements of a dedicated endovascular suite with immediately available trained staff has so far meant that EVAR for ruptured AAA is confined to large specialist vascular centres.

Conclusions

EVAR has made considerable progress in the last 15 years and has become established as a safe and viable alternative to open AAA repair, at least in the mid term [3]. Stent grafts will continue to evolve, with improved materials and fixation techniques, leading to lower rates of post-procedure complications. The development of lower profile stent grafts, with smaller delivery systems, will allow more patients to benefit from EVAR, make thoracic EVAR purely percutaneous and reduce the risks of device introduction.

Key points	Evidence level

- EVAR is a viable alternative to open repair of infrarenal AAA with significantly lower all-cause 30-day mortality and lower aneurysm-related mortality after four years. Ib/A

- Suprarenal stent-graft fixation confers greater endograft stability and does not significantly affect renal function in the short to mid term. IIa/B

- EVAR is feasible for ruptured AAA with results comparable to open surgical repair in stable patients. IIa/B

- Fenestrated endografts have yielded promising early results but longer follow-up is needed to assess potential renal complications; randomised trials are necessary to compare them to open repair. III/B

- Thoracic endografts can safely be used to treat a wide variety of thoracic aortic diseases, but controlled trials are needed to validate their use. III/B

References

1. Parodi JC, Palmaz JC, Barone HD. Transfemoral intraluminal graft implantation for abdominal aortic aneurysms. *Ann Vasc Surg* 1991; 5: 491-9.

2. Sayed S, Thompson MM. Endovascular repair of the descending thoracic aorta: evidence for the change in clinical practice. *Vascular* 2005; 13: 148-57.

3. Endovascular aneurysm repair versus open repair in patients with abdominal aortic aneurysm (EVAR Trial 1): randomised controlled trial. *Lancet* 2005; 365: 2179-86.

4. Lumsden AB, Allen RC, Chaikof EL, *et al*. Delayed rupture of aortic aneurysms following endovascular stent grafting. *Am J Surg* 1995; 170: 174-8.

5. Coppi G, Moratto R, Silingardi R, *et al*. The Italian trial of endovascular AAA exclusion using the Parodi endograft. *J Endovasc Surg* 1997; 4: 299-306.

6. May J, White GH, Yu W, *et al*. Importance of graft configuration in outcome of endoluminal aortic aneurysm repair: a 5-year analysis by the life table method. *Eur J Vasc Endovasc Surg* 1998; 15: 406-11.

7. Faries PL, Briggs VL, Rhee JY, *et al*. Failure of endovascular aortoaortic tube grafts: a plea for preferential use of bifurcated grafts. *J Vasc Surg* 2002; 35: 868-73.

8. Parodi JC, Criado FJ, Barone HD, *et al*. Endoluminal aortic aneurysm repair using a balloon-expandable stent-graft device: a progress report. *Ann Vasc Surg* 1994; 8: 523-9.

9. Yusuf SW, Whitaker SC, Chuter TA, *et al*. Early results of endovascular aortic aneurysm surgery with aortouniiliac graft, contralateral iliac occlusion, and femorofemoral bypass. *J Vasc Surg* 1997; 25: 165-72.

10. Thompson MM, Sayers RD, Nasim A, *et al*. Aortomonoiliac endovascular grafting: difficult solutions to difficult aneurysms. *J Endovasc Surg* 1997; 4: 174-81.

11. Thompson MM, Fishwick G, Bell PRF. Aorto-uni-iliac endovascular repair utilizing ePTFE and balloon expandable stents - The Leicester experience. In: *Indications in Vascular and Endovascular Surgery*. Greenhalgh RM, Ed. London: WB Saunders,1998: 229-40.

12. Moore WS, Brewster DC, Bernhard VM. Aorto-uni-iliac endograft for complex aortoiliac aneurysms compared with tube/bifurcation endografts: results of the EVT/Guidant trials. *J Vasc Surg* 2001; 33(2 Suppl): S11-20.

13. Walker SR, Braithwaite B, Tennant WG, *et al*. Early complications of femorofemoral crossover bypass grafts after aorta uni-iliac endovascular repair of abdominal aortic aneurysms. *J Vasc Surg* 1998; 28: 647-50.

14. Chuter TA, Donayre C, Wendt G. Bifurcated stent-grafts for endovascular repair of abdominal aortic aneurysm. Preliminary case reports. *Surg Endosc* 1994; 8: 800-2.

15. Chuter TA, Wendt G, Hopkinson BR, *et al*. European experience with a system for bifurcated stent-graft insertion. *J Endovasc Surg* 1997; 4: 13-22.

16. Lazarus HM. Endovascular grafting for the treatment of abdominal aortic aneurysms. *Surg Clin North Am* 1992; 72: 959-68.

17. Broeders I. The Endovascular Technologies system. In: *Endovascular surgery for aortic aneurysms*. Hopkinson BR, Yusef SW, Whitaker SC, Veith F, Eds. London, 1997: 104-21.

18. Carpenter JP. The Powerlink bifurcated system for endovascular aortic aneurysm repair: four-year results of the US multicenter trial. *J Cardiovasc Surg* (Torino) 2006; 47: 239-43.

19. Jacobs TS, Won J, Gravereaux EC, *et al*. Mechanical failure of prosthetic human implants: a 10-year experience with aortic stent graft devices. *J Vasc Surg* 2003; 37: 16-26.

20. Holtham SJ, Rose JD, Jackson RW, *et al*. The Vanguard endovascular stent-graft: mid-term results from a single centre. *Eur J Vasc Endovasc Surg* 2004; 27: 311-8.

21. van Marrewijk CJ, Leurs LJ, Vallabhaneni SR, et al. Risk-adjusted outcome analysis of endovascular abdominal aortic aneurysm repair in a large population: how do stent-grafts compare? *J Endovasc Ther* 2005; 12: 417-29.

22. Alric P, Hinchliffe RJ, Wenham PW, et al. Lessons learned from the long-term follow-up of a first-generation aortic stent graft. *J Vasc Surg* 2003; 37: 367-73.

23. Tonnessen BH, Sternbergh WC, 3rd, Money SR. Mid- and long-term device migration after endovascular abdominal aortic aneurysm repair: a comparison of AneuRx and Zenith endografts. *J Vasc Surg* 2005; 42: 392-400.

24. Alsac JM, Zarins CK, Heikkinen MA, et al. The impact of aortic endografts on renal function. *J Vasc Surg* 2005; 41: 926-30.

25. Parmer SS, Carpenter JP. Endovascular aneurysm repair with suprarenal vs infrarenal fixation: a study of renal effects. *J Vasc Surg* 2006; 43: 19-25.

26. Browne TF, Hartley D, Purchas S, et al. A fenestrated covered suprarenal aortic stent. *Eur J Vasc Endovasc Surg* 1999; 18: 445-9.

27. Volodos NL, Karpovich IP, Troyan VI, et al. Clinical experience of the use of self-fixing synthetic prostheses for remote endoprosthetics of the thoracic and the abdominal aorta and iliac arteries through the femoral artery and as intraoperative endoprosthesis for aorta reconstruction. *Vasa Suppl* 1991; 33: 93-5.

28. Matravers P, Morgan R, Belli A. The use of stent grafts for the treatment of aneurysms and dissections of the thoracic aorta: a single-centre experience. *Eur J Vasc Endovasc Surg* 2003; 26: 587-95.

29. Carpenter JP, Baum RA, Barker CF, et al. Impact of exclusion criteria on patient selection for endovascular abdominal aortic aneurysm repair. *J Vasc Surg* 2001; 34: 1050-4.

30. Stanley BM, Semmens JB, Mai Q, et al. Evaluation of patient selection guidelines for endoluminal AAA repair with the Zenith stent-graft: the Australasian experience. *J Endovasc Ther* 2001; 8: 457-64.

31. Sampaio SM, Panneton JM, Mozes GI, et al. Proximal Type I endoleak after endovascular abdominal aortic aneurysm repair: predictive factors. *Ann Vasc Surg* 2004; 18: 621-8.

32. Sternbergh WC, 3rd, Carter G, York JW, et al. Aortic neck angulation predicts adverse outcome with endovascular abdominal aortic aneurysm repair. *J Vasc Surg* 2002; 35: 482-6.

33. Wolf YG, Tillich M, Lee WA, et al. Impact of aortoiliac tortuosity on endovascular repair of abdominal aortic aneurysms: evaluation of 3D computer-based assessment. *J Vasc Surg* 2001; 34: 594-9.

34. Elefteriades JA. Natural history of thoracic aortic aneurysms: indications for surgery, and surgical versus nonsurgical risks. *Ann Thorac Surg* 2002; 74: S1877-80.

35. Chuter TA, Schneider DB, Reilly LM, et al. Modular branched stent graft for endovascular repair of aortic arch aneurysm and dissection. *J Vasc Surg* 2003; 38: 859-63.

36. Leurs LJ, Bell R, Degrieck Y, et al. Endovascular treatment of thoracic aortic diseases: combined experience from the EUROSTAR and United Kingdom Thoracic Endograft registries. *J Vasc Surg* 2004; 40: 670-9.

37. Rehders TC, Petzsch M, Ince H, et al. Intentional occlusion of the left subclavian artery during stent-graft implantation in the thoracic aorta: risk and relevance. *J Endovasc Ther* 2004; 11: 659-66.

38. Anderson JL, Adam DJ, Berce M, Hartley DE. Repair of thoracoabdominal aortic aneurysms with fenestrated and branched endovascular stent grafts. *J Vasc Surg* 2005; 42: 600-7.

39. Greenhalgh RM, Brown LC, Kwong GP, et al. Comparison of endovascular aneurysm repair with open repair in patients with abdominal aortic aneurysm (EVAR Trial 1), 30-day operative mortality results: randomised controlled trial. *Lancet* 2004; 364: 843-8.

40. Endovascular aneurysm repair and outcome in patients unfit for open repair of abdominal aortic aneurysm (EVAR Trial 2): randomised controlled trial. *Lancet* 2005; 365: 2187-92.

41. Drury D, Michaels JA, Jones L, et al. Systematic review of recent evidence for the safety and efficacy of elective endovascular repair in the management of infrarenal abdominal aortic aneurysm. *Br J Surg* 2005; 92: 937-46.

42. Peppelenbosch N, Buth J, Harris PL, et al. Diameter of abdominal aortic aneurysm and outcome of endovascular aneurysm repair: does size matter? A report from EUROSTAR. *J Vasc Surg* 2004; 39: 288-97.

43. Anderson JL, Berce M, Hartley DE. Endoluminal aortic grafting with renal and superior mesenteric artery incorporation by graft fenestration. *J Endovasc Ther* 2001; 8: 3-15.

44. Verhoeven EL, Prins TR, Tielliu IF, et al. Treatment of short-necked infrarenal aortic aneurysms with fenestrated stent-grafts: short-term results. *Eur J Vasc Endovasc Surg* 2004; 27: 477-83.

45. Greenberg RK, Haulon S, O'Neill S, et al. Primary endovascular repair of juxtarenal aneurysms with fenestrated endovascular grafting. *Eur J Vasc Endovasc Surg* 2004; 27: 484-91.

46. Haddad F, Greenberg RK, Walker E, et al. Fenestrated endovascular grafting: the renal side of the story. *J Vasc Surg* 2005; 41: 181-90.

47. Wheatley GH, 3rd, Gurbuz AT, Rodriguez-Lopez JA, et al. Midterm outcome in 158 consecutive Gore TAG thoracic endoprostheses: single-center experience. *Ann Thorac Surg* 2006; 81: 1570-7.

48. Rose DF, Davidson IR, Hinchliffe RJ, et al. Anatomical suitability of ruptured abdominal aortic aneurysms for endovascular repair. *J Endovasc Ther* 2003; 10: 453-7.

49. Reichart M, Geelkerken RH, Huisman AB, et al. Ruptured abdominal aortic aneurysm: endovascular repair is feasible in 40% of patients. *Eur J Vasc Endovasc Surg* 2003; 26: 479-86.

50. Hinchliffe RJ, Braithwaite BD, Hopkinson BR. The endovascular management of ruptured abdominal aortic aneurysms. *Eur J Vasc Endovasc Surg* 2003; 25: 191-201.

51. Peppelenbosch N, Geelkerken RH, Soong C, et al. Endograft treatment of ruptured abdominal aortic aneurysms using the Talent aortouniiliac system: an international multicenter study. *J Vasc Surg* 2006; 43: 1111-23.

Chapter 19

Safer thoraco-abdominal aneurysm repair

Marcus J Brooks FRCS MA MD, Specialist Registrar
John HN Wolfe FRCS MS, Consultant Vascular Surgeon
Regional Vascular Unit, St. Mary's Hospital, London, UK

Introduction

Thoraco-abdominal aneurysm (TAA) repair is a major undertaking, often in patients with limited organ reserve and concurrent disease. In addition to the mechanical trauma of an extensive tissue dissection are added the physiological insults of proximal aortic cross-clamping, massive blood loss, hypothermia and visceral ischaemia/reperfusion. Once ruptured, emergency repair of a TAA carries a mortality of at least 50-60% [1]. The results for elective repair are somewhat better, despite a significant incidence of respiratory failure, renal impairment, paraplegia, myocardial infarction and multiple organ dysfunction (Figure 1).

In the last few years, EVAR has offered an attractive alternative to open surgery for the management of TAA; there is no need for thoracotomy, extensive surgical dissection or aortic clamping. The challenge is maintaining perfusion of the intercostal, lumbar, visceral and renal arteries once the stent graft is deployed. There are two approaches: hybrid repairs, in which the visceral and/or renal arteries are revascularised retrogradely at an open operation and a stent is then deployed to exclude the aneurysm, and branched endografts (Chapter 18). Neither approach is yet able to maintain intercostal or lumbar artery patency and so both risk spinal cord ischaemia and paraplegia.

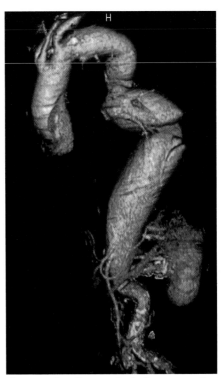

Figure 1. Computed tomography reconstruction of a thoraco-abdominal aortic aneurysm.

The keys to successful surgical management of TAA are an understanding of the risk factors that enable good patient selection and choice of the optimal procedure. This chapter reviews the evidence for safest practice, including a wealth of open trials, three randomised controlled trials and two meta-analyses [2-6].

Natural history

Most reports are based on observation of patients considered unfit for open surgery. Typically, they suggest that a TAA greater than 6cm has a poor prognosis, with survival as low as 40% at one year and 7% at five years [7]. In a prospective study from Yale of 1600 patients, the annual rupture risk at 6cm was <4% [8]. The annual mortality rate in these patients was 11% and most died from cardiac or cerebrovascular disease. In contrast, the risk of rupture of a 7cm aneurysm was 43%. The long-term outcome following successful surgery is consistent with these figures; survival is approximately 60% at five years and the majority of deaths are from cardiac causes [9]. Recently published studies have also considered quality of life after surgery. Worryingly, one report suggested that many of these patients never returned to independent living and that only half had a 'good' outcome at one year [10].

Pre-operative assessment

There are several risk factors known to affect the outcome after TAA repair. From the St. Mary's experience up to 1993 (130 patients), aneurysm rupture, aneurysm extent (Crawford Type II - see Figure 2), chronic aortic dissection, renal impairment and pulmonary disease were pre-operative risk factors associated with increased mortality [11]. In larger experiences from North America (Crawford 1446 patients, Coselli 1220 and Safi 841), aneurysms with symptoms, peptic ulcer disease and cerebrovascular disease were additional predictors of poor outcome [12-15] (Table 1).

Cardiac disease

Interestingly, cardiac factors were not predictive of outcome in any of the previous analyses. Suzuki *et al* studied 854 patients and found the only independent risk factor for mortality was a cardiac ejection fraction <50% [16]; most surgeons would not usually offer these patients TAA repair. Coronary artery bypass grafting has been performed safely in high-risk patients, and with reduced peri-operative mortality compared to patients with normal coronary anatomy [17].

Table 1. Multivariable analyses of pre-operative risk factors associated with death after open TAA repair. Values are odds ratios with 95% confidence intervals.

Pre-operative risk factor	Svensson *et al* (Houston)	Coselli *et al* (Houston)	Brooks *et al* (St. Mary's)
Number of TAA	1446	1108	272
Crawford type II (III)	2.54 (1.5-4.4)	2.06 (1.2-3.4)	3.32 (1.6-6.9)
Age	1.05 (1.0-1.1)	1.06 (1.0-1.1)	ns
Renal impairment	1.20 (1.1-1.3)	3.23 (1.9-5.7)	2.97 (1.6-5.4)
Coronary artery disease	1.66 (1.1-2.5)	ns	ns
Chronic lung disease	1.57 (1.1-2.3)	ns	4.72 (2.4-9.5)
Aneurysm symptoms	ns	2.47 (1.3-4.7)	ns
Systemic hypertension	ns	ns	2.17 (1.2-4.1)

ns = not significant

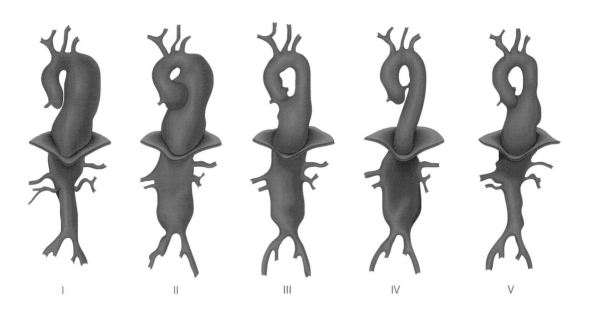

Figure 2. Crawford classification of TAA. *Reproduced with permission from Springer Science and Business Media. European Manual of Medicine. Liapis CD, Ed., 2006: Chapter 4.1.*

Pulmonary disease

Abnormal pre-operative spirometry is an independent and specific predictor of postoperative respiratory failure after TAA repair [12]. The correlation between respiratory reserve and the risk of respiratory failure is linear, so there is no clear threshold below which operation could be contraindicated. Spirometry may be employed to identify patients with poor respiratory reserve who may benefit from pre-operative physiotherapy and bronchodilator therapy. A recent randomised controlled study has shown that routine postoperative nasal continuous positive airways pressure ventilation can reduce the incidence of respiratory failure [5] **(Ib/A)**. Elective tracheostomy, at the time of aneurysm repair, may reduce sedation requirements in patients with poor respiratory function; alternatively, it can be done on the first postoperative day if the patient remains ventilator-dependent. Confining the surgical incision to the chest or abdomen alone may also reduce postoperative pulmonary complications [18].

Renal disease

Serum creatinine measurement, radio-nucleotide excretion renography and aortic angiography may be used to screen for renal artery stenoses, which may be present in up to one third of patients. It is important to remember to stop nephrotoxic drugs before surgery and to keep patients well hydrated. Renal artery stenoses are best corrected at the time of aortic reconstruction, rather than pre-operatively, since the 'stenosis' is frequently thrombus at the renal artery orifice within the aortic wall.

Operative technique

Open repair

The standard inlay technique has remained largely unchanged since originally described by Stanley Crawford (Figure 3). A number of techniques have been employed to reduce left ventricular strain and protect the viscera and spinal cord during cross-clamping in order to minimise the risks of surgery.

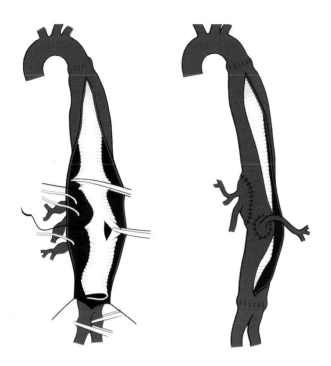

Figure 3. Aortic reconstruction using inlay technique described by Stanley Crawford.

Preserving spinal cord function

The incidence of paraplegia and paraparesis following TAA repair was initially almost 10% but has decreased over time to nearer 2% in expert hands. While publication bias may be a factor, it is likely that modified technical factors, such as intercostal artery re-implantation, hypothermia, left heart bypass, cerebrospinal fluid (CSF) drainage and cord monitoring have all played a part.

Intercostal / lumbar re-implantation

The spinal cord has a segmental blood supply from single anterior and paired posterior spinal arteries. In the middle third (T9-T12) the anterior spinal arteries are small and a single dominant artery (artery of Adamkiewicz) is believed to supply this segment, putting it at greatest risk. In an early retrospective study, intercostal re-implantation was associated with a significant reduction in the incidence of paraplegia after high-risk Type II TAA repair [19]. However, the benefit of intercostal re-implantation has since been questioned after postoperative angiography in the latter series revealed that three out of four of the implanted intercostals were occluded. Furthermore, comparable paraplegia rates have been reported without intercostal re-implantation [20]. In endovascular TAA repair, all intercostal arteries are lost and yet the rate of paraplegia appears lower than following open surgery.

It seems logical to incorporate large lumbar and intercostal arteries in either the proximal anastomosis or visceral patch, unless this excessively prolongs intra-operative spinal cord ischaemia **(IIb/B)**. In extensive repairs a 6mm side graft can be anastomosed to the artery of Adamkiewicz, or a similar large intercostal artery (Figure 4). Aneurysmal dilatation and rupture of the native aortic patches is a theoretical complication of this technique; every effort must be made to suture close to the visceral origins while leaving them widely patent.

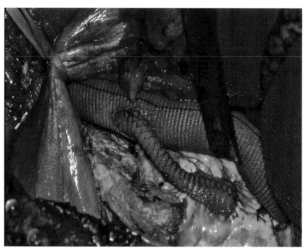

Figure 4. Jump graft from main aortic graft to a large intercostal artery.

Hypothermia

Hypothermia reduces tissue oxygen demand and can protect the spinal cord during ischaemia **(IIa/B)**. In a non-randomised comparison of 100 consecutive patients, hypothermia allowed longer cross-clamp times (47 minutes vs. 38 minutes) with no difference observed in the rate of paraplegia [21]. It has been suggested that even more aggressive cooling with hypothermic cardiopulmonary arrest is effective in protecting both the kidneys and spinal cord [22, 23], but the rate of respiratory complications is higher when this technique has been employed. An alternative to systemic cooling is local epidural cooling, although the technique is not easy to reproduce [24].

Distal perfusion

Left heart bypass reduces left heart strain during aortic cross-clamping, and has been reported to reduce postoperative paraplegia rates, although not all surgeons have shared this experience. A reduction in paraplegia rates has been described recently in retrospective studies of bypass of extensive TAA repairs [25, 26]. No randomised studies exist and the area remains controversial **(IIb/B)**.

Spinal cord monitoring and CSF drainage

Monitoring spinal cord function during operation is done using somatosensory evoked potential (SSEP) measurement; in one prospective and one retrospective study, loss of signal was highly predictive of the development of paraplegia [27, 28]. However, temperature, various anaesthetic agents and carbon dioxide retention all alter SSEP, and false positives are common. Transcranial motor-evoked potentials (MEP) have replaced SSEP in some centres as a method of detecting anterior motor horn ischaemia [29]. Studies using MEPs have highlighted the importance of the internal iliac arteries in maintaining spinal cord perfusion.

Spinal cord perfusion is the difference between local arterial, venous and CSF pressures. In experimental trials continuous CSF drainage to keep CSF pressure <10cm of water reduced the rate of paraplegia following proximal aortic cross-clamping [30, 31]. Several randomised trials have shown the benefit of CSF drainage in patients undergoing Crawford Type I and II repairs **(Ib/A)**. In a trial by Svensson et al that included 33 patients, intrathecal papaverine was administered to a CSF drainage group and compared

to controls by blinded independent assessors [32]. The study was stopped early because of the highly significant difference in paraplegia rates between the two patient groups. Coselli et al randomised 156 patients undergoing Crawford Type I or II aneurysm repair to CSF drainage or control groups and showed a benefit for both types of procedure [4]. In a third randomised trial, however, the paraplegia rate was not reduced by CSF drainage [33]. This study has been criticised as the volume of CSF drained was small and postoperative CSF pressure was not controlled. Several other studies using historical controls, some with additional pharmacological intervention in addition to CSF drainage, have shown a reduction in paraplegia rates in the intervention groups [34, 35]. It must, however, be remembered that CSF drainage carries the small risk of extradural haematoma, cerebral herniation and meningitis.

Two meta-analyses have presented contrasting reviews. A Cochrane meta-analysis by Khan and Stansby considered only the three randomised trials, and concluded that there were limited data supporting the role of CSF drainage in thoracic and thoraco-abdominal aneurysm surgery for prevention of neurological injury [2] **(Ia/A)**. This contrasts with Cina et al who included systematic review of non-randomised trials and cohort studies, and who supported the use of CSF drainage to prevent paraplegia, when used in expert centres [3] **(Ia/A)**.

Preserving renal function

Postoperative renal failure is strongly associated with mortality. In an experience of 657 repairs, 32% of patients with acute renal failure died [36]. Left heart bypass has been observed to reduce the risk of postoperative renal failure [12, 37]. In a recent trial, 30 patients undergoing Crawford Type TAA II repair with left heart bypass were randomised to renal artery perfusion with 4°C Ringer's lactate solution or normothermic blood from the bypass circuit: ten patients (63%) in the blood perfusion group and three patients (21%) in the cold crystalloid perfusion group developed acute renal failure (p=0.03) [6] **(Ib/A)**. Multivariable analysis confirmed that the use of cold crystalloid perfusion was independently protective against acute renal dysfunction.

Table 2. Case series published since 1996 reporting the outcome of open TAA repair.

Author, Year	n	Renal failure %	n	Paraplegia %	n	Mortality %	n
Grabitz, 1996	122	12.7	15	7.4	9	14.7	8
Mauney, 1996	91	11.0	10	9.9	9	13.2	12
Galloway, 1996	24	7.7	6	3.7	1	10.3	8
Cambria, 2002	337	13.5	45	6.6	22	8.3	28
Coselli, 2003 *	584	7.5	44	7.2	42	6.8	40
Schepens, 2004	123	16.9	21	16.1	20	14.1	17
Simple cross-clamp	**1281**	**11.0**	**141**	**8.0**	**103**	**8.8**	**113**
Grabitz, 1996	102	6.8	7	6.8	7	6.8	7
Galloway, 1996	54	7.7	6	4.2	2	10.3	8
Schepens, 1998	102	6.8	7	9.8	10	6.8	7
Coselli, 2003 *	666	5.2	35	3.9	26	5.0	33
Safi, 2003	741	-	-	2.4	18	-	-
Quinones-Baldrich, 1999	50	8.3	4	2.7	1	5.5	3
Lombardi, 2003	279	3.6	10	5.3	15	11.5	32
Chiesa, 2004	107	4.1	4	7.5	8	12.1	1
Left heart bypass	**2101**	**3.5**	**73**	**4.1**	**87**	**4.3**	**91**
Kunoiyoshi, 2004 **	52	0	0	0	0	9.6	5
Jacobs, 2004	279	1.0	3	2.1	6	8.6	24
Selective visceral perfusion	**331**	**0.9**	**3**	**2.2**	**6**	**8.8**	**29**

* Crawford Type I and II only

** 22/52 patients had selective visceral perfusion.

In a non-randomised prospective study of selective visceral perfusion, in which retrograde aortic flow was maintained by left heart bypass, and visceral flow by selective catheterisation of the visceral and renal arteries, renal impairment was minimised [38]. However, in a subsequent, smaller prospective non-randomised study using the same technique, renal failure was not reduced [39]. Achieving adequate flow rates through small distal catheters appears to have been the problem in the latter study. In a larger experience that included 279 patients managed with selective perfusion, the authors achieved an impressive 1% rate of renal failure that needed temporary haemodialysis [40]. In this study the flow through individual catheters was measured; the mean renal perfusion pressure was 69mmHg and the flow rate was 275mL/min, which exceeds that in previous studies and may help explain the apparent benefit.

Ischaemia / reperfusion injury

Visceral ischaemia/reperfusion injury is now believed to be a significant contributor to multiple organ dysfunction, spinal cord injury and renal failure after TAA repair. Ischaemia/reperfusion is associated with cellular dysfunction, leading to the build up of toxic products and the generation of pro-inflammatory cytokines, arachidonic acid breakdown products and oxygen-derived free radicals. Gut mucosal integrity is compromised and bacterial products (endotoxin and proteoglycans) can enter the circulation. Peak plasma endotoxin and neutrophil activation correlate with the development of organ dysfunction [41]. The cytokines tumour necrosis factor-alpha, and interleukins -6, -8 and -10 are also raised following TAA repair and appear to be important mediators of the systemic response [42]. It is too early to predict if these pathways can be moderated by therapeutic intervention, but the roles of endotoxin, neutrophil activation and endothelial adhesion warrant further study and a number of pharmacological agents capable of protecting organs are already under investigation.

Results of open surgery

The major case series reporting open TAA repair published in the last ten years are shown in Table 2. It should be remembered that these series are heterogeneous and subject to reporting bias; in a recent publication from the Nationwide Inpatient Sample, a stratified database of discharges from 20% of USA hospitals, 30-day mortality for elective TAA repair was 22% [43].

Endovascular repair for TAA

Very few patients have an hourglass-shape aneurysm to allow both thoracic and abdominal components of the aneurysm to be stented without visceral or renal revascularisation. In the majority a hybrid operation or branched stent graft is needed.

Hybrid repair

The St. Mary's approach for hybrid repair was described in 2003 [44]. The abdominal aorta, iliac arteries, coeliac axis, superior mesenteric artery (SMA) and renal arteries are exposed via a transperitoneal approach using an abdominal incision. Simultaneously a branched graft is constructed from an inverted 14 by 7mm Dacron graft with two additional 8mm side-grafts. Following heparin administration the branched graft is anastomosed to a pre-existing or a newly inserted infrarenal aortic graft, the distal aorta, or the proximal iliac arteries. In patients who have had previous repair of the infrarenal aorta, the existing graft provides a safe distal landing zone for the stent graft and take-off point for the retrograde bypass. The graft to the coeliac axis is tunnelled retroperitoneally, in front of the pancreas and anastomosed end-to-side to the origin of the hepatic artery. The graft to the SMA is anastomosed proximally to avoid damage to the middle colic branch and lies as a loose 'Lazy C' curve so that it does not kink when the small bowel is returned to the abdomen (Figure 5).

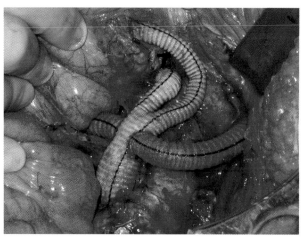

Figure 5. Retrograde visceral and renal artery revascularisation demonstrating the 'lazy C' curve on the superior mesenteric artery bypass.

The renal arteries are sequentially anastomosed end-to-side with the graft to the right renal artery tunnelled through the base of the small bowel mesentery. The origins of these arteries are ligated on completion of the anastomosis. Next, a suitable access site is chosen for endovascular stent deployment, usually via a 10mm side-graft sewn onto the retrograde bypass. For proximal stent fixation it is safe to cover the origin of the left subclavian artery; carotid-carotid bypass allows fixation even more proximally in the arch. A hybrid approach allows the entire aorta from the left subclavian origin to the bifurcation to be excluded, leaving the viscera and renal arteries perfused from the proximal iliac arteries (Figure 6). Deploying the stent at the time of open surgery has advantages since any disruption of flow in the visceral grafts can be corrected immediately.

In a consecutive series of 29 patients in whom the hybrid approach was attempted (Crawford Type I in 3, II in 18, III in 7 and IV in 1), 30-day mortality was 13% and no patient suffered paraplegia, although this complication may be expected at some point as experience increases [45]. At a median follow-up of eight months, graft patency is encouraging (98%) but the Type I endoleak rate (26%) is a concern. Many other surgeons have adopted a similar approach, though usually only in patients considered high risk for open repair, having re-do surgery or with a heavily calcified aorta [46-48]. At St. Mary's this procedure is

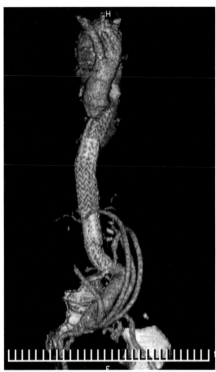

Figure 6. CT reconstruction of completed hybrid procedure showing the aortic stent and grafts to the coeliac, superior mesenteric and renal arteries.

now done preferentially for most TAAs, except Crawford Type IV.

Branched endografts

Developments in endograft technology have led to the availability of commercial custom endografts that can branch into the coeliac, SMA and renal arteries. These endografts allow a totally endovascular approach to the treatment of TAA [49, 50]. The only reported case series is from the Cleveland Clinic, where nine patients with TAA and 20 with a suprarenal aneurysm have been treated [51]. Thirty-day mortality was 2%, but there were three late aneurysm-related deaths, presumably due to failed aneurysm exclusion. Branched endografts may replace the hybrid approach as technology improves, though the cost of the different procedures may affect uptake.

Conclusions

Patients with TAA already have a reduced life expectancy from cardiovascular, pulmonary and renal disease. Open surgical repair can reduce the risk of rupture, but at a significant risk of renal failure, paraplegia or death. The results of open repair appear to have improved with the use of adjuvant techniques, despite the fact that there is rarely direct evidence of the efficacy of these interventions. It must not be forgotten that the excellent results reported in the literature may not reflect prospective national audit data. Currently, most centres reserve hybrid and branched endovascular techniques for patients considered at high risk for open repair.

Strategies to prevent paraplegia, renal failure and multiple organ failure are crucial to the success of these complex operations. Left heart bypass, CSF drainage and intercostal re-implantation are now established methods used in many major centres. Spinal cord monitoring, local epidural cooling and selective visceral perfusion are technically challenging and have only been adopted by a minority of centres. It is likely that in the future TAA repair will be performed in a limited number of specialist centres offering full technical support and the option of endovascular intervention.

Key points	Evidence level
◆ The annual rupture risk for a 6cm TAA is <5%.	IIa/B
◆ Results of open repair, in terms of renal impairment, paraplegia and mortality have improved over the last 20 years.	III/B
◆ The following are used selectively by surgeons to minimise the risks of paraplegia:	
• left heart bypass;	IIa/B
• hypothermia;	IIa/B
• spinal cord monitoring and CSF drainage;	Ia/A
• selective visceral perfusion; and	IIb/B
• re-implantation of lumbar and intercostal arteries.	IIb/B
◆ The introduction of endovascular procedures, including hybrid and branched endografts, may reduce mortality and paraplegia rates, but patients who undergo these procedures should have careful follow-up to ensure their durability.	IV/C

References

1. Cowan JA, Jr., Dimick JB, Wainess RM, *et al*. Ruptured thoracoabdominal aortic aneurysm treatment in the United States: 1988 to 1998. *J Vasc Surg* 2003; 38: 319-22.

2. Khan SN, Stansby G. Cerebrospinal fluid drainage for thoracic and thoracoabdominal aortic aneurysm surgery. *Cochrane Database Syst Rev* 2004; 1: CD003635.

3. Cina CS, Abouzahr L, Arena GO, *et al*. Cerebrospinal fluid drainage to prevent paraplegia during thoracic and thoracoabdominal aortic aneurysm surgery: a systematic review and meta-analysis. *J Vasc Surg* 2004; 40: 36-44.

4. Coselli JS, Lemaire SA, Koksoy C, *et al*. Cerebrospinal fluid drainage reduces paraplegia after thoracoabdominal aortic aneurysm repair: results of a randomized clinical trial. *J Vasc Surg* 2002; 35: 631-9.

5. Kindgen-Milles D, Muller E, Buhl R, *et al*. Nasal-continuous positive airway pressure reduces pulmonary morbidity and length of hospital stay following thoracoabdominal aortic surgery. *Chest* 2005; 128: 821-8.

6. Koksoy C, LeMaire SA, Curling PE, *et al*. Renal perfusion during thoracoabdominal aortic operations: cold crystalloid is superior to normothermic blood. *Ann Thorac Surg* 2002; 73: 730-8.

7. Juvonen T, Ergin M, Galla J, *et al*. Prospective study of the natural history of thoracic aortic aneurysms. *Ann Thorac Surg* 1997; 63: 1533-45.

8. Elefteriades JA. Natural history of thoracic aortic aneurysms: indications for surgery, and surgical versus nonsurgical risks. *Ann Thorac Surg* 2002; 74: S1877-80.

9. Miller CC, 3rd, Porat EE, Estrera AL, *et al*. Number needed to treat: analyzing of the effectiveness of thoracoabdominal aortic repair. *Eur J Vasc Endovasc Surg* 2004; 28: 154-7.

10. Rectenwald J, Huber TS, Martin TD, *et al*. Functional outcome after thoracoabdominal aortic aneurysm repair. *J Vasc Surg* 2002; 35: 640-7.

11. Gilling-Smith GL, Worswick L, Knight PF, *et al*. Surgical repair of thoracoabdominal aortic aneurysm: 10 years' experience. *Br J Surg* 1995; 82: 624-9.

12. Svensson LG, Crawford ES, Hess KR, *et al*. Experience with 1509 patients undergoing thoracoabdominal aortic operations. *J Vasc Surg* 1993; 17: 357-68.

13. Coselli JS, LeMaire SA, Miller CC, 3rd, *et al*. Mortality and paraplegia after thoracoabdominal aortic aneurysm repair: a risk factor analysis. *Ann Thorac Surg* 2000; 69: 409-14.

14. Brooks MJ, Kerle M, Cheshire NJ, *et al*. Thoracoabdominal aortic aneurysm: evaluation of pre-operative assessment in 257 elective repairs. *Br J Surg* 2000; 87: 1-92.

15. Miller CC, 3rd, Porat EE, Estrera AL, *et al*. Analysis of short-term multivariate competing risks data following thoracic and thoracoabdominal aortic repair. *Eur J Cardiothorac Surg* 2003; 23: 1023-7.

16. Suzuki S, Davis CA, 3rd, Miller CC, 3rd, *et al*. Cardiac function predicts mortality following thoracoabdominal and descending thoracic aortic aneurysm repair. *Eur J Cardiothorac Surg* 2003; 24: 119-24.

17. Cox GS, O'Hara PJ, Hertzer NR, *et al*. Thoracoabdominal aneurysm repair: a representative experience. *J Vasc Surg* 1992; 15: 780-7.

18. Brooks MJ, Bradbury A, Wolfe HN. Elective repair of type IV thoraco-abdominal aortic aneurysms; experience of a

subcostal (transabdominal) approach. *Eur J Vasc Endovasc Surg* 1999; 18: 290-3.

19. Svensson LG, Patel V, Robinson MF, *et al.* Influence of preservation or perfusion of intraoperatively identified spinal cord blood supply on spinal motor evoked potentials and paraplegia after aortic surgery. *J Vasc Surg* 1991; 13: 355-65.

20. Cambria RP, Davison JK, Zannetti S, *et al.* Thoracoabdominal aneurysm repair: perspectives over a decade with the clamp-and-sew technique. *Ann Surg* 1997; 226: 294-303.

21. von Segesser LK, Marty B, Mueller X, *et al.* Active cooling during open repair of thoraco-abdominal aortic aneurysms improves outcome. *Eur J Cardiothorac Surg* 2001; 19: 411-5.

22. Kouchoukos NT, Masetti P, Rokkas CK, *et al.* Hypothermic cardiopulmonary bypass and circulatory arrest for operations on the descending thoracic and thoracoabdominal aorta. *Ann Thorac Surg* 2002; 74: S1885-7.

23. Soukiasian HJ, Raissi SS, Kleisli T, *et al.* Total circulatory arrest for the replacement of the descending and thoracoabdominal aorta. *Arch Surg* 2005; 140: 394-8.

24. Motoyoshi N, Takahashi G, Sakurai M, *et al.* Safety and efficacy of epidural cooling for regional spinal cord hypothermia during thoracoabdominal aneurysm repair. *Eur J Cardiothorac Surg* 2004; 25: 139-41.

25. Coselli JS. The use of left heart bypass in the repair of thoracoabdominal aortic aneurysms: current techniques and results. *Semin Thorac Cardiovasc Surg* 2003; 15: 326-32.

26. Safi HJ, Hess KR, Randel M, *et al.* Cerebrospinal fluid drainage and distal aortic perfusion: reducing neurologic complications in repair of thoracoabdominal aortic aneurysm types I and II. *J Vasc Surg* 1996; 23: 223-8.

27. Laschinger JC, Cunningham JN, Jr, Catinella FP, *et al.* Detection and prevention of intraoperative spinal cord ischemia after cross-clamping of the thoracic aorta: use of somatosensory evoked potentials. *Surgery* 1982; 92: 1109-17.

28. Grabitz K, Sandmann W, Stuhmeier K, *et al.* The risk of ischemic spinal cord injury in patients undergoing graft replacement for thoracoabdominal aortic aneurysms. *J Vasc Surg* 1996; 23: 230-40.

29. Jacobs MJ, Mess W, Mochtar B, *et al.* The value of motor evoked potentials in reducing paraplegia during thoracoabdominal aneurysm repair. *J Vasc Surg* 2006; 43: 239-46.

30. Elmore JR, Gloviczki P, Harper CM, Jr., *et al.* Spinal cord injury in experimental thoracic aortic occlusion: investigation of combined methods of protection. *J Vasc Surg* 1992; 15: 789-98.

31. McCullough JL, Hollier LH, Nugent M. Paraplegia after thoracic aortic occlusion: influence of cerebrospinal fluid drainage. Experimental and early clinical results. *J Vasc Surg* 1988; 7: 153-60.

32. Svensson LG, Hess KR, D'Agostino RS, *et al.* Reduction of neurologic injury after high-risk thoracoabdominal aortic operation. *Ann Thorac Surg* 1998; 66: 132-8.

33. Crawford ES, Svensson LG, Hess KR, *et al.* A prospective randomized study of cerebrospinal fluid drainage to prevent paraplegia after high-risk surgery on the thoracoabdominal aorta. *J Vasc Surg* 1991; 13: 36-45.

34. Acher CW, Wynn MM, Hoch JR, *et al.* Combined use of cerebral spinal fluid drainage and naloxone reduces the risk of paraplegia in thoracoabdominal aneurysm repair. *J Vasc Surg* 1994; 19: 236-46.

35. Estrera AL, Rubenstein FS, Miller CC, 3rd, *et al.* Descending thoracic aortic aneurysm: surgical approach and treatment using the adjuncts cerebrospinal fluid drainage and distal aortic perfusion. *Ann Thorac Surg* 2001; 72: 481-6.

36. Hassoun HT, Miller CC, 3rd, Huynh TT, *et al.* Cold visceral perfusion improves early survival in patients with acute renal failure after thoracoabdominal aortic aneurysm repair. *J Vasc Surg* 2004; 39: 506-12.

37. von Segesser LK, Killer I, Jenni R, *et al.* Improved distal circulatory support for repair of descending thoracic aortic aneurysms. *Ann Thorac Surg* 1993; 56: 1373-80.

38. Najafi H. 1980: descending aortic aneurysmectomy without adjuncts to avoid ischemia. 1993 update. *Ann Thorac Surg* 1993; 55: 1042-5.

39. Leijdekkers VJ, Wirds JW, Vahl AC, *et al.* The visceral perfusion system and distal bypass during thoracoabdominal aneurysm surgery: an alternative for physiological blood flow? *Cardiovasc Surg* 1999; 7: 219-24.

40. Jacobs MJ, van Eps RG, de Jong DS, *et al.* Prevention of renal failure in patients undergoing thoracoabdominal aortic aneurysm repair. *J Vasc Surg* 2004; 40: 1067-73.

41. Foulds S, Cheshire NJ, Schachter M, *et al.* Endotoxin related early neutrophil activation is associated with outcome after thoracoabdominal aortic aneurysm repair. *Br J Surg* 1997; 84: 172-7.

42. Welborn MB, Oldenburg HS, Hess PJ, *et al.* The relationship between visceral ischemia, proinflammatory cytokines, and organ injury in patients undergoing thoracoabdominal aortic aneurysm repair. *Crit Care Med* 2000; 28: 3191-7.

43. Cowan JA, Jr., Dimick JB, Henke PK, *et al.* Surgical treatment of intact thoracoabdominal aortic aneurysms in the United States: hospital and surgeon volume-related outcomes. *J Vasc Surg* 2003; 37: 1169-74.

44. Rimmer J, Wolfe JH. Type III thoracoabdominal aortic aneurysm repair: a combined surgical and endovascular approach. *Eur J Vasc Endovasc Surg* 2003; 26: 677-9.

45. Black SA, Wolfe JH, Clark M, *et al.* Complex thoracoabdominal aortic aneurysms: endovascular exclusion with visceral revascularization. *J Vasc Surg* 2006; 43: 1081-9.

46. Flye MW, Choi ET, Sanchez LA, *et al.* Retrograde visceral vessel revascularization followed by endovascular aneurysm exclusion as an alternative to open surgical repair of thoracoabdominal aortic aneurysm. *J Vasc Surg* 2004; 39: 454-8.

47. Iguro Y, Yotsumoto G, Ishizaki N, *et al.* Endovascular stent-graft repair for thoracoabdominal aneurysm after reconstruction of the superior mesenteric and celiac arteries. *J Thorac Cardiovasc Surg* 2003; 125: 956-8.

48. Ruppert V, Salewski J, Wintersperger BJ, *et al*. Endovascular repair of thoracoabdominal aortic aneurysm with multivisceral revascularization. *J Vasc Surg* 2005; 42: 368.

49. Anderson JL, Adam DJ, Berce M, *et al*. Repair of thoracoabdominal aortic aneurysms with fenestrated and branched endovascular stent grafts. *J Vasc Surg* 2005; 42: 600-7.

50. Bleyn J, Schol F, Vanhandenhove I, *et al*. Side-branched modular endograft system for thoracoabdominal aortic aneurysm repair. *J Endovasc Ther* 2002; 9: 838-41.

51. Greenberg RK, West K, Pfaff K, *et al*. Beyond the aortic bifurcation: branched endovascular grafts for thoracoabdominal and aortoiliac aneurysms. *J Vasc Surg* 2006; 43: 879-86.

Chapter 20

Duplex imaging for varicose veins

Timothy A Lees MD FRCS, Consultant Vascular Surgeon, Freeman Hospital, Newcastle upon Tyne, UK

Crispian Oates MSc MIPEM AVS, Consultant Physicist, Newcastle General Hospital, Newcastle upon Tyne, UK

Sanjay Nalachandran FRCS, Clinical Fellow, Freeman Hospital, Newcastle upon Tyne, UK

Introduction

Continuous wave Doppler ultrasound was first used clinically to detect blood flow in the 1950s. The use of pulsed Doppler ultrasound and, subsequently, duplex imaging became widespread in the 1970s, predominantly for arteries. Duplex imaging of veins only really developed significantly in the 1980s, but considerable expansion has occurred since then with the advent of more powerful scanning machines with higher resolution. Duplex ultrasonography is now the most frequently used investigation for venous disorders.

Duplex imaging combines a B-mode grey scale image with a Doppler waveform trace, which allows a vessel to be examined for flow direction and velocity. A colour display can be superimposed on the B-mode image to show areas where echoes are Doppler shifted, providing an easy method of evaluating venous flow and its direction. This colour technique may be referred to as 'colour flow imaging', 'colour duplex' or 'colour Doppler ultrasonography'.

Diagnostic capability of duplex imaging

Duplex imaging can be used to examine the following features of the venous circulation.

Anatomy:

◆ presence or absence of a vein;
◆ presence of duplicate veins;
◆ number of veins, e.g. perforating veins;
◆ diameter of veins;
◆ presence or absence of venous valves;
◆ presence of thrombus and recanalised channels;
◆ position of veins, e.g. position of the saphenopopliteal junction.

Function:

◆ which veins or which segments of vein are incompetent;
◆ source of filling of incompetent veins;
◆ duration of reflux;
◆ quantity of reflux (although there is doubt about accuracy).

The ability of duplex imaging to detect blood flow and its direction is particularly useful in the diagnosis of abnormalities in venous flow, especially reflux. Duplex imaging can also guide treatment. For example, it is used widely in radiofrequency and laser ablation of veins and in foam sclerotherapy (see Chapter 22).

Indications for duplex imaging

Whether or not duplex imaging should be used routinely in the investigation of varicose veins is controversial; to some extent this will depend on the resources available. Many surgeons consider a selective policy of scanning to be appropriate and that simple varicose veins are adequately investigated using only a hand-held Doppler device. The evidence for this view is discussed later but, whatever the clinical viewpoint, the following conditions are certainly suitable for duplex investigation.

◆ primary varicose veins affecting the long or short saphenous systems;
◆ primary non-saphenous varicose veins;
◆ recurrent varicose veins;
◆ suspected deep vein disease and chronic venous disorders (e.g. post-thrombotic limb);
◆ vascular malformations.

Duplex imaging is also useful in assessing the effect of treatment and for surface marking of veins before both venous and arterial operations.

Equipment and techniques

Details of the techniques used for venous duplex imaging are available in a European Consensus Document published on behalf of the Union Internationale de Phlebologie **(IV/C)** [1]. If the equipment has sufficient sensitivity to image and show colour flow, varicose veins may be assessed using a small portable scanner. The alternative is a full-sized machine of higher specification (Figure 1). Scanning is performed using a 7.5-12MHz linear array probe so that in longitudinal section veins are viewed at a constant angle to the probe face. A 3.5-5MHz linear array transducer can be useful for obese or oedematous limbs and a curvilinear array transducer for pelvic veins.

Standard procedure is to image the thigh veins with the patient standing in front of the sonographer, who is seated on a chair in a position to view the screen and operate the controls. The vein of interest is imaged in cross-section with the probe angled

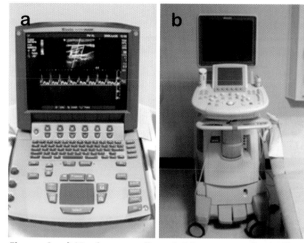

Figure 1. a) Modern small portable scanner including Doppler colour flow imaging. b) Modern full-sized machine of higher specification. Both machines are suitable for the examination of venous anatomy and function in patients with varicose veins.

towards the patient's head and the colour Doppler box positioned over the vein. Care must be taken not to compress the vein. The colour scale is set low to enable the slow flow typical of veins to be imaged. Venous flow is elicited by requesting the patient to dorsiflex the foot, keeping the heel on the floor, and then resting the foot down again; any reflux is observed on the colour display. Examination of the popliteal fossa may also be made with the patient standing, but this time facing away from the sonographer. Flow is elicited by compression of the calf, either by hand or by rapid inflation of a pneumatic cuff. An alternative method for the popliteal fossa (which is used routinely for calf veins) is for the patient to sit on the edge of a raised couch with the forefoot resting on the sonographer's chair. The calf can then be compressed with one hand and the probe manipulated with the other. This method avoids awkward bending and back strain. Finally, to confirm the site of the saphenopopliteal junction the patient is asked to stand with their back to the sonographer.

Diagnosing reflux

The presence of reflux is usually obvious on the colour image, but can also be examined using the

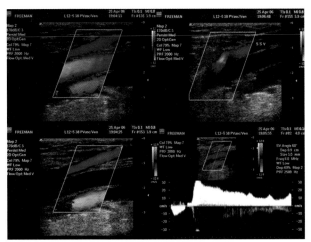

Figure 2. Doppler waveform displaying reflux.

Doppler waveform display (Figure 2). The duration of reflux that indicates a pathological situation is uncertain. Van Bemmelen *et al* [2] demonstrated that normal popliteal valves close within 0.66s and so a level of 1s seems a reasonable indication of pathology. If reflux is encountered at an unusual site, its source should be sought by tracking up what may be a very tortuous and branching vessel. In the case of reflux in the gastrocnemius system, there is nearly always a perforator connecting to superficial veins and this should be located. Similarly, reflux in a deep vein of the calf may run to a single perforator that may be dealt with surgically. If there is short saphenous reflux, the position of the saphenopopliteal junction, which is variable, can be marked before surgery. Perforators may also be marked. A useful technique is to apply dark 'water colour' pencil through the coupling gel, with the centre of the probe over the point to be identified. The gel can then be wiped away and the mark made secure using a permanent marker pen.

Evidence

Duplex imaging and anatomy

Duplex imaging has allowed considerable new understanding of normal anatomy and its variations (which are encountered often). A consensus document from the Union Internationale de Phlebologie has detailed the anatomy of the lower limb venous system as defined by duplex; this work relies on a combination of data from previous studies and the opinions of recognised experts [3] **(III-IV/B)**.

The long saphenous vein (LSV) runs from in front of the medial malleolus up the medial side of the calf and thigh to terminate at its junction with the common femoral vein, the saphenofemoral junction. In the thigh there may be anterior and posterior accessory saphenous veins (AASV and PASV), and anterior and posterior thigh circumflex veins (tributaries of the LSV, or of the AASV and PASV, respectively). The short saphenous vein (SSV) runs from behind the lateral malleolus up the posterior aspect of the calf to terminate in the popliteal fossa at the saphenopopliteal junction (SPJ). The location of this junction varies, but in 60% of people it lies between 2-7cm above the skin crease of the knee [4] **(IIb/B)**. A continuation of the SSV (thigh extension of the SSV) may branch in the thigh to join the LSV and this is known as the Vein of Giacomini. There may also be a lateral venous system on the lateral side of the thigh and calf, and various intersaphenous veins that connect the LSV to the SSV. Finally, there are four principal groups of perforating veins in both calf and thigh that connect the deep veins to the superficial veins. These may be delineated as medial, anterior, lateral and posterior perforators.

Duplex imaging versus hand-held Doppler and clinical examination

Studies that have compared duplex imaging with other more simple methods of venous assessment fall into two main groups: those that assess the findings of the other methods compared to duplex, and those that assess the potential or actual clinical outcome of treatments based on the different methods of investigation. These trials are summarised in Table 1. In summary, the sensitivity of hand-held Doppler compared to duplex imaging at the SFJ is between 60-100% and at the SPJ it is 25-90%; the specificity is between 70-100% at the SFJ and between 90-100% at the SPJ. Inadequate surgery will be performed on between 1-10% of patients if planned on the basis of hand-held Doppler and clinical examination alone, without the aid of duplex imaging.

Table 1. Summary of published results from trials comparing duplex imaging to other methods.				
Author	**Type of evidence**	**Imaging**	**Number**	**Results of limbs**
Singh 1996 [5]	IIa/B	3 independent surgical assessments: CE, CE+ HHD, CE+D	71	When compared with D, inappropriate surgery would have been performed on 20% on the basis of CE and on 13% on the basis of HHD
Campbell 1997 [6]	IIa/B	All limbs had HHD followed by D by an independent operator	122	When compared with D, HHD missed 11 instances of popliteal fossa reflux of which 4 involved the SSV. Overall, HHD missed 11% of LSV or SSV reflux
Darke 1997 [7]	IIa/B	All limbs had HHD followed by D by an independent operator	100	In diagnosis of LSV incompetence (87 limbs), compared with D, HHD had sensitivity of 95% and specificity of 100%. For the SSV (21 limbs) the sensitivity was 90% and the specificity 93%
Wills 1998 [8]	IIa/B	All limbs had HHD followed by D by an independent operator	315	38% had recurrent disease. Sensitivity of CE with HHD compared to D was 71% at SFJ, 36% at SPJ, 44% in perforating veins, and 29% in deep veins. 29% of patients felt to have sole SFJ incompetence, if treated by saphenofemoral disconnection, strip and phlebectomies would have had sites of reflux untreated
Mercer 1998 [9]	IIa/B	All limbs had HHD followed by D by an independent operator	89	Sensitivity of HHD compared to D was 73% at SFJ, 77% at SPJ, and 51% for perforating veins. For primary varicose veins, planned surgery on the basis of HHD and CE would have left sites of reflux in 24%
Kent 1998 [10]	IIa/B	All limbs had HHD followed by D by an independent operator	108	A policy of selective D for suspected SSV incompetence, no identifiable sites of reflux, or posterior thigh perforator reflux on HHD would have resulted in appropriate surgery in 94%, excess surgery in 5% and inadequate surgery in 1%
Kim 2000 [11]	IIa/B	All limbs had HHD followed by D by an independent operator	70	The sensitivity of HHD compared to D was 97% at the SFJ, 82% in the LSV and 80% at the SPJ
Smith 2002 [12]	Ib/A	RCT of D marking of varicose veins compared to CE or HHD marking before surgery. 12-month CE and D follow-up	149	Marking with D for the LSV system conferred no benefit in terms of satisfactory vein surgery or recurrence at 1 year. Quality of life improved in all groups. Benefit for the SSV not clear
Rautio 2002 [13]	IIa/B	All limbs had CE and HHD followed by D by an independent operator. Plan for treatment was recorded after each of CE, HHD and D	142	Sensitivity of HHD compared to D was 56% at SFJ and 23% at SPJ; specificity 97% and 96%, respectively. CE failed in 51% for perforating veins. Primary varicose vein surgery on the basis of HHD and CE would have left sites of reflux in 24%
Campbell 2005 [14]	IIa/B	Patients within a RCT were evaluated with HHD and then D. Clinicians were asked to state after HHD examination when they would order D	1218	D would not have been requested in 645 of 1052 (62%) limbs. Among these, HHD missed significant reflux in the LSV in 18 (3%) and the SSV in 25 (4%). Reasons for requesting D were popliteal fossa reflux (202), recurrent (94) or atypical (86) varicose veins, and possible previous thrombosis (67)

CE = clinical examination; HHD = hand-held Doppler; D = duplex imaging; LSV = long saphenous vein; SSV = short saphenous vein; RCT = randomised controlled trial

Blomgren *et al* [15] performed a randomised controlled trial of surgery for varicose veins with, or without pre-operative duplex imaging **(Ib/A)**. Re-operation rates, and clinical and duplex findings, were compared at two months and two years after surgery. In Group 1, 166 legs were operated after duplex imaging; in Group 2, 177 legs were operated without such imaging. In 44 legs (26.5%), duplex examination suggested a different surgical procedure than had been considered on clinical grounds and the operation was changed accordingly for 29 legs. At two months, incompetence was detected at the SFJ or SPJ (or both) in 14 legs (8.8%) in Group 1 and in 44 legs (26.5%) in Group 2 (p<0.001). At two years, two legs (1.4%) had undergone or were awaiting re-operation in Group 1 and 14 (9.5%) in Group 2 (p=0.002). In the remainder, major incompetence was found in 19 legs (15.0%) in Group 1 and in 53 (41.1%) in Group 2 (p<0.001). This is one of a few trials that shows that routine pre-operative duplex examination leads to an improvement in surgical results for patients with primary varicose veins.

In light of the above, a good argument can be made for performing duplex imaging in all patients with varicose veins for whom treatment is planned. The counter argument is that scanning is expensive and time-consuming for already stretched vascular laboratories. A compromise is to scan all patients except those with simple LSV incompetence, as such a policy minimises (but does not eradicate) errors of diagnosis.

Duplex versus other functional investigations

A few studies have compared duplex imaging with functional investigations other than hand-held Doppler for the diagnosis and quantification of venous reflux. Payne *et al* [16] compared air plethysmography with clinical assessment, ambulatory venous pressure measurement and duplex ultrasonography in 103 unselected legs with venous disease and ten normal control legs. Measurements of venous function obtained by air plethysmography showed considerable overlap between groups of limbs classified on the basis of clinical condition or by the presence of popliteal incompetence detected by duplex imaging **(IIa/B)**.

Duplex for recurrent varicose veins

Duplex imaging has been used widely in the assessment of recurrent varicose veins and it appears to be a reliable non-invasive method of detecting a residual LSV stump with incompetence of the SFJ [17] **(IIa/B)**. A further study has assessed whether duplex imaging one year after SFJ ligation might predict results after five years. This involved 100 legs and the scan had a sensitivity of 80%, with a specificity of 91%, a positive predictive value of 70% and a negative predictive value of 95% in predicting recurrent disease at five years [18] **(IIa/B)**.

Conclusions

Duplex imaging has become the most frequently used investigation for varicose veins. It is simple, relatively cheap, non-invasive, and provides considerable information on anatomy and function of varicose veins. Studies have demonstrated it to be a reliable and accurate investigation that can help to direct surgery for varicose veins, thereby improving the clinical outcome of such surgery.

Key points	Evidence level

◆ Duplex imaging has become the standard method of assessing venous haemodynamics of the leg, with an agreed methodology - European consensus document. — IV/C

◆ Knowledge of anatomy has increased as a result of duplex imaging. Methodology for assessing venous anatomy using duplex imaging has been defined - European consensus document. — III/B

◆ Pre-operative duplex imaging identifies sites of reflux more accurately than hand-held Doppler or clinical examination. — IIa/B

◆ Pre-operative duplex imaging allows more appropriate planning of surgery. — IIa/B

◆ Pre-operative duplex imaging improves outcome after varicose vein surgery. — Ib/A

◆ Pre-operative duplex marking of the LSV confers no benefit over other methods of marking; evidence for the SSV is unclear. — Ib/A

◆ Duplex imaging reliably detects sites of reflux in recurrence disease and may be useful in predicting recurrence following varicose vein surgery. — IIa/B

References

1. Coleridge-Smith P, Labropoulos N, Partsch H, et al. Duplex ultrasound investigation of the veins in chronic venous disease of the lower limbs - UIP consensus document. Part I. Basic principles. Eur J Vasc Endovasc Surg 2006; 31: 83-92.

2. Van Bemmelen PS, Beach K, Bedford G, Strandness DE Jr. The mechanism of venous valve closure. Its relationship to the velocity of reverse flow. Arch Surg 1990; 125: 617-9.

3. Cavezzi A, Labropoulos N, Partsch H, et al. Duplex ultrasound investigation of the veins in chronic venous disease of the lower limbs - UIP consensus document. Part II. Anatomy. Eur J Vasc Endovasc Surg 2006; 31: 288-99.

4. Vasdekis SN, Clarke GH, Hobbs JT, Nicolaides AN. Evaluation of non-invasive and invasive methods in the assessment of short saphenous vein termination. Br J Surg 1989; 76: 929-32.

5. Singh S, Lees TA, Donlon M, et al. Improving preoperative assessment of varicose veins. Br J Surg 1997; 84: 801-2.

6. Campbell WB, Niblett PG, Ridler BM, et al. Hand-held Doppler as a screening test in primary varicose veins. Br J Surg 1997; 84: 1541-3.

7. Darke SG, Vetrivel S, Foy DM, et al. A comparison of duplex scanning and continuous wave Doppler in the assessment of primary and uncomplicated varicose veins. Eur J Vasc Endovasc Surg 1997; 14: 457-61.

8. Wills V, Moylan D, Chambers J. The use of routine duplex scanning in the assessment of varicose veins. ANZ J Surg 1998; 68: 41-4.

9. Mercer KG, Scott DJ, Berridge DC. Preoperative duplex imaging is required before all operations for primary varicose veins. Br J Surg 1998; 85: 1495-7.

10. Kent PJ, Weston MJ. Duplex scanning may be used selectively in patients with primary varicose veins. Ann R Coll Surg Engl 1998; 80: 388-93.

11. Kim J, Richards S, Kent PJ. Clinical examination of varicose veins - a validation study. Ann R Coll Surg Engl 2000; 82: 171-5.

12. Smith JJ, Brown L, Greenhalgh RM, Davies AH. Randomised trial of pre-operative colour duplex marking in primary varicose vein surgery: outcome is not improved. Eur J Vasc Endovasc Surg 2002; 23: 336-43.

13. Rautio T, Perälä J, Biancari F, et al. Accuracy of hand-held Doppler in planning the operation for primary varicose veins. Eur J Vasc Endovasc Surg 2002; 24: 450-5.

14. Campbell WB, Niblett PG, Peters AS, et al. The clinical effectiveness of hand-held Doppler examination for diagnosis of reflux in patients with varicose veins. Eur J Vasc Endovasc Surg 2005; 30: 664-9.

15. Blomgren L, Johansson G, Bergqvist D. Randomized clinical trial of routine preoperative duplex imaging before varicose vein surgery. Br J Surg 2005; 92: 688-94.

16. Payne SP, Thrush AJ, London NJ, et al. Venous assessment using air plethysmography: a comparison with clinical examination, ambulatory venous pressure measurement and duplex scanning. Br J Surg 1993; 80: 967-70.

17. Berbabou JE, Molnar LJ. Duplex sonographic evaluation of saphenofemoral junction in patients with recurrent varicose veins after surgery. J Clin Ultrasound 1998; 26: 401-4.

18. DeMaeseneer MG, Vanderbroeck CP. Accuracy of duplex evaluation 1 year after varicose vein surgery to predict recurrence at the saphenofemoral junction after 5 years. Eur J Vasc Endovasc Surg 2005; 29: 308-12.

Chapter 21

Optimal varicose vein surgery

Jonothan J Earnshaw DM FRCS, Consultant Vascular Surgeon

Gloucestershire Royal Hospital, Gloucester, UK

Introduction

Over the past 50 years, apart from a brief enthusiasm for liquid sclerotherapy in the 1970s, surgery has remained the pre-eminent treatment for varicose veins. Currently, however, several new endovenous techniques are being promoted (Chapter 22), although formal comparisons with conventional surgery do not yet exist. The time is right for a re-evaluation of the strengths and weaknesses of standard operations for varicose veins [1].

Surgical specialisation over the last 20 years has led to trained vascular surgeons performing an increasing amount of the venous surgery in the UK. Furthermore, the science of varicose vein surgery has advanced rapidly with the advent of duplex imaging (Chapter 20), resulting in the accurate, non-invasive diagnosis of both anatomical and haemodynamic venous abnormalities. Despite this, the general perception is that the results of operations for varicose veins remain poor. This is reflected in the pessimism (or realism) among family doctors who refer patients for a specialist opinion. While few other elective surgical operations bear such a high perceived risk of disease recurrence, there is very little objective information about actual recurrence rates. The main problem is that it is difficult to agree a general classification for recurrent veins. Yet improving the results of varicose vein surgery is an important challenge, not least because approximately 20% of all venous surgery is for recurrent varicosities. Not only is recurrence a disappointment for the patient, re-operation is more difficult for the surgeon and attended by more complications.

The cause of recurrent varicose veins

Early studies blamed high recurrence rates on inadequate groin dissection by poorly trained or inexperienced surgeons [2, 3]. It was believed that the increase in venous surgery undertaken by specialist vascular surgeons who have the confidence to operate at the saphenofemoral junction (SFJ) would minimise recurrence, although the few long-term studies available have proved disappointing in this regard. Campbell et al reported recurrence rates ten years after operation; only 30% of patients were completely free from recurrent varicose veins, 44% had 'just a few' varicosities and 26% had varicose veins 'as badly as before'. Twenty-four patients (34%) were not 'generally pleased' at ten years [4]. Winterborn et al similarly described recurrence rates of 62% and a re-operation rate of up to 20% 11 years after primary operation [5].

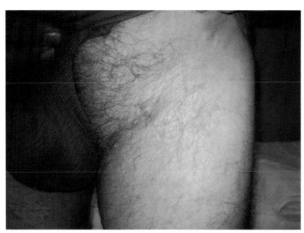

Figure 1. Dilated vein under the groin scar nine months after saphenofemoral disconnection: tributary or neovascularisation?

Most patients with recurrent veins have incompetence in the long saphenous vein (LSV) due either to a mid-thigh perforating vein or recurrent incompetence at the SFJ. At re-operation it is common to find a leash of veins connecting the SFJ and the LSV. The question is whether these are new veins that have grown at the SFJ by angiogenesis (neovascularisation) or expansion of existing small collateral veins in response to saphenofemoral ligation (Figure 1). One histological study found that the veins excised from the groin during re-operative surgery were immature and thin-walled, and therefore likely to be due to neovascularisation [6], but this has been disputed [7]. Still less is known about disease recurrence after operation for varicosities relating to the short saphenous vein, but it is thought to be an even greater problem than after LSV operation. Neovascularisation is also recognised in the popliteal fossa.

A rather poorly investigated cause of recurrent veins after successful ligation in the superficial venous system is altered venous haemodynamics. In a study from Leeds, routine duplex imaging six weeks after varicose vein surgery documented new sites of superficial incompetence in 20% of legs [8]. It was assumed that the operation had altered venous haemodynamics and rendered weak valves incompetent.

Strategies to reduce recurrent disease

Two main factors in minimising disease recurrence after surgery are, first, an accurate pre-operative diagnosis and, second, an appropriate and technically successful operation. Recurrence rates seem not to be related to the indication for primary surgery (symptomatic or complicated), although re-recurrence is more frequent after re-operative surgery.

Clearly, recurrence is more likely if an incorrect operation is performed. Improving the accuracy of pre-operative diagnosis should be beneficial, although the evidence is conflicting. The level of venous reflux is usually diagnosed by a combination of clinical examination and hand-held Doppler ultrasonography by a vascular surgeon in the outpatient clinic. The advent of colour duplex imaging has brought new controversy. Venous disorders may now be diagnosed anatomically and haemodynamically, and mapped before operation. While this increases the workload of vascular laboratories, it may be justified if clinical results are improved. A pilot randomised trial found no advantage from routine duplex imaging, but the definitive trial was never carried out [9]. A later study from Scandinavia reported improved results two years after operation in association with routine pre-operative duplex imaging [10]. This study has, however, been criticised because some of the participants were general surgeons, not vascular specialists. It is possible that a routine pre-operative duplex imaging would be of less value to a vascular specialist experienced in the use of the hand-held Doppler instrument. A cost-effective compromise is to screen patients with a hand-held Doppler device and to use duplex imaging solely for those with recurrent varicosities, complicated situations and/or a reflux signal in the popliteal fossa (see Chapter 20).

Surgery for long saphenous vein disease

For some operations it has been convincingly shown that having the procedure done by a specialist with a high volume of cases improves outcome. No such evidence is yet available for venous surgery, partly because of the difficulty in defining and measuring recurrence. It is believed that careful saphenofemoral ligation is the most important part of LSV surgery, yet this concept has been challenged by the results of new endovenous techniques that ignore the SFJ and simply obliterate the LSV. Certainly the SFJ is the area with the highest potential for local recurrence and it is the most technically challenging site of varicose vein surgery for an inexperienced operator.

If it is accepted that neovascularisation is a significant problem after saphenofemoral ligation, it would seem important to remove any veins near the SFJ such that there is nothing for neovascular veins to rejoin. Tributaries should not simply be tied adjacent to the SFJ but should be dissected back to their first branch before ligation. The author employs diathermy avulsion of tributaries back to, and beyond the first branch, which has the advantage of speed and simplicity. The medial deep perforating branch remains a conundrum. Some surgeons deny that this has any role in recurrent veins, while others believe it should always be divided. Most surgeons simply suture ligate the SFJ. Frings *et al* explored the effect of oversewing the SFJ to avoid leaving exposed endothelium as a potential source of neovascularisation. In a randomised trial, flush oversewing reduced the rate of recurrent groin reflux from 11% to 3% compared with standard ligation (p<0.025) [11].

One component of the LSV operation that clearly affects outcome is routine stripping of the LSV to knee level **(Ia/A)**. Several randomised trials have now demonstrated unequivocally that stripping reduces the risk of recurrence and improves venous haemodynamics [5, 12-18]. In the Gloucester study of 100 patients undergoing LSV surgery, 20 of 69 legs randomised to routine stripping required re-operation by 11 years, compared to seven of 64 legs that had saphenofemoral ligation alone (p=0.012) [5]. Stripping has several potentially beneficial effects. It abolishes any connection with mid-thigh perforating veins that might subsequently become incompetent. In addition, if neovascularisation does occur in the groin, it has nothing to join to and thereby cause recurrence. For the latter reason it is also important to remove any other residual thigh veins. The LSV may be bifid and, if so, both vessels should be removed. The anterolateral thigh vein is commonly identified during

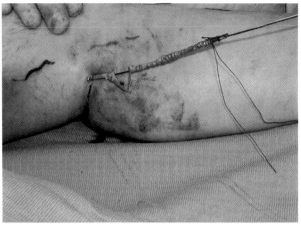

Figure 2. Inversion stripping using the standard plain metal stripper.

groin exploration for LSV varicosities; it may be stripped, but it is often possible to remove 10-15cm by careful avulsion through the groin wound.

The morbidity associated with routine stripping has discouraged some surgeons, but this may be minimised by perforate invagination (PIN), or inversion stripping [19], or sequential avulsion [20]. Simple inversion stripping can be achieved with a bare wire stripper (Figure 2). Some argue that the LSV vein should be preserved for future use in arterial bypass surgery, but a varicose vein is rarely a useable conduit. Selective retention of a non-varicose, competent LSV (on duplex imaging) might be advantageous in this respect, but at the risk of increased probability of recurrence [21].

Barrier technology

The creation of a barrier over the ligated SFJ has been suggested as a way of reducing recurrence due to neovascularisation. Sheppard first described the use of pectineus fascia, dissected free, turned back and sutured over the SFJ [22]. Glass was one of the first to describe the use of prosthetic (Mersilene) mesh in the groin to try to prevent recurrent varicosities [23]. His work was reported before the introduction of duplex imaging, but use of a mesh sutured over the ligated SFJ reduced the rate of clinical recurrence from 25% to 1% after four years. Most venous surgeons remain to be convinced about the practical relevance of these

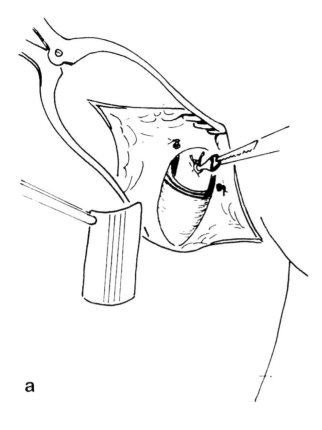

a

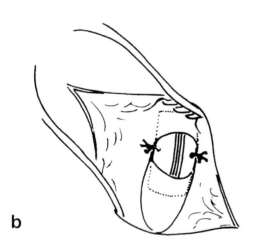

b

Figure 3. Polytetrafluoroethylene patch saphenoplasty. a) Flush saphenofemoral ligation with the patch ready for insertion. b) Patch sutured to tissue either side of the common femoral vein; the upper and lower ends are then tucked underneath the cribriform fascia. *Reproduced with permission from Phlebology* [24].

results. There is concern both about making a simple operation complicated and the potential for infection of artificial material in the groin (Figure 3). Early results of patching for primary varicose veins have been reported, but no randomised trial exists [24].

Surgery for short saphenous vein disease

Short saphenous vein (SSV) surgery is technically more challenging. The aim is to ligate the SSV at the saphenopopliteal junction (SPJ). Careful dissection is needed to avoid damage to neurovascular structures in the popliteal fossa. All patients should be warned explicitly about this potential complication before operation. The anatomy of the SPJ, which is deep to the superficial fascia, is very variable; it may lie several centimetres above the skin crease of the knee. Because of this variability, it is helpful to have the junction marked before operation using duplex imaging. It is recommended that the site of the junction and the site at which the SSV passes through the fascia should be marked separately. Patients with recurrent SSV disease often have a leash of veins emanating from the popliteal fossa to join the SSV, analogous to neovascularisation in the groin.

As for the LSV, stripping of the SSV might seem to be a logical way of reducing recurrence, but the incidence of damage to the sural nerve seemed high in historical series. Despite this, in a recent prospective, non-randomised series of 234 SSV procedures from the members of the Joint Vascular Research Group (JVRG) routine stripping of the SSV did not increase the rate of nerve damage, but did reduce the rate of recurrent saphenopopliteal incompetence on duplex imaging one year after surgery, from 33% to 13% (p<0.01) (unpublished data). One common problem in the popliteal fossa is the presence of gastrocnemius veins. These may be confused with the SSV unless dissection is thorough. Gastrocnemius veins are thin-walled and fragile, and do not avulse well. They should be ligated and divided, as they are a significant cause of recurrent varicosities. Surprisingly little is known about the incidence of recurrent SSV disease. In the JVRG study, after one year 27% of patients had visible recurrence and this may increase over time. Recurrent SSV disease should prove a fruitful area for future investigation.

Operations for recurrent veins

Recurrence rates after re-operation are likely to be higher than after surgery for primary varicosities. Morbidity is also higher, principally due to wound complications, such as infection or seroma. Accurate pre-operative diagnosis with duplex imaging is essential.

For recurrent saphenofemoral incompetence, the aim should be to clear 2-3cm of the common femoral vein at the SFJ. A variety of surgical methods exist based on dissection through virgin tissue and the lateral approach from the direction of the common femoral artery is the most popular of these. Flush re-ligation is important, as is stripping of any residual LSV. The LSV may need to be marked using duplex before operation if it is not visible or palpable.

Barrier methods have also been investigated in the treatment of recurrent varicosities. Prosthetic material (Dacron or polytetrafluoroethylene) has been placed

over the SFJ. Autologous tissue has also been used, but a pectineus flap did not appear to reduce subsequent recurrence in a randomised controlled trial [25]. In Gloucester, a PTFE patch has been used in 81 legs in 50 patients who have been followed-up for a median of 19 months. Sixteen (23%) legs had visible recurrent veins, although only eight were symptomatic. In ten legs (12%) recurrence was attributed to failure of the patch [26]. In a randomised trial from Belgium, placement of a silicone patch reduced the rate of neovascularisation at the SFJ from 16% to 6% at one year after surgery for recurrent veins [27]. Although it does not totally prevent recurrent groin incompetence (Figure 4), the late results of barrier technology are such that this concept seems worth pursuing, especially as the outcome of surgery in this group of patients is generally poorer than that encountered in those with primary varicose veins **(Ib/A)**.

Minimising complications

Optimising results also entails minimising complications. The common complications of venous surgery are infection, haematoma and bruising; the most feared is deep vein thrombosis (DVT). No study has ever shown that routine antibiotic prophylaxis is worthwhile for varicose vein surgery. Nevertheless, infection is commoner when a venous ulcer is present and it is the author's practice to give a single dose of intravenous co-amoxiclav (Augmentin) in this situation. The commonest site for haematoma is in the stripper track in the thigh. While reducing the size of the stripper head or using a PIN stripper reduces the size of the stripper exit site, it does not decrease the size of any haematoma [19]. Operating under a tourniquet, on the other hand, not only reduces blood loss and the duration of the procedure, it also decreases the size of any postoperative haematoma [28] **(Ib/A)**. Many different regimens for postoperative bandaging exist but there does not seem to be any advantage in prolonging this beyond one week after surgery [29].

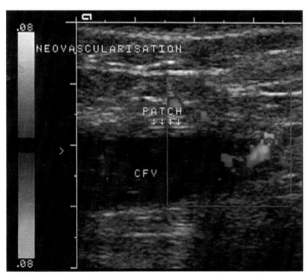

Figure 4. Duplex scan of neovascular vein curling round a polytetrafluoroethylene patch to cause recurrent saphenofemoral incompetence.

The possibility of DVT after varicose vein surgery arouses much anxiety in both patient and surgeon, yet prospective studies have shown the risk to be very low [30]. A survey by Campbell and Ridler showed that fewer than 12% of surgeons use antithrombotic prophylaxis with heparin for all patients undergoing varicose vein surgery. Most employ heparin selectively, based on other risk factors such as previous DVT and contraceptive pill use [31].

Effect of surgery on quality of life

There is much debate about the effectiveness of routine surgery for varicose veins. In health services where there is competition for funding, uncomplicated (and even complicated) varicose veins may be regarded as trivial and their treatment unworthy of purchase. Yet in the past few years routine varicose vein surgery has been shown to reduce the rate of ulcer recurrence in patients with varicose ulceration [32]. For uncomplicated varicosities, surgery has been shown to have a beneficial effect on quality of life [33], and at a cost usually funded within the UK healthcare system according to National Institute for Clinical Excellence guidelines [34] **(Ib/A)**.

Conclusions

Varicose vein surgery is routine and often delegated to non-consultant staff, yet it has stood the test of time. A thoughtful and specialist approach can yield optimal results. Attractive modern non-invasive treatments that simply obliterate the LSV or SSV may sacrifice long-term results for short-term expediency. It is likely that the greatest challenge to conventional operation will come from foam sclerotherapy (Chapter 22) for which short-term results may be equivalent, but with a less costly and easier (for both patient and surgeon) procedure. Over the next few years venous specialists should accept the challenge of comparing these treatments formally.

Key points	Evidence level
◆ Standard varicose vein surgery improves quality of life and is cost-effective.	Ib/A
◆ Surgery reduces the rate of ulcer recurrence in patients with varicose ulceration.	Ib/A
◆ Stripping the LSV reduces the rate of re-operation.	Ia/A
◆ Barrier methods have a positive effect in the short term but it is unknown if they prevent late recurrence.	Ib/A
◆ It is uncertain if stripping should be routine for the SSV.	IV/C
◆ New endovenous techniques must be compared formally with standard surgery and not introduced solely for reasons of expediency and/or cost.	IV/C

References

1. Winterborn R, Earnshaw JJ. Crossectomy and great saphenous vein stripping. *J Cardiovasc Surg* 2006; 47: 19-33.
2. Redwood NFW, Lambert D. Patterns of reflux in recurrent veins assessed by duplex scanning. *Br J Surg* 1994; 81: 1450-1.
3. Labropoulos N, Touloupakis E, Giannoukas AD, *et al.* Recurrent varicose veins: investigation of the pattern and extent of reflux with colour flow duplex scanning. *Surgery* 1996; 119: 406-9.
4. Campbell WB, Vijay Kumar A, Collin TW, *et al.* The outcome of varicose vein surgery at 10 years: clinical findings, symptoms and patient satisfaction. *Ann R Coll Surg Engl* 2003; 85: 52-7.
5. Winterborn RJ, Foy C, Earnshaw JJ. Causes of varicose vein recurrence: late results of a randomized controlled trial of stripping the long saphenous vein. *J Vasc Surg* 2004; 40: 634-9.
6. Nyamekye I, Shephard NA, Davies B, *et al.* Clinicopathological evidence that neovascularisation is a cause of recurrent varicose veins. *Eur J Vasc Endovasc Surg* 1998; 15: 412-5.

7. El Wajeh Y, Giannoukas AD, Gulliford CJ, et al. Saphenofemoral venous channels associated with recurrent varicose veins are not neovascular. Eur J Vasc Endovasc Surg 2004; 28: 590-4.

8. Turton EPL, Scott DJA, Richards SP, et al. Duplex-derived evidence of reflux after varicose vein surgery: neoreflux or neovascularisation. Eur J Vasc Endovasc Surg 1999; 17: 230-3.

9. Smith JJ, Brown L, Greenhalgh RM, Davies AH. Randomised trial of preoperative colour duplex marking in primary varicose vein surgery: outcome is not improved. Eur J Vasc Endovasc Surg 2002; 23: 336-43.

10. Blomgren L, Johansson G, Bergqvist D. Randomized clinical trial of routine preoperative duplex imaging before varicose vein surgery. Br J Surg 2005; 92: 688-94.

11. Frings N, Nelle A, Tran PH, et al. Reduction of neoreflux after correctly performed ligation of the saphenofemoral junction. A randomized trial. Eur J Vasc Endovasc Surg 2004; 28: 246-52.

12. Jackobsen BH. The value of different forms of treatment for varicose veins. Br J Surg 1979; 66: 182-4.

13. Munn Sr, Morton JB, Macbeth WAAG, McLeish AR. To strip or not to strip the long saphenous vein. A varicose vein trial. Br J Surg 1981; 68: 426-8.

14. Woodyer AB, Reddy PJ, Dormandy JA. Should we strip the long saphenous vein? Phlebology 1986; 1: 221-4.

15. Hammersten J, Pederson P, Cederlund C-G, Campanello M. Long saphenous vein-saving surgery for varicose veins. A long-term follow-up. Eur J Vasc Surg 1990; 4: 361-4.

16. Nelgen P, Einarsson E, Eklof B. The functional long-term value of different types of treatment for saphenous vein incompetence. J Cardiovasc Surg (Torino) 1993; 34: 295-301.

17. Rutgers PH, Kitslaar PJEHM. Randomised trial of stripping versus high ligation combined with sclerotherapy in the treatment of the incompetent greater saphenous vein. Am J Surg 1994; 168: 311-5.

18. Sarin S, Scurr JH, Coleridge-Smith PD. Stripping of the long saphenous vein in the treatment of primary varicose veins. Br J Surg 1994; 81: 1455-8.

19. Durkin MT, Turton EPL, Scott DJA, Berridge DC. A prospective randomised trial of PIN versus conventional stripping in varicose vein surgery. Ann R Coll Surg Engl 1999; 81: 171-4.

20. Khan RBN, Khan SN, Greaney MG, Blair SD. Prospective randomized trial comparing sequential avulsions with stripping of the long saphenous vein. Br J Surg 1996; 83: 1559-62.

21. Zamboni P, Marcellino MG, Capelli M, et al. Saphenous vein sparing surgery: principles, techniques and results. Cardiovasc Surg 1998; 39: 151-62.

22. Sheppard M. A procedure for the prevention of recurrent saphenofemoral incompetence. ANZ J Surg 1978; 48: 322-6.

23. Glass GM. Prevention of recurrent saphenofemoral incompetence after surgery for varicose veins. Br J Surg 1989; 76: 1210.

24. Earnshaw JJ, Davies B, Harradine K, Heather BP. Preliminary results of PTFE patch saphenoplasty to prevent neovascularisation leading to recurrent varicose veins. Phlebology 1998; 13: 10-3.

25. Gibbs PJ, Foy DM, Darke SG. Reoperation for recurrent saphenofemoral incompetence: a prospective randomised trial using a reflected flap of pectineus fascia. Eur J Vasc Endovasc Surg 1999; 18: 494-8.

26. Bhatti TS, Whitman B, Harradine K, et al. Causes of re-recurrence after polytetrafluoroethylene patch saphenoplasty for recurrent varicose veins. Br J Surg 2000; 87: 1356-60.

27. De Maeseneer MG, Vandenbroeck CP, Van Schil PE. Silicone patch saphenoplasty to prevent repeat recurrence after surgery to treat recurrent saphenofemoral incompetence: long-term follow-up study. J Vasc Surg 2004; 40: 98-110.

28. Sykes TCF, Brookes P, Hickey NC. A prospective randomized trial of tourniquet in varicose vein surgery. Ann R Coll Surg Engl 2000; 82: 280-2.

29. Raraty MGT, Greaney MG, Blair SD. There is no benefit from 6 weeks of compression after varicose vein surgery: a prospective randomized trial. Br J Surg 1997; 84: A574.

30. Van Rij AM, Chai J, Hill GB, Christie RA. The incidence of deep vein thrombosis after varicose vein surgery. Br J Surg 2004; 91: 1582-5.

31. Campbell WB, Ridler BM. Varicose vein surgery and deep vein thrombosis. Br J Surg 1995; 82: 1494-7.

32. Barwell JR, Davies CE, Deacon J, et al. Comparison of surgery and compression with compression alone in chronic venous ulceration (ESCHAR study): randomised controlled trial. Lancet 2004; 363: 1854-9.

33. Michaels JA, Brazier JE, Campbell WB, et al. Randomized controlled trial comparing surgery with conservative treatment for uncomplicated varicose veins. Br J Surg 2006; 92: 175-81.

34. Ratcliffe J, Brazier JE, Campbell WB, et al. Cost-effectiveness analysis of surgery versus conservative treatment for uncomplicated varicose veins in a randomized clinical trial. Br J Surg 2006; 93: 182-6.

Chapter 22

New interventions for varicose veins

Bruce Campbell MS FRCP FRCS, Consultant Surgeon and Professor
Royal Devon and Exeter Hospital and Peninsula Medical School, Exeter, UK

Introduction

The established treatment for most symptomatic varicose veins is surgery (Chapter 21). Appropriate surgery on properly selected patients has been shown to be both a clinically **(Ib/A)** and cost-effective **(Ib/A)** treatment, and it is the gold standard by which new treatments must be judged [1, 2]. Conventional sclerotherapy is also effective in the medium term for treating smaller varicose veins that are not associated with saphenous reflux **(Ib/A)**, but this will not be considered further here [1].

In recent years, three new types of treatment for varicose veins have started to become popular: radiofrequency ablation (RFA), laser ablation and foam sclerotherapy. A fourth new method - transilluminated powered phlebectomy - enjoyed a brief period of publicity, but its dissemination has been quite limited and the available evidence suggests that it has no important advantages over standard surgical phlebectomy **(Ib/A)** [3, 4]. This chapter outlines the evidence available on the new techniques, together with those gaps in evidence that must be filled if they are to find their proper places in the treatment of varicose veins.

The aims of new interventions

The main aim of all the new interventions is to reduce trauma to the patient and to hasten full recovery. Aspects of this may include avoidance of general anaesthesia, of groin incisions, and of thigh haematoma, which sometimes follows stripping of the long saphenous vein (LSV). Phlebectomy wounds and associated haematoma may also be avoided, specifically by foam sclerotherapy. Avoidance of surgical dissection in the groin or popliteal fossa might reduce the incidence of recurrence due to neovascularisation and, finally, the new techniques may reduce the incidence of complications, such as nerve damage.

It is worth noting that the aim of treatment seems to vary from surgeon to surgeon. Some aim not only to ablate truncal reflux and to relieve symptoms, but also to abolish all visible varicosities (the author's preference). Others are content to deal with the worst of the varicose veins and the main symptoms, accepting that some varicose veins may remain, especially if treatment is for lipodermatosclerosis. The inevitably different perceptions of success are often poorly defined in published reports.

Efficacy, safety and cost

For the new techniques to be clinically effective, they need not only to ablate incompetent veins in the short term, but also to produce long-term recurrence rates that are not significantly greater than those observed after conventional surgery. It is also most important that the new treatments do not have serious side effects, which would influence their use for a condition that seldom threatens life or limb.

The matter of cost is complex and depends on several factors, which may vary between specialists and hospitals. Table 1 shows some of these considerations. Particularly relevant is the extent of varicosities and whether they involve one or both legs. If there are extensive varicose veins affecting both legs, only a procedure under general anaesthesia will deal with all of the problem in a predictable way and at a single session; usually this consists of removal or ablation of both LSVs and multiple phlebectomies. This fundamental concept seems often to be forgotten in the current atmosphere of enthusiasm for less invasive treatments. Repeat treatment sessions may have an important bearing on cost and patient preference. There is currently little good information about these issues.

Patient selection

There seems to be consensus that certain groups of patients may be especially suitable for the new interventions, in particular those with recurrent reflux

---

Table 1. Practical considerations when setting up services using the new treatments. Variations influence both cost and cost-effectiveness; good data are lacking to inform choice about most of these issues.

Issue	Considerations
Where treatment is delivered (office, outpatient suite, operating theatre)	Main requirement is adequate space. Operating theatre facilities may not be necessary, even though theatre may be the easiest starting place in health service practice
Capital costs of equipment and costs of disposables (specifically costs of RFA and laser equipment, plus cost of any additional duplex scanner)	Will the duplex scanner be used for other purposes; might expense be shared? What benefits will accrue as a result of moving to RFA or laser therapy? How many patients will be treated?
Staff required	Will a vascular technologist be needed for duplex imaging? Some surgeons perform scanning themselves. How many other assistants are necessary? Who should they be?
How long each treatment takes	Will RFA or laser ablation take longer than conventional surgery? How many patients can be treated by foam sclerotherapy in an allocated session? How to anticipate if further treatment will be needed?
How many treatment sessions are required	May be difficult to predict. More than one attendance is likely, unless patients have had thorough surgery under general anaesthesia, or have veins of limited extent
Coding and remuneration	How will procedures be coded? How will remuneration work for repeat sessions? How will purchasers respond?

after previous surgery at the saphenofemoral or saphenopopliteal junctions. There are numerous other considerations, such as:

- the extent of varicose veins (surgery may be the treatment of choice for extensive bilateral varicose veins);
- whether any communication with the deep veins is large or small (if small then surgery may be an unattractive option) or easy/difficult for surgical ligation;
- the size of the varicose veins (huge veins may be uncomfortably thrombosed for many weeks after foam sclerotherapy);
- the build of the patient (specifically, obesity);
- medical comorbidities (increased risk for general anaesthesia); DVT history might make foam sclerotherapy less appropriate.

Any evidence that helps to define more clearly those patients more or less suitable for each of the new interventions would be helpful.

Combinations of treatments

These deserve mention, because they are not well described in some studies and they complicate the interpretation of others. Furthermore, combinations may make translation of published data into everyday practice difficult. A good example is the randomised controlled trial by Bountouroglou *et al* of foam sclerotherapy versus surgery [5]. These authors combined foam treatment with saphenofemoral ligation, inevitably confounding interpretation of their results and setting their study out of context with most clinical practice. There are many other potential combinations, for example radiofrequency or laser ablation under local, regional or general anaesthesia, and combined with either multiple phlebectomy or foam sclerotherapy, either synchronously or at a later date.

Can the thermal ablation techniques be considered together?

RFA and laser ablation each has its advocates, who are understandably reluctant to see the results of one

technique extrapolated to the other. However, there are some important similarities and reviews already exist that place them alongside each other [6]. Both work by thermal ablation of truncal veins and aim to replace only the saphenofemoral (or saphenopopliteal) ligation and stripping elements of varicose vein operations; adjunctive procedures are usually required to deal with other varicose veins, although these may not always be necessary [7] **(III/B)**. Both interventions may be done under general or extensive local anaesthesia. Their early success rates might differ, but it would be reasonable to suppose that, if a similar segment of truncal vein can be obliterated in the short term by both techniques, the long-term outcomes might well be similar. By contrast, important differences might be found in their early efficacy and their side effect profiles.

No direct comparisons have been done of RFA versus laser ablation, but Puggioni *et al* have made a historical comparison of 53 limbs treated by RFA with 77 treated later by laser **(III/B)** [8]. Duplex follow-up was particularly poor in the RFA group but suggested similar ablation rates in excess of 90% after about one week. There was a trend suggesting a greater incidence of minor complications in the group treated by laser ablation **(III/B)**.

Finally, it should be noted that the amount of thermal energy delivered during treatment may be very variable. With laser in particular, different wavelenths, power settings and exposure times have been used; these have not always been clearly specified. Such differences might affect both safety and efficacy [9].

The published evidence

The quality of evidence

The quality of evidence for these new techniques is poor or, at best, modest. RFA has, perhaps, the best evidence base. The results of two randomised studies [10-13] **(Ib/A)** and one registry of fair size [14-16] **(III/B)** have been published, including follow-up of some patients for up to five years. It is difficult to ascertain if some duplicate reporting of patients has taken place, because authors reappear with different co-authors in different publications [14-16]. Case series have also been published, for example that of Weiss *et al* [17] **(III/B)**.

For laser ablation there is one very small within-patient randomised study [18] **(Ib/A)**. The remaining evidence on this technique is limited to case series [8, 9, 19-23] **(III/B)**. A systematic review published in 2005 found only 13 studies and pressed the case for well designed randomised trials of laser ablation versus conventional surgery [24].

The quality of evidence on foam sclerotherapy is particularly disappointing, especially as it has been in use for a decade by enthusiasts and is now widely used around the world on large numbers of patients. Apart from the RCT by Bountouroglou *et al* [5] **(Ib/A)** discussed above and another by Belcaro *et al* [25] (which, although randomised, is complex and difficult to draw clear conclusions from), the evidence consists solely of case series [26-30] **(III/B)**. While some of these papers contain interesting observations and descriptions of technique, they do not provide the hard scientific data required to allow a confident judgement to be made about the place of foam sclerotherapy in the treatment of varicose veins.

Efficacy

Radiofrequency ablation (Figure 1)

Complete or near-complete occlusion of the long saphenous trunk has been reported in over 90% of patients in the early weeks after RFA **(III/B)**. Some results have been published on five-year follow-up [16], but the bulk of information reflecting the longer term is for two to three years [11, 13, 15, 17] **(mostly III/B)**. These papers generally describe occlusion rates of 80% to 90%. When short unoccluded segments are present, for example 17% at three years [15] **(III/B)**, they are not usually associated with symptoms, but it is not clear what implications they harbour for future years.

The one well reported but small randomised comparison against surgical ligation and stripping showed no early differences, apart from shorter

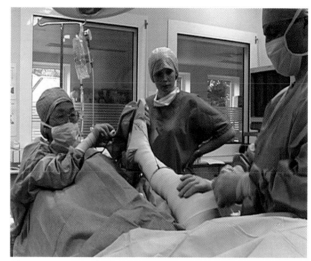

Figure 1. Radiofrequency ablation. The limb is compressed to encourage closure of the lumen during each episode of heating by radiofrequency. *Courtesy of Mr. Mark Whiteley, Guildford.*

postoperative sick leave with RFA [10] **(Ib/A)**. Direct medical costs of RFA were somewhat higher than for stripping. Follow-up at three years revealed no recanalisations after RFA and one duplicate long saphenous trunk after stripping [11] **(Ib/A)**. There were 33% residual/recurrent veins after RFA and 23% after stripping - a statistically insignificant trend.

Laser ablation (Figure 2)

As for RFA, reported early results all describe occlusion rates of at least 90%. At one to three-year follow-up, persistent occlusion of the LSV occurs in about 76% to 100% of limbs [9, 20-23]. Veins which appear occluded on duplex imaging after three months tend to remain occluded [20, 22]. One small randomised study, in which 20 patients had stripping of one LSV and laser ablation of the other, found no difference between the limbs in terms of pain, but swelling and bruising were less on the laser treated side [18] **(Ib/A)**. There was one recanalisation after laser ablation and no serious adverse event after either technique. Finally, there is some evidence that failure rates are higher for both laser ablation and RFA in patients with high body mass index [9, 16].

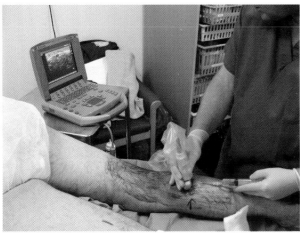

Figure 2. Preparing to ablate the short saphenous vein by laser under ultrasound control. *Courtesy of Mr. Michael Gough, Leeds.*

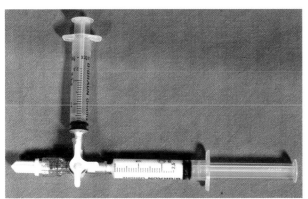

Figure 3. Preparation of sclerosant foam by the Tessari method.

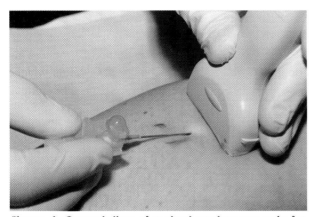

Figure 4. Cannulation of a short saphenous vein for foam sclerotherapy under ultrasound guidance.

Foam sclerotherapy (Figures 3 and 4)

The data for foam sclerotherapy are more difficult to assess because, unlike RFA or laser treatment, non-ablation of the LSV during a single treatment session is not generally regarded as a 'failure', but rather as a 'feature' of the technique. A recent report by Darke *et al* [30], which defined complete occlusion as occlusion of the saphenous trunk and/or 85% of the varicosities, described such complete occlusion in 100% of legs with incompetent short saphenous trunks after a single treatment, compared with only 66% of legs with incompetent long saphenous trunks. Good information about the longer term is sparse; occlusion seems to persist in over 70% of treated legs [26, 27, 29] **(III/B)**. Results may be less satisfactory in veins with a diameter exceeding 10mm [28] **(III/B)**.

A study that randomised 60 patients to stripping under general anaesthesia or to foam treatment under local anaesthesia (all had saphenofemoral ligation) found a significantly earlier return to normal activity (median two versus eight days) in the latter group. Cost was also lower in the foam-treated group, despite four patients developing recanalisation that required further treatment [5] **(Ib/A)**.

Safety

Reported side effects have been generally minor for all three techniques. For RFA, haematoma, paraesthesia, superficial thrombophlebitis and skin burns [10, 12, 14] seem all to occur infrequently and there are no reports of important long-term morbidity. For laser treatment, occasional skin burns have also been reported, and haematoma, superficial phlebitis and paraesthesia are all perhaps a little more frequent than with RFA; induration of the treated vein may be painful [8, 19-21, 23]. There is great variation in reporting of adverse events. DVT has occurred in association with both techniques, with an incidence in the region of 1%; occasional reports of pulmonary embolism exist, but this is very rare [6].

Local complications of foam sclerotherapy include tender induration of the injected veins, pigmentation, thrombophlebitis, skin necrosis [27, 28, 31] and, rarely,

DVT [30] **(II-III/B)**. Visual disturbance and confusion are of major concern [31, 32], as is the possibility that bubbles of foam might enter the arterial circulation through a patent foramen ovale and provoke a stroke. Indeed, one instance of stroke has now been reported in association with foam treatment [32], but an unusually large volume of foam (20ml) had been injected. The absence of any other reported strokes among the large numbers of patients who have received the more usual smaller volumes of foam provide fair reassurance that this complication is very rare. There seems little justification for the suggestion that patients should be scanned for patent foramen ovale before treatment. Finally, a single myocardial infarction associated with foam treatment has been cited in the National Institute for Health and Clinial Excellence (NICE) guidance, based on unpublished data [33].

Introducing the new treatments into clinical practice

Table 1 shows what needs to be considered when introducing new treatments into everyday practice, particularly when negotiating with hospitals and healthcare purchasers. Training is important; any surgeon who starts to use a new technology without receiving formal instruction and mentoring risks censure, especially if adverse events occur.

Whenever possible, patients should be entered into research studies to achieve a better understanding of outcome and to assess the best place for these new methods of treating varicose veins. It should be appreciated that patient selection is not yet well defined. Table 2 sets out suggestions for research,

Table 2. Suggestions for future research, audit and debate.	
Type of research/ audit/debate	**Suggested aims**
Randomised controlled trials	Particularly of foam sclerotherapy and of laser versus surgery Cost-effectiveness of different methods and models of care Clinically significant outcomes (in addition to duplex scan data) Long-term follow-up (at least 5 years)
Other controlled studies	Patient preferences about repeated treatments under local anaesthesia for extensive varicose veins against single treatment under general or regional anaesthesia
Case series and reports	Surgeons treating substantial numbers of patients and who are unwilling to be involved in RCTs should publish their experience - thoroughly and explicitly Serious adverse events should be published
Debate at meetings	Exchange of ideas and experience is important in developing models of treatment There should be debate about patient selection (influence of bilateral varicose veins, size of veins, obesity), organisation of services (treatment settings, types of anaesthesia, what staff are involved, number of treatment sessions, duration of compression), and patient preferences (with regard to anaesthesia, need for more than one treatment session, inconvenience of compression)
National audit	Reporting of all serious adverse events to the National Patient Safety Agency
Local audit	Surgeons should keep good records of patients treated and review these to inform future practice. How services are delivered should be considered carefully

audit and debate that would help to resolve current uncertainties. In July 2006 the Health Technology Assessment Programme of the NHS advertised for commissioned research in the form of a randomised controlled trial of foam sclerotherapy versus conventional surgery.

NICE has issued guidance on each of the new techniques. While, this recommends that both RFA and laser ablation may be used with normal arrangements for clinical governance, consent and audit, it also highlights the need for more long-term data [34-35]. Recent guidance on foam sclerotherapy has been more cautious, requiring special arrangements for clinical governance, consent and audit; this will be reviewed after a systematic review, commissioned by NICE [33].

Conclusions

There is adequate evidence that RFA and laser ablation are both reasonable alternatives to conventional ligation and stripping of saphenous veins. However, it is uncertain whether the gain from avoiding a groin incision and some reduction in bruising in the thigh is adequately offset by the increased cost, possible increase in operating time and the need for further treatment of residual varicosities (particularly after treatment under local anaesthesia). Foam sclerotherapy is spreading rapidly into everyday clinical practice, despite evidence of relatively poor scientific quality. While it appears to offer an attractive and radical alternative to traditional surgery, good randomised comparisons of clinical and cost-effectiveness are missing. Better data are also required to guide patient selection. The long-term results of all of the new treatments discussed in this chapter are eagerly awaited. Randomised comparisons with conventional surgery would be particularly useful.

Key points	Evidence level

♦ RFA and laser ablation both occlude saphenous trunks (long and short) in >80% of patients, without significant recanalisation up to three years. Both are reasonable alternatives to conventional operation but usually require adjunctive treatments to remove varicosities. **Ib/A**

♦ Outpatient foam sclerotherapy has been used for many patients. Repeat sessions are sometimes needed for ablation of saphenous trunks and extensive varicosities. This treatment is a promising alternative to conventional operation. **III/B**

♦ Conventional operation, or RFA or laser ablation with multiple phlebectomy, under general or regional anaesthesia is the only way of treating extensive bilateral varicose veins at a single session. Foam sclerotherapy may have an advantage for recurrent varicose veins and for the short saphenous system. **IV/C**

♦ Return to normal activity is earlier after RFA, laser ablation and foam sclerotherapy than after conventional operation. Differences in analgesia requirements are statistically, but not clinically, significant. Any differences between treatments do not affect direct healthcare costs, an issue when considering investing in equipment for RFA or laser treatment. **Ib/A**

♦ How the service is organised (outpatient suite or operating theatre, and particularly the need for further treatment sessions) influences cost.

♦ Conscientious reporting of adverse events is necessary to confirm a low incidence of serious side effects, in particular to establish if stroke ever occurs when using conventional volumes of sclerosant foam.

♦ Good randomised controlled trials are needed of all the new treatments (particularly foam sclerotherapy and laser) versus conventional operation. Clinical and cost-effectiveness must be examined in the long term.

References

1. Michaels JA, Brazier JE, Campbell WB, et al. Randomised controlled trial comparing surgery with conservative treatment for uncomplicated varicose veins. Br J Surg 2006; 93: 175-81.

2. Ratcliffe J, Brazier JE, Campbell WB, et al. Cost-effectiveness analysis of surgery versus conservative treatment for uncomplicated varicose veins in a randomised controlled. Br J Surg 2006; 93: 182-6.

3. Aremu MA, Magendran B, Butcher W, et al. Prospective randomized controlled trial: conventional versus powered phlebectomy. J Vasc Surg 2004; 39: 88-94.

4. Chetter IC, Mylankal KJ, Hughes H, Fitridge R. Randomised controlled trial comparing multiple stab incision phlebectomy with transilluminated powered phlebectomy for varicose veins. Br J Surg 2006; 93: 169-74.

5. Bountouroglou DG, Azzam M, Kakkos SK, et al. Ultrasound-guided foam sclerotherapy combined with sapheno-femoral ligation compared to surgical treatment of varicose veins: early results of a randomised controlled clinical trial. Eur J Vasc Endovasc Surg 2006; 31: 93-100.

6. Pannier F, Rabe E. Endovenous laser therapy and radiofrequency ablation of saphenous varicose veins. J Cardiovasc Surg 2006; 47: 3-8.

7. Monaghan D. Can phlebectomy be deferred in the treatment of varicose veins? J Vasc Surg 2005; 42: 1145-9.

8. Puggioni A, Kalra M, Carmo M, *et al.* Endovenous laser therapy and radiofrequency ablation of the greater saphenous vein: analysis of early efficacy and complications. *J Vasc Surg* 2005; 42: 488-93.

9. Timperman P. Prospective evaluation of higher energy great saphenous vein endovenous laser treatment. *J Vasc Intervent Radiol* 2005; 16: 791-4.

10. Rautio T, Ohinmaa A, Perala J, *et al.* Endovenous obliteration versus conventional stripping operation in the treatment of primary varicose veins: a randomised controlled trial with comparison of the costs. *J Vasc Surg* 2002; 53: 958-65.

11. Perala J, Rautio T, Biancari F, *et al.* Radiofrequency endovenous obliteration versus stripping of the long saphenous vein in the management of primary varicose veins: 3-year outcome of a randomized study. *Ann Vasc Surg* 2005; 19: 669-72.

12. Lurie F, Creton D, Eklof B, *et al.* Prospective randomized study of endovenous radiofrequency ablation (Closure procedure) versus ligation and vein stripping in a selected patient population (EVOLVeS). *J Vasc Surg* 2003; 38: 207-14.

13. Lurie F, Creton D, Eklof B, *et al.* Prospective randomized study of endovenous radiofrequency ablation (closure procedure) versus ligation and vein stripping (EVOLVeS): two-year follow-up. *Eur J Vasc Endovasc Surg* 2005; 29: 67-73.

14. Merchant RF, DePalma RG, Kabnick LS. Endovascular obliteration of saphenous reflux: a multicenter study. *J Vasc Surg* 2002; 35: 1190-6.

15. Nicolini PH and the Closure Group. Treatment of primary varicose veins by endovenous obliteration with the VNUS closure system: results of a multicentre study. *Eur J Vasc Endovasc Surg* 2005; 29: 433-9.

16. Merchant RF, Pichot O; Closure Study Group. Long-term outcomes of endovenous radiofrequency obliteration of saphenous reflux as a treatment for venous insufficiency. *J Vasc Surg* 2005; 42: 502-9.

17. Weiss RA, Weiss MA. Controlled radiofrequency endovenous occlusion using a unique radiofrequency catheter under duplex guidance to eliminate saphenous varicose vein reflux: a 2-year follow-up. *Dermatol Surg* 2002; 28: 38-42.

18. de Medeiros CA, Luccas GC. Comparison of endovenous treatment with an 810nm laser versus conventional stripping of the great saphenous vein in patients with primary varicose veins. *Dermatol Surg* 2005; 31: 1685-94.

19. Chang CJ, Chua JJ. Endovenous laser photocoagulation (EVLP) for varicose veins. *Laser Med Surg* 2002; 31: 257-62.

20. Min RJ, Khilnani N, Zimmet SE. Endovenous laser treatment of saphenous vein reflux: long-term results. *J Vasc Interv Radiol* 2003; 14: 991-6.

21. Proebstle T, Gul D, Lehr HA, *et al.* Infrequent early recanalization of greater saphenous vein after endovenous laser treatment. *J Vasc Surg* 2003; 38: 511-6.

22. Disseldoff BC, der Kinderen DJ, Moll FL. Is there recanalisation of the great saphenous vein 2 years after endovenous laser treatment? *J Endovasc Ther* 2005; 12: 731-8.

23. Sharif MA, Soong CV, Lau LL, *et al.* Endovenous laser treatment for long saphenous incompetence. *Br J Surg* 2006; 93: 831-5.

24. Mundy L, Merlin TL, Fitridge RA, Hillier JE. Systematic review of endovenous laser treatment for varicose veins. *Br J Surg* 2005; 92: 1189-94.

25. Belcaro G, Cesarone MR, Di Renzo R, *et al.* Foam-sclerotherapy, surgery, sclerotherapy, and combined treatment for varicose veins: a 10-year, prospective, randomized, controlled trial VEDICO trial). *Angiology* 2003; 54: 307-15.

26. Cabrera J, Cabrera Jr J, Garcia-Olmedo MA. Treatment of varicose long saphenous veins with sclerosant in microfoam form: long-term outcomes. *Phlebology* 2000; 15: 19-23.

27. Frullini A, Cavezzi A. Sclerosing foam in the treatment of varicose veins and telangiectases: history and analysis of safety and complications. *Dermatol Surg* 2002; 28: 11-5.

28. Barrett J, Allen B, Ockelford A, Goldman MP. Microfoam ultrasound-guided sclerotherapy treatment for varicose veins in a subgroup with diameters at the junction of 10mm or greater compared with a subgroup of less than 10mm. *Dermatol Surg* 2004; 30: 1386-90.

29. Bergan J, Pascarella L, Mekenas L. Venous disorders: treatment with sclerosant foam. *J Cardiovasc Surg* 2006; 47: 9-18.

30. Darke SG, Baker SJ. Ultrasound-guided foam sclerotherapy for the treatment of varicose veins. *Br J Surg* 2006; 93: 969-74.

31. Alos J, Carreno P, Lopez JA, *et al.* Efficacy and safety of sclerotherapy using polidocanol foam: a controlled clinical trial. *Eur J Vasc Endovasc Surg* 2006; 31: 101-7.

32. Forlee MV, Grouden M, Moore DJ, Shanik G. Stroke after varicose vein foam injection sclerotherapy. *J Vasc Surg* 2006; 43: 162-4.

33. National Institute for Health and Clinical Excellence. Ultrasound-guided foam sclerotherapy for varicose veins. NICE interventional procedures guidance number 182. London: National Institute for Health and Clinical Excellence, 2006. www.nice.org.uk/IPG.

34. National Institute for Clinical Excellence. Radiofrequency ablation of varicose veins. NICE interventional procedures guidance number 8. London: National Institute for Clinical Excellence, 2003. www.nice.org.uk/IPG.

35. National Institute for Clinical Excellence. Endovenous laser treatment of the long saphenous vein. NICE interventional procedures guidance number 52. London: National Institute for Clinical Excellence, 2004. www.nice.org.uk/IPG.

Chapter 23

The significance of perforating vein disease

Simon G Darke MS FRCS, Consultant Surgeon
Royal Bournemouth Hospital, Bournemouth, UK

Introduction

The significance of perforating veins in the pathogenesis of primary and recurrent varicose veins is established and is not addressed here. This chapter focuses exclusively on the more contentious issue of their role in venous ulceration. A number of recent publications have described duplex imaging to assess the morphological significance of perforators and there have been case series on the outcome of perforator ligation but, as yet, no randomised controlled trials. So, opinions remain divided. Respected American authors express the view that routine perforator ligation is appropriate in the treatment of leg ulcer until more evidence is available [1], while others feel it should be reserved for those rare patients whose only demonstrable venous abnormality is incompetent perforators [2]. Why should such uncertainty exist? In part this is due to the difficulties that complicate research into venous ulcer:

- uncertainty that an ulcer is venous in origin;
- unpredictable natural history of leg ulcer;
- wide variation in venous morphology and difficulty in quantifying it;
- difficulty in recruiting comparable patients;
- long follow-up needed to confirm benefit.

Historical perspective

Ninety years ago, without the advantages of modern investigative technology, John Homans wrote a prescient review on the management of leg ulcer [3]. He noted: "It is a very general rule, if not a law, that the more prominent and tortuous the surface veins the simpler the cure; the less noticeable the surface veins the more malignant and resistant their attendant ulcers and the more radical the operative procedure required for cure." In other words, if there was a big incompetent saphenous system, the management was straightforward. The difficulty arose when superficial reflux was less impressive. From this came the concept that ankle perforator ligation might be the solution. This notion was based on a number of observations:

- perforating veins can be shown to be 'incompetent', meaning that blood passes from the deep to the superficial system;
- some of these veins are anatomically situated at the predominant sites of venous ulceration;
- incompetent perforating veins can be demonstrated in some patients with a venous ulcer;
- ligation of these incompetent veins might lead to ulcer healing.

This view was promoted in subsequent years by Cockett in the UK and Linton in the US, and the concept that perforator ligation was an essential part of the management of venous ulcer remained unquestioned until the late 1970s. At this time the prevailing view was challenged because it was recognised that some ulcers healed after saphenous ablation alone, without additional perforator ligation, irrespective of whether the perforators were incompetent or not. There was also disillusionment with the conventional surgical methods because of the morbidity that often accompanied them. Furthermore, certain groups of patients failed to heal their ulcers or developed recurrence, despite operation [4].

Further doubts followed the introduction of duplex ultrasound imaging and these culminated in the view that surgery should be tailored more precisely to the specific venous abnormalities of an individual patient [5]. Ironically, however, just as perforator ligation was falling into disrepute, enthusiasm was rekindled by the development of a new and less invasive surgical technique, now known widely as subfascial endoscopic perforator surgery (SEPS) [6]. It is noteworthy that this occurred even though the early protagonists of SEPS seemed to have no clear view about the clinical circumstances in which it was indicated [7] (Figure 1).

Venous morphology

Venous abnormalities that might contribute to the pathogenesis of leg ulceration are:

- reflux in the superficial systems: long and/or short saphenous systems (ligation / stripping / surgical ablation of which will be termed here as 'superficial surgery');
- reflux in the deep systems: femoral veins, popliteal veins, calf veins (rarely recorded). It should be noted that reflux in the deep system can be confined to segments (segmental) or involve the whole system (total);
- reflux in the perforating veins.

In a leg there may be any combination of these abnormalities, a situation further complicated by whether they are primary, or secondary to previous

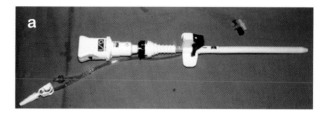

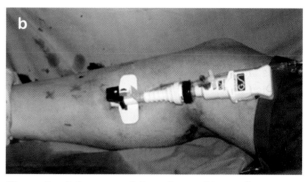

Figure 1. a) Commercial equipment to perform SEPS. b) The device *in situ* for perforator ligation. *Courtesy of Mr. Tim Lees, Newcastle upon Tyne.*

thrombosis. In the latter instance there may be an additional obstructive element.

Several authors have described the broad categories of venous morphology that can be found in association with venous ulcer. Their findings show remarkably little variance in terms of the proportions [2, 5, 8-11]: superficial reflux alone - 55%, superficial plus deep reflux - 40% (approximately two thirds segmental and one third total) and deep system alone - 5%. In addition, some authors specify post-thrombotic elements [8-10, 12]. Most of the affected limbs also have incompetent perforators, but it is rare for these to occur in isolation.

The significance of incompetent perforating veins

Numerous studies have shown that the number and size of perforating veins in the calf varies [13]. These veins are incompetent in some clinically normal legs as well as in those with venous hypertension. Cadaveric dissection has revealed that valves are present in only the larger vessels (>1mm diameter) and that some of these valves are configured to direct blood from the deep to the superficial system, that is to say in an 'incompetent' direction [14]. These matters notwithstanding, in those with leg ulceration due to chronic venous insufficiency, incompetent ankle perforators are found predominantly in the medial aspect of the middle third of the calf, becoming more prevalent, enlarged and incompetent with increasing clinical severity of venous insufficiency [15-17]. A particular difficulty in the evaluation of the clinical significance of incompetent ankle perforating veins is the lack of a haemodynamic test to demonstrate their purported effect. This also makes it difficult to judge the effect of their ligation. Indeed the latter can only be estimated by the demonstration of clinical benefit.

Seminal work on the pathophysiology of perforating veins was conducted before the era of duplex imaging by Bjordal [18], who employed simultaneous pressure measurements and electromagnetic flowmetry in patients undergoing primary varicose vein surgery under local anaesthetic to confirm outward, that is to say 'incompetent', flow in ankle perforating veins.

This work was the first to show in primary venous insufficiency that perforator incompetence was secondary to saphenous reflux. Several others have since confirmed this with duplex studies, showing recovery of competence and a reduction in diameter of the perforators when re-examined after superficial surgery [15, 19-21]. Although some have described this recovery as not as complete in the presence of coexisting deep incompetence [15], others have found significant, if not complete, reversal, irrespective of coexisting segmental or total deep vein reflux [20, 21]. Several authors have also noted that incompetent deep veins too regain competence after correction of superficial reflux [22-24]; some found that this reached significant levels only in segmental reflux, recovery in the face of total reflux being less apparent [25, 26].

To summarise, while incompetent ankle perforating veins can be demonstrated in clinically normal legs, they are more evident with increasing severity of both venous insufficiency and coexistent reflux in saphenous and deep veins. Incompetent ankle perforators are associated with, and possibly secondary to, saphenous incompetence. Even if the deep system is incompetent, perforating veins tend to recover their competence after saphenous ablation, as do - to some degree at least - the deep veins.

Does ligation of incompetent ankle perforating veins heal venous ulcers?

Perforator incompetence as a cause of venous ulceration without associated superficial and/or deep vein incompetence is rare; indeed it might never occur. As perforator incompetence is so often accompanied by superficial incompetence, assessing the clinical effect of perforator ligation is complicated by the influence of any simultaneous correction of saphenous reflux. Early reports of perforator ligation are particularly difficult to evaluate as they are invariably contaminated by synchronous saphenous ligation. The first useful report was by Negus and Friedgood in 1983 [27]. In a series of 109 ulcerated legs there was a 76% healing rate at three years following open subfascial ligation of perforating veins. Half the patients had simultaneous saphenous ligation but, unfortunately, no specific data were given on the influence of synchronous saphenous ligation on ulcer healing.

All the more recent reports on perforator ligation have involved SEPS and this experience has been summarised recently in a review of 20 publications [1]. All were simple case series but they amount to a combined experience of over 1000 limbs, two thirds having synchronous superficial surgery **(IIa/B)**. Overall, in the short term ulcers healed in 88% and recurred in 13%. The review cited four studies in which concomitant superficial surgery appeared to be associated with healing, but while combining the data from three of these studies showed a lower risk of non-healing, this did not reach statistical significance. Factors that did influence healing were ulcer diameter >2cm and secondary (post-thrombotic) disease. Associated deep incompetence did not seem to affect outcome. The authors of the review concluded that, while the continued use of SEPS was appropriate, more information was needed to define its benefits.

To summarise, isolated ankle perforator incompetence is rare in patients with venous ulceration. There are no randomised trials on the outcome of perforator ligation; all available reports have limitations due to confounding by the established benefits of synchronous superficial surgery.

Does superficial venous surgery alone heal venous ulceration?

Recek was, in 1971, the first to report successful treatment by saphenous ligation alone in patients with primary incompetence in the saphenous and perforating veins plus a normal deep system [28]. Subsequently, Hoare *et al* described such surgery in a group of patients with normal deep veins, saphenous incompetence and associated perforator reflux in some [29]. Sethia *et al* measured dorsal foot vein pressures in 12 patients with combined saphenous and perforator incompetence who had normal deep veins on ascending and descending venography [30]. Venous pressures were normalised by an above-knee tourniquet, simulating the effect of long saphenous ligation. Postoperative pressure studies were in line with the pre-operative findings and all the ulcers healed.

Later case series have also shown healing after superficial surgery [16], the more recent based on duplex assessment [25, 31]. A significant reduction in recurrence rate at 12 months has also been demonstrated in a comparative (non-randomised) study: recurrence was 14% in patients treated with superficial surgery and compression compared with 28% in those treated with compression alone, although there was no difference in healing rate [32]. Others have had a similar experience [33] and, in a review of over 1000 leg ulcers, failure to operate on superficial reflux was recognised as a significant independent variable in promoting recurrence [34].

Two recent randomised trials are relevant. In one small trial the recurrence at three years was 9% after superficial surgery compared with 38% after compression alone [35]. In the larger ESCHAR trial patients were followed-up for one year [2]. For isolated superficial incompetence, the recurrence rate was 9% after superficial surgery and compression and 38% after compression alone, although there was no significant difference in healing rate.

In conclusion, patients with isolated superficial and perforator reflux benefit from superficial surgery alone, although not all ulcers heal **(Ia/A)**. Whether additional perforator ligation confers extra benefit is uncertain, but it seems unlikely as perforator reflux recovers anyway.

Management of patients with a combination of superficial, perforator and deep incompetence

In a personal study, after excluding post-thrombotic change using ascending venography, 52 ulcerated legs were recognised with apparently primary superficial, perforator and deep incompetence on descending venography. These were treated by superficial surgery alone and at four-year follow-up only 21 (40%) had healed [36]. This was a disappointing outcome compared to that of patients with isolated superficial reflux [8]. The ESCHAR trial reported recurrence in those with segmental reflux as 9% after surgery compared with 25% after compression alone, which was statistically significant. The respective figures for those with total deep incompetence were 19% and 31%, which was not significant. There were no differences in healing rates in either group [2]. This is in accord with Adam *et al* [25] who described reasonable levels of healing in a series of patients with segmental deep reflux. In a detailed study of 11 legs with this morphology Padberg *et al* showed improved haemodynamic and clinical status after surgery with no recurrent ulceration [37].

It can be concluded that superficial surgery benefits this group, but to a lesser extent than those with normal deep veins. Failure to show a statistically significant reduction in recurrence rate in those with total deep incompetence may be related to patient numbers, but data in general suggest that the more widespread the deep incompetence, the worse the clinical outcome (and the less likely that perforator and deep vein competence will be regained after superficial surgery) **(Ib/A)**.

Post-thrombotic disease

From the evidence presented above, it is apparent that some patients may not benefit even if both the saphenous and perforating veins are ligated, and one such group is those with post-thrombotic disease.

Although about 90% of thrombosed deep veins recanalise, most develop incompetence; this has been shown by a number of prospective duplex follow-up studies. Of the 10-15% of known post-thrombotic patients who subsequently develop an ulcer, most also have superficial reflux [38-40]. Burnand et al were the first to report the influence of post-thrombotic obstructive damage on outcome [4]. They used ascending venography to determine post-thrombotic changes. Forty-one patients with venous ulceration all underwent open subfascial ligation with saphenous ligation. After five years, recurrent ulceration had occurred in all 23 patients who had evidence of previous deep vein thrombosis. In contrast, only one of those with normal deep veins had a recurrent ulcer. Similar results of poor outcome have been reported in later studies [41], including the recent review of SEPS [1].

Conclusions

As yet there is no evidence that perforator ligation benefits leg ulcer disease and what information there is suggests to the contrary. Its use should not be employed routinely, therefore, and could only be justified in patients with persistent ulceration thought to be of venous origin and in whom any superficial reflux has already been ablated and post-thrombotic changes excluded.

Key points	Evidence level
◆ Calf perforators are more common, larger and more incompetent in ulcerated legs.	IIb/B
◆ They become smaller and regain competence after superficial venous surgery.	Ib/A
◆ Some, but not all, patients benefit clinically from superficial surgery. Associated deep vein incompetence probably has adverse effects.	Ib/A
◆ Superficial surgery promotes some recovery of deep vein reflux.	IIa/B
◆ Post-thrombotic ulcer, in particular, is unlikely to benefit from superficial/perforator surgery. It should be identified, if possible, and regarded as a separate category.	
◆ No evidence yet exists that perforator ligation confers any benefit.	Ib/A
◆ A randomised controlled trial is required to study superficial surgery, with and without perforator ligation. This trial ideally should exclude post-thrombotic legs.	
◆ The characteristics of those patients who do, and do not, benefit from superficial surgery need to be identified (for instance, saphenous vein diameter may be relevant, as suggested 90 years ago).	

References

1. Tenbrook JA, Iafrati MD, O'Donnell TF, et al. Systematic review of outcomes after surgical management of venous disease incorporating subfascial endoscopic perforator surgery. *J Vasc Surg* 2004; 39: 583-9.

2. Barwell JR, Davies CE, Deacon J, et al. Comparison of surgery and compression with compression alone in chronic venous ulceration (ESCHAR study): randomized controlled trial. *Lancet* 2004; 363: 1854-9.

3. Homans J. The operative treatment of varicose veins and ulcers, based upon a classification of these lesions. *Surg Gynecol Obstet* 1916; 22: 143-58.

4. Burnand KG, Lea Thomas M, O'Donnell TF, Browse NL. The relationship between post-phlebitic changes in the deep veins and results of surgical treatment of venous ulcers. *Lancet* 1976; 1: 936-8.

5. Adam DJ, Naik J, Hartshorne T, *et al.* The diagnosis and management of 689 chronic leg ulcers in a single visit assessment clinic. *Eur J Vasc Endovasc Surg* 2003; 25: 462-8.

6. Rhodes JM, Gloviczki P, Canton L, *et al.* Endoscopic perforator vein division with ablation of superficial reflux improves venous hemodynamics. *J Vasc Surg* 1998; 28: 839-47.

7. Whiteley MS, Galland RB, Smith JJ. Subfascial endoscopic perforator vein surgery (SEPS): current practice among British surgeons. *Ann R Coll Surg Engl* 1998; 80: 104-7.

8. Grabs AJ, Wakely MC, Nyamekye I, *et al.* Colour duplex ultrasonography in the rational management of chronic venous leg ulcers. *Br J Surg* 1996; 83: 1380-2.

9. Sciven JM, Hartshorne T, Bell PRF, *et al.* Single visit venous ulcer assessment clinic: the first year. *Br J Surg* 1997; 84: 334-6.

10. Labropoulos N. Clinical correlation to various patterns of reflux. *J Vasc Surg* 1997; 31: 242-7.

11. Labropoulos, N Tassiopoulos AK, Kang SS, *et al.* Prevalence of deep venous reflux in patients with primary superficial incompetence. *J Vasc Surg* 2000; 32: 663-8.

12. Darke SG, Penfold C. Venous ulceration and saphenous ligation. *Eur J Surg* 1992; 6: 4-9.

13. Sarin S, Scurr JH, Coleridge-Smith PD. Medial calf perforators in venous disease; the significance of outward flow. *J Vasc Surg* 1992; 16: 40-6.

14. Barber RF, Shatara FI. The varicose disease. *NY State J Med* 1925; 25: 162-6.

15. Stuart WP, Adam DJ, Allan PL, *et al.* Saphenous surgery does not correct perforator incompetence in the presence of deep venous reflux. *J Vasc Surg* 1998; 28: 834-8.

16. Delis KT, Ibgegbuna V, Nicolaides AN, *et al.* Prevalence and distribution of incompetent perforating veins in chronic venous insufficiency. *J Vasc Surg* 1998; 28: 815-25.

17. Stuart WP, Adam DJ, Allan PL, *et al.* The relationship between the number, competence and diameter of the medial calf perforating veins and the clinical status in healthy subjects and patients with lower-limb venous disease. *J Vasc Surg* 2000; 32: 138-43.

18. Bjordal R. Simultaneous pressure and flow recordings in varicose veins of the lower extremity. *Acta Chir Scand* 1970; 136: 309-17.

19. Stuart WP, Lee AJ, Allan PL, *et al.* Most incompetent calf perforating veins are found in association with superficial venous reflux. *J Vasc Surg* 2001; 34: 774-8.

20. Gohel MS, Barewell JR, Wakely C, *et al.* The influence of superficial venous surgery and compression on incompetent calf perforators in chronic leg ulceration. *Eur J Vasc Endovasc Surg* 2005; 29: 78-82.

21. Blomgren L, Johansson G, Dahlberg-Akerman A, *et al.* Changes in superficial and perforating vein reflux after varicose vein surgery. *J Vasc Surg* 2005; 42: 315-20.

22. Walsh JC, Bergan JJ, Beeman S, Commen TP. Femoral venous reflux abolished by greater saphenous vein stripping. *Ann Vasc Surg* 1994; 8: 566-9.

23. Sales CM, Bilof ML, Petrillo KA, Luka NL. Correction of lower extremity deep venous incompetence by ablation of superficial venous reflux. *Ann Vasc Surg* 1996; 10: 186-9.

24. Ciostek P, Michalak J, Noszczyk W. Improvement in deep vein haemodynamics following surgery for varicose veins. *Eur J Vasc Endovasc Surg* 2004; 28: 473-8.

25. Adam DJ, Bello M, Hartshorne T, London NJ. Role of superficial venous surgery in patients with combined superficial and segmental deep venous reflux. *Eur J Vasc Endovasc Surg* 2003; 25: 469-72.

26. Gohel MS, Barwell JR, Earnshaw JJ, *et al.* Randomised clinical trial of compression plus surgery versus compression alone in chronic venous ulceration (ESCHAR study) - haemodynamic and anatomical changes. *Br J Surg* 2005; 92: 291-7.

27. Negus D, Friedgood A. The effective management of venous ulceration. *Br J Surg* 1983; 70: 623-7.

28. Recek C. A critical appraisal of the role of ankle perforators for the genesis of venous ulcers in the lower leg. *J Cardiovasc Surg* 1971; 12: 45-9.

29. Hoare MC, Nicolaides AN, Miles CR, *et al.* The role of primary varicose veins in venous ulceration. *Surgery* 1983; 92: 450-3.

30. Sethia KK, Darke SG. Long saphenous incompetence as a cause of venous ulceration. *Br J Surg* 1984; 71: 754-5.

31. Bello M, Scriven M, Hartshorne T, *et al.* The role of superficial venous surgery in the treatment of venous ulceration. *Br J Surg* 1999; 86: 755-9.

32. Barwell JR, Taylor M, Deacon J, *et al.* Surgical correction of isolated superficial venous reflux reduces long-term recurrence rate in chronic venous leg ulcers. *Eur J Vasc Endovasc Surg* 2000; 20: 363-8.

33. Ghauri ASK, Taylor MC, Deacon JE, *et al.* Influence of specialized leg ulcer service on management and outcome. *Br J Surg* 2000; 87: 1048-56.

34. Gohel MS, Taylor M, Earnshaw JJ, *et al.* Risk factors from delayed healing and recurrence of chronic venous leg ulcers - an analysis of 1324 legs. *Eur J Vasc Endovasc Surg* 2005; 29: 74-7.

35. Zamboni P, Cisno C, Marchetti F, *et al.* Minimally invasive surgical management of primary venous leg ulcers versus compression treatment: a randomized clinical trial. *Eur J Vasc Endovasc Surg* 2003; 25: 313-8.

36. Darke SG. Can we tailor surgery to the venous abnormality? In: *Venous disease, epidemiology management and delivery of care.* Ruckley CV, Fowkes FGR, Bradbury AW, Eds. London: Springer, 1998.

37. Padberg FT, Pappas PJ, Araki CT, *et al.* Hemodynamic and clinical improvement after superficial vein ablation in primary combined venous insufficiency with ulceration. *J Vasc Surg* 1996; 24: 711-8.

38. Caprini JA, Arcelus JI, Hoffman KN, *et al.* Venous duplex imaging follow-up of acute symptomatic deep vein thrombosis. *J Vasc Surg* 1995; 21: 472-6.

39. Johnson BF, Manzo RA, Bergelin RO, Standness DE. Relationship between changes in the deep venous system and the development of the post-thrombotic syndrome after an acute episode of lower limb deep vein thrombosis: a one to six-year follow-up. *J Vasc Surg* 1995; 21: 307-12.

40. Labropoulos N, Leon M, Nicolaides AN, *et al.* Venous reflux in patients with previous deep venous thrombosis: correlation with ulceration and other symptoms. *J Vasc Surg* 1994; 20: 20-6.

41. Stacey MC, Burnand KG, Lea Thomas M, Pattison M. Influence of phlebographic abnormalities on the natural history of venous ulceration. *Br J Surg* 1991; 78: 868-71.

Chapter 24

The management of venous ulceration

Katy AL Darvall MB ChB MRCS, Research Fellow
Andrew W Bradbury BSc MB ChB MD MBA FRCSEd, Professor of Vascular Surgery
Birmingham University Department of Vascular Surgery
Heart of England NHS Trust, Birmingham, UK

Introduction

In Northern Europe, the life-time risk of developing chronic venous ulceration (CVU) is estimated at 1%, with 10% of those affected having an open ulcer at any one time (estimated point prevalence 0.1%). It is also generally accepted that the treatment of lower limb venous disease consumes 1-2% of UK National Health Service spending. Although limb loss from CVU is rare, ulceration is associated with a marked reduction in quality of life. Despite this, the problem continues to receive a low priority for research funding and, as a result, there remains a lack of evidence regarding optimal management. Although reliable data are scarce, in the UK most patients with CVU are managed in the community and the general impression is that such treatment is often associated with suboptimal rates of healing and recurrence. Several different bodies have attempted to address this by preparing evidence-based guidelines.

Clinical assessment

The patient

CVU can be defined as a breach in the skin between the ankle and knee joint, of presumed venous aetiology, which has been present for at least four weeks. Before focusing on the ulcer, it is important to assess the patient as a whole. Many 'venous' ulcers, particularly those that are refractory to treatment, are multi-factorial in aetiology. Sustained healing will only be achieved once both systemic and local aetiological factors have been addressed; for example, diabetes mellitus, obesity, rheumatoid arthritis, peripheral arterial disease, cardiac failure, anaemia and renal disease. Certain lifestyle and socio-economic factors, such as occupation, quality/type of housing, heating, nutrition and mobility may also have an important bearing on both aetiology and prognosis. Carers need to take a holistic approach to CVU, managing the ulcer in the context of the whole leg, the leg in the context of the whole patient, and the patient in the context of their social and cultural circumstances.

The leg

The aetiology of a leg ulcer can usually be determined through careful history and examination. Particular attention should be paid to the locomotor system, the presence and distribution of oedema and, of course, the symptoms and signs of venous and arterial disease. Flat feet, a fixed ankle, and reduced mobility at the hips and/or knees all result in calf muscle pump dysfunction and so increase venous hypertension. Oedema (due to one or more of the following: venous disease, lymphoedema, cardiac failure, renal disease and hypoproteinaemia) significantly increases skin tension and impairs skin perfusion. The oedema fluid takes the path of least resistance, which is through the ulcer bed, thereby preventing re-epithelialisation. CVU will not heal unless oedema is controlled by elevation and compression.

The skin changes of chronic venous insufficiency are usually readily apparent but, in the obese, heavily scarred, ulcerated leg, even gross (surgically correctable) superficial venous reflux may be missed on clinical examination alone. All patients with CVU should be assessed at least by hand-held Doppler (HHD) examination; a full duplex ultrasound assessment is ideal.

Up to 20% of patients with CVU have significant arterial disease that both precludes the use of (full) compression therapy and impairs wound healing. Measurement of the ankle brachial pressure index (ABPI) by HHD is the most reliable way of detecting arterial insufficiency [1, 2] and this should be done for all patients with CVU **(IIa/B)**. Compression is generally considered safe if the ABPI is >0.8, but absolute pressure (rather than the ratio) may be more informative. Caution is required in patients with neuropathy and in the presence of incompressible vessels; both of these features are found most commonly in association with diabetes **(III/B)**.

The ulcer

A full and structured description of the ulcer is important for both diagnosis and assessment of healing. The following should be noted:

- position: gaiter area, foot or atypical;
- base: necrotic, sloughy or granulating;
- margin: regular or irregular, epithelialising or not;
- surrounding tissue: infected, indurated, oedematous, friable;

- depth: shallow, deep, punched-out, tendon or bone exposed.

The surface area of the ulcer should be measured serially **(IIb/B)** and calibrated clinical photographs are valuable in assessing response to treatment. Most venous ulcers are colonised by bacteria rather than being infected in a causative sense and routine bacteriological swabbing is not indicated unless there are clinical signs of active infection [3] **(IIb/B)**.

Treatment

Compression

Compression therapy has been the mainstay of treatment for more than two thousand years. Bandaging is preferred initially to stockings to obtain healing of the ulcer, as stockings are difficult to apply over dressings and become soiled with exudate. However, compression hosiery can be used once the ulcer has healed to reduce the risk of recurrence or in ulcers that have little exudate. It is well-established that compression should be graduated, that is to say it should be highest at the ankle, diminishing towards the knee [4, 5] **(Ia/A)**.

Bandages can provide elastic or non-elastic compression. A systematic review of five randomised controlled trials comparing multi-layered systems has shown that elastic compression is more effective than non-elastic compression [6] **(Ia/A)**. Furthermore, while no difference in healing rates was observed between four-layer bandaging and other high compression multi-layer bandaging systems, multi-layered high compression appears significantly more effective than single-layer compression [6] **(Ia/A)**. No evidence is available on the cost-effectiveness of different bandaging systems. Importantly, whichever form of compression is chosen, it must be applied correctly and appropriate training is necessary for the best results.

Intermittent pneumatic compression has been the subject of a systematic review of four randomised controlled trials. One trial found increased ulcer healing with this technique [7] but the other three studies found no advantage over the methods described in the previous paragraph [8].

Debridement and cleaning

There have been no methodologically robust trials of the effects on healing of different types of chemical and/or mechanical debridement. The Venus II trial that is currently underway aims to define the clinical and cost-effectiveness of larval therapy in venous and mixed arterial-venous ulcers [9]. One randomised study has shown that the rate of infection in acute, traumatic wounds is lower when they are washed in tap water than when they are washed in sterile water [10] **(Ib/A)**.

Dressings

It is generally accepted that the type of primary dressing has little effect on healing. A systematic review of five randomised controlled trials comparing semi-occlusive dressings (e.g. foam, film and alginates) with simple low adherent dressings (e.g. paraffin-tulle or knitted viscose), and of nine randomised controlled trials comparing hydrocolloid (occlusive) dressings with simple dressings, found no significant differences in healing rates between any of these [11] **(Ia/A)**. It is, however, worth noting that the power of the studies was such that only a large difference would have been detected. A randomised controlled trial (VULCAN) is currently underway to assess whether antimicrobial dressings are cost-effective [12].

Painful ulcers

There is some evidence that hydrocolloid and/or foam dressings are better than simple dressings in particularly painful ulcers, but a Cochrane review of the subject found no randomised controlled trials [13].

Topical agents

No topical agent has yet been shown to improve healing. Topical antibiotics are often allergy sensitisers and also promote the emergence of resistant organisms. They should not be used [14] **(III/B)**.

Systemic therapy

The evidence (or lack of it) for a benefit from systemic pharmacotherapy in the treatment of CVU is summarised in Table 1 [15-21]. A recent systematic review of eight randomised controlled trials suggested that oral pentoxifylline (Trental) was more effective than placebo in terms of healing, although not all studies have shown benefit and the benefit, if any, is small [15] **(Ia/A)**. A recent systematic review of 59 randomised controlled trials concluded that there was insufficient evidence to support the use of flavonoids [17]. A systematic review (five randomised controlled trials) found no evidence of benefit from oral zinc supplements [22]. The use of systemic antibiotics in clinically uninfected CVU is widely accepted to be ineffective and risks the emergence of resistant organisms as well as other antibiotic-related complications; their use should be reserved for wounds with documented infection and based on sensitivities **(Ib/A)**.

Surgery

A recent randomised controlled trial comparing compression with compression plus varicose vein surgery found no difference in healing rates [23]. However, recurrence was significantly lower in the surgery group (see below). On the basis of personal experience, numerous published uncontrolled studies and this trial, most surgeons believe that, in the absence of post-thrombotic deep venous disease, eradication of superficial venous reflux by operation (or some other method, such as foam sclerotherapy) is of benefit **(IIb/B)**. Many surgeons, including the authors, do not now wait for ulcer healing before considering intervention. Although advocated by some, there is no convincing evidence that perforator surgery (open or endoscopic), superficial valve repair, deep venous reconstruction or autologous skin grafting alters the natural history of CVU [24-27]. However, a systematic review of two randomised controlled trials found significantly better healing rates with tissue-engineered skin

Table 1. Systemic pharmacotherapy for chronic leg ulceration.		
Drug	Proposed mode of action	Comment
Pentoxifylline	Improves microcirculatory blood flow and increases oxygenation of ischaemic tissues	Recently shown to be more effective than placebo in healing ulcers when used with compression [15]
Stanozolol	Enhances fibrinolysis to 'dissolve' fibrin cuff	Reduces lipodermatosclerosis but no effect on healing rates [16]
Flavonoids	May improve venous tone or decrease capillary hyperpermeability	Symptomatic improvement in chronic venous insufficiency, but limited evidence of an effect on ulcer healing [17]
Aspirin	Reduces the thrombocytosis and increased platelet volume associated with venous hypertension	Small studies have suggested an increase in healing rates [18, 19]
Ergotamine	Causes vein wall contraction leading to reduced vein diameter and reduced reflux	May improve healing rates, but toxic with a narrow therapeutic index; not recommended [20]
Prostaglandin E1	Inhibits platelet aggregation and neutrophil activation which may have an effect on 'white cell trapping'	May improve healing, but only available as an expensive intravenous preparation [21]

containing epidermal and dermal components than with non-adherent dressing [27].

Arterial surgery

Various forms of modified compression have been advocated when the ABPI is between 0.6 and 0.8, although their use is not, strictly speaking, evidence-based. If the ABPI is less than 0.6 it is generally accepted that compression of any form is contraindicated. In such circumstances, arterial intervention may relieve pain, allow the safe use of compression, improve healing and reduce recurrence. Although such an approach makes intuitive sense, it has not been the subject of rigorous scientific study.

Other modalities

A systematic review of seven randomised controlled trials comparing ultrasound with either sham ultrasound (four studies) or standard therapy revealed no significant difference in healing rates, but it is worth noting that there was a small treatment effect in favour of ultrasound in all studies [28]. A larger, multi-centre, randomised controlled trial (VenUS III) is currently underway to try to resolve the issue [29]. A systematic review and two further randomised studies failed to provide evidence in favour of laser treatment [30-32]. Finally, a further systematic review of three randomised controlled trials failed to show any benefit from electromagnetic therapy, although the studies were all small and powered only to detect large (probably unrealistic) differences in healing rates [33].

Secondary prevention

Compression

Two randomised controlled trials have found that below-knee graduated compression stockings reduce the recurrence rate over five years [34, 35]. Class III stockings appear to be more effective than Class II overall, even when the higher rate of non-compliance with the stronger compression is taken into account (Table 2). It is widely accepted that not wearing any compression is strongly associated with ulcer recurrence. It is recommended that correctly fitted graduated compression hosiery be prescribed for at least five years (probably 'for life') for all patients who have successfully healed a venous leg ulcer **(Ib/A)**.

Table 2. Classes of compression hosiery.	
Class	Pressure at the ankle
I	<25mmHg
II	25-35mmHg
III	35-45mmHg
IV	>45mmHg

Surgery

Two recent randomised controlled trials have shown that the eradication of superficial venous reflux by superficial venous surgery reduces ulcer recurrence; one found that the 12-month recurrence rate of CVU was reduced from 28% to 12% [23], and the other that the recurrence rate over three years was 10% with surgery and compression, compared with 38% for compression alone [36]. Superficial venous surgery in patients with CVU is significantly different from that in patients with uncomplicated varicose veins. Those with CVU tend to be older and to have comorbidity, increasing the risk of general anaesthesia. They may also be at greater risk of postoperative thrombo-embolic complications, particularly if the ulcer is associated with post-thrombotic syndrome. The ulcer and surrounding skin are often colonised with bacteria, so prophylaxis against surgical wound infection seems wise. Although not specifically studied to date, this may be a situation

in which a minimally invasive alternative to a conventional operation, such as ultrasound-guided foam sclerotherapy, may be of particular benefit (Figures 1 and 2). No drugs or other therapies have been shown to have any role in the prevention of ulcer recurrence [37].

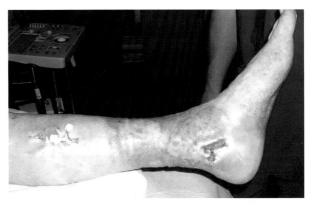

Figure 1. Chronic venous ulcer in the medial gaiter area in association with long saphenous varicose veins. The deep veins appeared normal on duplex ultrasound imaging. A cannula has been placed in the long saphenous vein below the knee under duplex guidance in preparation for ultrasound-guided foam sclerotherapy.

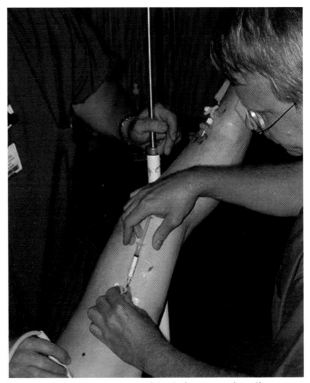

Figure 2. Ultrasound-guided foam sclerotherapy. Cannulas have been placed in the long saphenous vein above and below the knee under duplex guidance. Foam is being introduced into the long saphenous vein to occlude it.

Provision of care

Much has been written about different models of care for the provision of leg ulcer services and, in particular, the problems of establishing a patient-focused, community-based service, and quality assurance [38]. A recent survey of practice in the UK has revealed [39]:

- 92% of areas of the UK have a dedicated venous ulcer service;
- 54% of these are managed by acute hospitals and 28% in the community;
- 64% are supervised by doctors and 33% by nurses.

The provision of care inevitably varies with location, but many experts in the field believe that the following are important components of any model:

- the overall treatment package should be delivered by an interdisciplinary team of doctors and nurses who communicate readily with each other and have easy access to the skills of other disciplines, such as physiotherapists and occupational therapists;
- carers should understand the multi-factorial aetiology of leg ulcers and be capable of identifying, early in the course of the disease, patients who might benefit from surgical correction of underlying venous and arterial disease and/or other specialist input (Table 3);
- patients are treated according to evidence-based guidelines derived from a systematic review of the available literature;
- the patients' treatment is viewed as a joint effort between primary and secondary care.

Conclusions

CVU remains a common and debilitating condition that consumes a large amount of health care resources. Although research into new (often high-tech) treatments, such as artificial skin substitutes, is interesting, it is actually failure to apply the knowledge that is already available that has the most adverse impact on patients' lives. Every week in clinic the authors see patients with ulcers that have been

Table 3. Suggested criteria for specialist referral.
◆ Uncertain aetiology
◆ Atypical ulcer distribution
◆ Suspicion of malignancy
◆ Peripheral arterial disease (ABPI <0.8)
◆ Surgically correctable superficial venous reflux
◆ Diabetes mellitus
◆ Rheumatoid arthritis or other suspected vasculitis
◆ Dermatitis refractory to topical steroids
◆ Failure to respond to conventional therapy

present for months, if not years, in association with obvious varicose veins who have never enjoyed the benefits of compression and have never had an adequate vascular assessment. Not surprisingly, once provided with properly applied graduated, multi-layer compression, and once their superficial reflux has been corrected, these patients usually heal their ulcers rapidly and have a low rate of recurrence. Of course, it is not always so simple. Every ulcer service must deal with a difficult, but relatively small, group of patients with complex ulcers that are often associated with arterial disease and extensive deep vein reflux. In such circumstances, symptom relief rather than healing is the main goal and, rarely, such patients may actually be well served by primary amputation and fitting with a prosthesis.

If it is accepted that most on-going care for CVU should be delivered in the community then, as the Scottish Leg Ulcer Project and other similar research has shown, it needs to be delivered by specialist nurses who are properly trained and who have a case-load sufficient to maintain their skills [38]. It is also important that those who develop leg ulcers of whatever aetiology are referred as soon as possible (within weeks) for a full vascular assessment, which will usually be carried out in a hospital outpatient setting. In this way those with correctable superficial reflux and significant arterial disease can be identified and treated appropriately. It is regrettable, therefore, that in many parts of the UK, rationing of venous surgery and services effectively means that patients are referred for such an assessment only after ulceration has developed and persisted for a prolonged interval in the community. The haphazard and unsatisfactory treatment that many with CVU still receive cannot be justified in terms of cost or clinical effectiveness and it is certainly not evidence-based.

Key points	Evidence level

Assessment

- Measurement of the ankle brachial pressure index (ABPI) by hand-held Doppler is essential in the assessment of chronic leg ulcer. — IIa/B
- Patients with an ABPI <0.8 should be assumed to have arterial disease. — III/B
- The surface area of the ulcer should be measured serially. — IIb/B
- Bacteriological swabs should be taken only when there is clinical evidence of active infection. — IIb/B

Treatment

- Graduated compression should be used for healing uncomplicated venous ulcers. — Ia/A
- Elastic compression is the treatment of choice for uncomplicated venous leg ulcers. — Ia/A
- Multilayer bandaging is recommended. — Ia/A
- Ulcerated legs should be washed in tap water and dried carefully. — Ib/A
- Simple non-adherent dressings are recommended in the treatment of venous ulcers, as no specific dressing has been shown to improve healing rates. — Ia/A
- Antibiotics should be used only when there is evidence of active infection (e.g. cellulitis). — Ib/A
- Topical antibiotics are frequent sensitisers and should be avoided. — III/B
- Systemic therapy in the treatment of leg ulcers is not recommended. — Ia/A
- Venous surgery followed by graduated compression should be considered in patients with chronic venous ulceration. — IIb/B

Secondary prevention

- Correctly fitted graduated compression hosiery should be prescribed for at least five years for all patients who have successfully healed a venous leg ulcer. — Ib/A

References

1. Caruana MF, Bradbury AW, Adam DJ. The validity, reliability, reproducibility and extended utility of ankle to brachial pressure index in current vascular surgical practice. *Eur J Vasc Endovasc Surg* 2005; 29: 443-51.

2. Moffatt CJ, Oldroyd MI, Greenhalgh RM, Franks PJ. Palpating ankle pulses is insufficient in detecting arterial insufficiency in patients with leg ulceration. *Phlebology* 1994; 9: 170-2.

3. Hansson C, Hoborn J, Moller A, Swanbeck G. The microbial flora in venous leg ulcers without clinical signs of infection. Repeated culture using a validated standardised microbiological technique. *Acta Derm Venereol* 1995; 75: 24-30.

4. Fletcher A, Cullum N, Sheldon TA. A systematic review of compression treatment for venous leg ulcers. *Br Med J* 1997; 315: 576-80.

5. Palfreyman SJ, Lochiel R, Michaels JA. A systematic review of compression therapy for venous leg ulcers. *Vasc Med* 1998; 3: 301-13.

6. Cullum N, Nelson EA, Fletcher AW, Sheldon TA. Compression for venous leg ulcers. *The Cochrane Database of Systematic Reviews* 2001; Issue 2: Art. No. CD000265. DOI: 10.1002/14651858.

7. Coleridge Smith P, Sarin S, Hasty J, Scurr JH. Sequential gradient pneumatic compression enhances venous ulcer healing: a randomized trial. *Surgery* 1990; 108: 871-5.

8. Mani R, Vowden K, Nelson EA. Intermittent pneumatic compression for treating venous leg ulcers. *The Cochrane Database of Systematic Reviews* 2001; Issue 4: Art. No. CD001899. DOI: 10.1002/14651858.CD001899.

9. Cullum N. Venus II: larval therapy venous ulcer study. http://www.hta.ac.uk/project.asp?PjtId=1339.

10. Hall Angeras M, Brandberg A, Falk A, Seeman T. Comparison between sterile saline and tap water for the cleaning of acute traumatic soft tissue wounds. *Eur J Surg* 1992; 158: 347-50.

11. Bradley M, Cullum N, Nelson EA, *et al*. Dressings and topical agents for healing of chronic wounds: a systematic review. *Health Technol Assess* 1999; 3: 17 Pt2.

12. Michaels J. Randomised controlled trial and economic modelling to evaluate the place of anti-microbial agents in the management of venous leg ulcers (VULCAN). http://www.hta.ac.uk/project.asp?PjtId=1380.

13. Briggs M, Nelson EA. Topical agents or dressings for pain in venous leg ulcers. *The Cochrane Database of Systematic Reviews* 2003; Issue 1: Art. No. CD001177. DOI: 10.1002/14651858.CD001177.

14. Zaki I, Shall L, Dalziel KL. Bacitracin: a significant sensitizer in leg ulcer patients? *Contact Dermatitis* 1994; 31: 92-4.

15. Jull AB, Waters J, Arroll B. Pentoxifylline for treating venous leg ulcers. *The Cochrane Database of Systematic Reviews* 2002; Issue 1: Art. No. CD001733. DOI: 10.1002/14651858.CD001733.

16. McMullin G, Watkin GT, Coleridge Smith PD. The efficacy of fibrinolytic enhancement with stanozolol in the treatment of venous insufficiency. *Phlebology* 1991; 6: 233-8.

17. Martinez MJ, Bonfill X, Moreno RM, *et al*. Phlebotonics for venous insufficiency. *The Cochrane Database of Systematic Reviews* 2005; Issue 3: Art. No. CD003229.pub2. DOI: 10.1002/14651858.CD003229.pub2.

18. Layton AM, Ibbotson SH, Davies JA, Goodfield MJD. The effect of oral aspirin in the treatment of chronic venous leg ulcers. *Lancet* 1994; 344: 164-5.

19. Ibbotson SH, Layton AM, Davies JA, Goodfield MJD. The effect of aspirin on haemostatic activity in the treatment of chronic venous leg ulceration. *Br J Dermatol* 1995; 132: 422-6.

20. Bjerle P. Treatment of venous insufficiency with dihydroergotamine. *VASA* 1979; 8: 158-62.

21. Rudofsky G. Intravenous prostaglandin E1 in the treatment of venous ulcers in a double-blind, placebo-controlled trial. *VASA* 1989; Suppl 28: 39-43.

22. Wilkinson EAJ, Hawke C. Oral zinc for arterial and venous leg ulcers. *The Cochrane Database of Systematic Reviews* 1998; Issue 4: Art. No. CD001273. DOI: 10.1002/14651858. CD001273.

23. Barwell JR, Davies CE, Deacon J, *et al*. Comparison of surgery and compression with compression alone in chronic venous ulceration (ESCHAR study): randomised controlled trial. *Lancet* 2004; 363: 1854-9.

24. Stuart WP. Perforator surgery; what is its role? In: *The epidemiology and management of venous disease*. Ruckley CV, Fowkes FGR, Bradbury AW, Eds. London: Springer Verlag, 1998: 132-8.

25. Warburg FE, Danielsen L, Madsen SM, *et al*. Vein surgery with or without skin grafting versus conservative treatment for leg ulcers. *Acta Dermatol Venereol* 1994; 74: 307-9.

26. Hardy SC, Riding G, Abidia A. Surgery for deep venous incompetence. *The Cochrane Database of Systematic Reviews* 2004; Issue 3: Art. No. CD001097.pub2. DOI: 10.1002/14651858.CD001097.pub2.

27. Jones JE, Nelson EA. Skin grafting for venous leg ulcers. *The Cochrane Database of Systematic Reviews* 2000, Issue 2: Art. No. CD001737.pub2. DOI: 10.1002/14651858. CD001737.pub2.

28. Flemming K, Cullum N. Therapeutic ultrasound for venous leg ulcers. *The Cochrane Database of Systematic Reviews* 2000; Issue 4: Art. No. CD001180. DOI: 10.1002/14651858. CD001180.

29. Nelson EA. VenUS III - Venous Ulcer Studies III: ultrasound for venous leg ulcers. http://www.hta.ac.uk/project.asp?PjtId=1451.

30. Flemming K, Cullum N. Laser therapy for venous leg ulcers. *The Cochrane Database of Systematic Reviews* 1999; Issue 1: Art. No. CD001182. DOI: 10.1002/14651858. CD001182.

31. Lagan KM, McKenna T, Witherow A, *et al*. Low-intensity laser therapy/combined phototherapy in the management of chronic venous ulceration: a placebo-controlled study. *J Clin Laser Med Surg* 2002; 20: 109-16.

32. Franek A, Krol P, Kucharzewski M. Does low output laser stimulation enhance the healing of crural ulceration? Some critical remarks. *Med Eng Phys* 2002; 24: 607-15.

33. Ravaghi H, Flemming K, Cullum N, Olyaee Manesh A. Electromagnetic therapy for treating venous leg ulcers. *The*

Cochrane Database of Systematic Reviews 2006; Issue 2: Art. No. CD002933.pub3. DOI: 10.1002/14651858. CD002933.pub3.

34. Nelson EA, Bell-Syer SEM, Cullum NA. Compression for preventing recurrence of venous ulcers. *The Cochrane Database of Systematic Reviews* 2000; Issue 4: Art. No. CD002303. DOI: 10.1002/14651858.CD002303.

35. Harper DR, Nelson EA, Gibson B, *et al.* A prospective randomised trial of class 2 and class 3 elastic compression in the prevention of venous ulceration. In: *Phlebology '95.* Negus D, Jantet G, Coleridge Smith PD, Eds. London: Springer Verlag, 1995: 872-3.

36. Zamboni P, Cisno C, Marchetti F, *et al.* Minimally invasive surgical management of primary venous ulcers vs. compression treatment: a randomised clinical trial. *Eur J Vasc Endovasc Surg* 2003; 25: 313-8.

37. Taylor HM, Rose KE, Twycross RG. A double-blind clinical RCT of hydroxyethylrutosides in obstructive arm lymphoedema. *Phlebology* 1993; 8 (suppl 1): 22-8.

38. Scottish leg ulcer project: a randomized trial evaluating the implementation of national guidelines *Br J Surg* 2001; 88: 607-8

39. Campbell WB, Thomson H, MacIntyre JB, *et al.* Venous ulcer services in the United Kingdom. *Eur J Vasc Endovasc Surg* 2005; 30: 437-40.

Chapter 25

Renal revascularisation

George Hamilton FRCS, Professor of Vascular Surgery

Vascular Unit, University Department of Surgery, Royal Free Hampstead NHS Trust

Royal Free & University College School of Medicine, London, UK

Introduction

The clinical significance of renal artery stenosis is its association with hypertension and renal dysfunction, particularly in the elderly patient. Renovascular disease accounts for over 90% of renal artery stenoses in European countries, with fibromuscular disease accounting for the remaining 10%. Fibromuscular dysplasia was previously thought to be uncommon, but has recently been shown to have a prevalence of 1-2% in an autopsy study of western patients [1]. Takayasu's arteritis is much more common in the Indian sub-continent and the Far East, where it accounts for up to 60% of all cases of renal artery stenosis. In western aging populations prone to progressive atherosclerosis and hypertension, up to 6.8% of patients over the age of 65 years have a renal artery stenosis >60% [2].

Pathophysiology and epidemiology

Until this last decade, stenosis of the main stem renal artery has been the primary focus of attention in studies on the pathophysiology of atherosclerotic renovascular disease (ARVD). A significant renal artery stenosis can result in renal ischaemia that causes hypertension with, or without salt and water retention, and the eventual development of renal failure which may or may not be reversible. There has been debate regarding the definition of a significant renal artery stenosis. Based on experimental studies, a significant stenosis is defined as being greater than 60%, but in the clinical setting assessment by angiography is not always that accurate. Several recent studies using isotopic measurement of single-kidney glomerular filtration have highlighted the lack of any relationship between the severity of renal artery stenosis and the degree of renal dysfunction. Indeed these studies have often shown similar or even worse renal dysfunction in the contralateral kidney with a normal renal artery on imaging [3]. The clinical scenario of an isolated, tight renal artery stenosis resulting in impaired renal function undoubtedly occurs, but only in a minority of patients with ARVD. These clinical findings highlight the importance of intrarenal or parenchymal disease in the aetiology of renal failure in many patients [4]. Renal artery stenosis secondary to fibromuscular dysplasia rarely results in renal failure, while the opposite is true of renal artery stenosis secondary to atherosclerosis. Therefore, renovascular disease is now preferred to describe renal artery stenosis in combination with atherosclerosis.

Atherosclerotic disease is progressive in nature; a recent prospective study using duplex ultrasound imaging documented an average rate of 7% per year, with stenoses of over 60% progressing by 30% at one year and 40% at three years [5]. A similar study performed in the 1990s using angiography reported significant renal artery stenosis progression in over 11% of patients during a mean of 2.6 years [6]. Best medical therapy has changed dramatically in the last few years, and it is not clear whether this will mitigate the progression of renal artery stenosis in these patients.

A decision to intervene in patients with ARVD must be taken in the light of their poor overall prognosis. Connolly et al showed that their survival correlated with initial angiographic findings [7]. Two-year actuarial survival was 96% in patients with unilateral renal artery stenosis, reducing to 74% for bilateral stenoses and only 47% for unilateral occlusion. Mailloux et al reported that once on dialysis as a result of atherosclerotic renal artery stenosis, patients had an average five-year survival of only 12% [8].

Atherosclerotic renal vascular disease is associated with other cardiac and vascular conditions including coronary artery disease, peripheral vascular disease, aortic aneurysms and cerebral vascular disease. Up to 15% of patients undergoing coronary angiography have been shown to have significant renal artery stenosis; a further 15% had insignificant stenoses [9]. Patients with extensive coronary artery disease and renal artery stenosis are a particularly high-risk group. Similarly, ARVD is common in patients with peripheral vascular disease. Significant renal artery stenosis was found in 38% of patients with an abdominal aortic aneurysm, 33% in patients with aorto-occlusive disease and 39% of patients with peripheral vascular disease undergoing angiography for these indications [10].

Clinical presentation and investigation

Over 90% of patients with ARVD are hypertensive in the presence of other risk factors for atherosclerosis. Patients with fibromuscular dysplasia or Takayasu's disease involving the renal arteries invariably present with hypertension, but rarely with renal failure. In contrast, patients with ARVD present with a combination of hypertension and/or renal failure. Acute renal failure is an uncommon presentation but may result from causes such as hypovolaemia (often complicating diuretic use), or complicating the administration of angiotensin converting enzyme (ACE) inhibitors or angiotensin II receptor blockers. Acute renal failure may also develop as a result of intrarenal cholesterol embolisation, which can complicate angiography/angioplasty. More commonly ARVD is associated with chronic kidney disease, a condition sometimes also termed ischaemic nephropathy. This disease is characterised by severe hypertensive damage, intrarenal vascular disease, cholesterol embolisation and sclerosing glomerular lesions. Progressive renal atrophy leads to end-stage disease, with 15-25% of older patients progressing to renal replacement therapy [11].

An important complication is the sudden onset of pulmonary oedema, usually with no previous cardiac history. These patients have bilateral renal artery disease, and flash pulmonary oedema is an increasingly recognised presentation, occurring in up to 10% of patients with ARVD [12]. Renal artery stenosis is also common in elderly patients with congestive cardiac failure. A study looking at cardiac function that compared patients with ARVD and chronic kidney disease to those with chronic kidney disease from other causes, found a significantly higher prevalence of left ventricular hypertrophy, (78.5% compared with 46%), and left ventricular diastolic dysfunction, (40.5% compared with 12%). Only 5% of patients with ARVD and chronic kidney disease had a normal heart [13]. The key clinical features of ARVD are listed in Table 1.

Table 1. Clinical features of renal artery stenosis.
Hypertension   Abrupt onset in young (fibromuscular disease) or >50 years (ARVD)   Accelerated or malignant hypertension   Refractory to antihypertensive therapy
Renal function   Unexplained renal failure in >50 years   Renal failure following ACE or Angiotensin II receptor inhibitors   Asymmetrical kidneys
Other features   Flash pulmonary oedema   Clinical features of systemic atherosclerosis (bruits etc)   Neurofibromatosis

Investigation

Investigation should be undertaken in patients with the above features and abnormal renal function. Identification of renal artery stenosis involves assessment of renal function and imaging for the presence of renal artery disease. Intra-arterial angiography (DSA), previously the gold standard, is now being supplanted by less invasive methods of assessment with angiography being reserved for those patients selected for intervention.

Renal ultrasonography

Duplex ultrasound assessment of renal length and asymmetry is used in many specialist centres but there are problems with its reproducibility and operator dependency. Direct imaging of the renal artery and detection of stenosis is possible in skilled hands, but is a lengthy procedure. More practical is measurement of the resistive index (RI=peak systolic flow velocity minus minimum diastolic flow velocity/peak systolic flow velocity), and pulsatility index (PI=peak systolic flow velocity minus minimum diastolic flow velocity/mean flow velocity), by imaging of the intrarenal vessels. In particular, RI has been studied as a method of assessing renal disease; a high RI predicted a poor renal functional response to angioplasty [14]. There is ongoing debate about whether RI is a useful marker of intrarenal disease or simply a marker of generalised atherosclerosis.

Renal scintigraphy

Renal scintigraphy is a widely available test that allows measurement of differential function to identify poorly functioning and non-functioning kidneys. Captopril (stress) renography is rarely used currently because of its poor sensitivity and specificity, except in high-grade stenoses, and because of the complications of administration. The isotopic measurement of single kidney glomerular filtration rate (GFR) may help inform the decision regarding revascularisation, particularly where a kidney with a renal artery stenosis is shown to have a very low GFR. This investigation is not widely available, however.

Magnetic resonance imaging

Gadolinium-enhanced magnetic resonance angiography (MRA) is more widely available and has become the favoured imaging technique for renal artery disease. In comparison with contrast angiography, MRA demonstrated 87% sensitivity, 69% specificity, 85% accuracy, 95% negative predictive value and 51% positive predictive value in the diagnosis of renal artery stenosis [15]. There continue to be problems with inter-observer agreement; MRA can result in significant over-estimation of renal artery stenosis in up to one third of patients. It also must be stressed that Gadolinium is itself nephrotoxic in high doses.

Spiral CT angiography

CT angiography has similar sensitivity and specificity to MRA. There have been major advances in CT angiography but as yet little evidence for any improved accuracy. A recent assessment of multi-detector-row CT angiography compared with DSA in 50 patients with renal artery stenosis showed sensitivity of 100%, specificity of 98.6% and accuracy of 96.9% [16]. If this accuracy was confirmed in larger studies spiral CT angiography would be an alternative to DSA **(IIa/B)**.

Digital subtraction angiography

This remains the gold standard but because of its invasive nature and the significant risk of contrast nephrotoxicity, it has a place only in patients where non-invasive assessment gives equivocal results, or as a preliminary to angioplasty revascularisation. The value of peri-operative hydration in preventing contrast-induced nephropathy is now established, with the addition of N-acetylcysteine or sodium bicarbonate [17].

Management

The priorities in the management of ARVD are control of hypertension, optimisation of renal function, avoiding the need for renal replacement therapy, and improving cardiovascular morbidity. Renal artery stenosis and ARVD are now treated medically, with best therapy including vigorous control of hypertension, hyperlipidaemia and diabetes, if present, antiplatelet therapy, smoking cessation and lifestyle modifications such as reduced salt intake and increased exercise (Chapter 5). All these patients should have statin therapy, based on the favourable outcomes of the randomised trials, although there is little specific clinical evidence regarding the value of statins for ARVD. Many different agents are now available for antihypertensive therapy; ACE inhibitors in particular have proved to be effective, although great care must be taken to monitor renal function in these patients, who are at risk of drug-related renal failure.

In most units only symptomatic patients with ARVD are currently offered intervention by renal revascularisation; however, each patient needs to be considered individually by a multidisciplinary team. Options for intervention include angioplasty with, or without stenting, surgical revascularisation or nephrectomy.

The main indications for intervention in renal artery stenosis are shown in Table 2. There remains debate about what constitutes successful intervention in these patients. Successful treatment is defined as improved or stabilised renal function, together with a 15% reduction in diastolic blood pressure, or the same blood pressure with less medication. A 'cure' constitutes a diastolic blood pressure <90mmHg with no medication.

Renal revascularisation

Endovascular revascularisation

Surgical revascularisation has largely been replaced by percutaneous techniques, initially simple renal angioplasty, but increasingly with the addition of a renal stent (Figure 1). Recent analysis of the trends in Medicare patients in the USA showed that stent angioplasty now accounts for over 95% of all revascularisation procedures [18].

Excellent results can be obtained with simple angioplasty for stenosis due to fibromuscular

Table 2. Indications for revascularisation in patients with renal artery stenosis.
◆ Refractory hypertension despite best medical therapy
◆ Deteriorating renal function despite best medical therapy
◆ Recent or rapid onset end-stage renal failure
◆ Acute renal failure after ACE inhibitor or angiotensin receptor blocker therapy
◆ Diminishing renal mass on best medical therapy
◆ Progression of stenosis
◆ Flash and recurrent pulmonary oedema

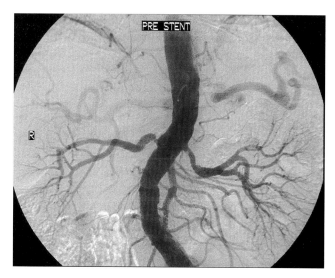

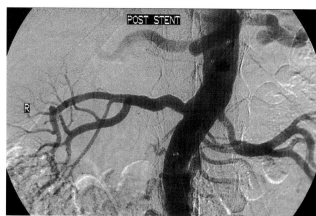

Figure 1. Angiograms demonstrating the result of renal artery stent insertion. *Courtesy of Professor A. Watkinson, Exeter.*

dysplasia; in 314 patients, 43% were cured, 42% improved and in only 15% did the procedure fail [19, 20] (IIa/B). Over 50% of patients with initially successful treatment did not require further antihypertensive medication, and recurrence was rare.

In contrast, there are few randomised controlled trials relating to the efficacy of renal angioplasty for atherosclerotic renal artery stenosis. Stenting, in addition to angioplasty, is now favoured for ostial disease because of the improved technical success rate. Most experience has been gained using balloon expandable stents such as the Palmaz stent. Self-expanding stents are also available, such as the Wallstent and the Memotherm. Renal stent angioplasty is technically demanding due to the associated severe aortic atheroma, renal artery angulation and the occasional need for a brachial approach to position the stent accurately. Subsequent surgery, following occlusion of a metallic renal stent, can be challenging. It is therefore important that stents should not be used in the distal renal artery where surgical rescue techniques may be rendered impossible. The technical success rate of renal stenting is high, with primary patency rates typically in excess of 95%. Renal stent angioplasty is associated with a (mostly minor) complication rate of about 10%, but with a mortality rate of 1.2% (range 0-4.2%) [21].

Reviews of the outcome of renal stent angioplasty have indicated that approximately a quarter of patients improve, 50% stabilise but a further quarter will continue to have deterioration in their renal function (IIa/B). Stabilisation of renal function has been deemed as an acceptable outcome; this is probably so in patients with minor to moderate renal failure, but cannot be considered a success in patients at risk of needing renal replacement therapy. In patients with severe pre-operative renal insufficiency, stabilisation of renal function was associated with a similar risk of dialysis and death as in patients whose renal function deteriorated [22].

Filters

In some reports, surgical revascularisation has lower rates of deterioration after intervention, which are typically about 10% after angioplasty. This difference has been attributed to contrast nephropathy, but increasingly, athero-embolism caused by endovascular manipulation is being implicated. The recent introduction of filter protection devices has confirmed that there is a significant release of athero-embolic material, even with stent angioplasty. Unfortunately the currently available filter devices capture only larger particles and thus do not offer complete protection. The use of distal embolic protection by temporary balloon occlusion and aspiration instead may minimise the athero-embolism [23]. There remains no controlled evidence to support the use of filters, although the recently started CORAL trial in the USA comparing stent angioplasty with embolic protection devices and best medical therapy should provide some answers.

Restenosis

In-stent restenosis is a significant complication of stent angioplasty. In a recent review, an average of 19% restenosis was found for lesions classified as >50% after follow-up of 12.5 months, and 13.4% for >60% stenosis after 13 months [24]. In-stent restenosis can be treated with repeat balloon angioplasty, but a re-recurrence rate of over 20% is reported. In addition, other methods such as the use of cutting balloons, brachytherapy and drug-eluting stents have also been reported but as yet there is no evidence to suggest objective benefit for these interventions [25].

The current evidence for endovascular treatment of ARVD

There remains a lack of data from randomised trials on the value of percutaneous techniques in the management of ARVD, with only four published clinical trials. The Scottish and Newcastle Renal Artery Stenosis group compared angioplasty with medical therapy in hypertensive patients with both unilateral and bilateral disease [26]. They concluded that angioplasty resulted in a statistically significant improvement in systolic blood pressure, but this benefit was seen only in patients with bilateral disease. There was no significant difference in renal function or major outcome events such as death, cardiovascular or cerebrovascular events, or dialysis. There was, however, a complication rate of 27.5% following endovascular intervention. The difficulty of performing randomised controlled trials in this disease was highlighted by the fact that this study only recruited 55 patients **(Ib/A)**.

Two other studies that compared angioplasty and best medical therapy both described only modest improvements in blood pressure control after revascularisation, and no improvement in renal function [27, 28]. In the Dutch randomised trial of arterial stenting (n=43) versus balloon angioplasty (n=42) for ostial atherosclerotic renovascular lesions, the primary success rate for angioplasty alone was 57% compared to 88% for stents. Angiography six months later showed restenosis rates of 48% and 14%, respectively. Multivariate analysis did not find any difference in clinical results between angioplasty or stenting with respect to creatinine concentration, mean blood pressure and median number of antihypertensive drugs taken [29] **(Ib/A)**.

Placement of renal artery stents in a solitary poorly functioning kidney has not been subject to a randomised trial. In a retrospective analysis of 21 patients, renal function had improved or stabilised in 15 (71%), six to 25 months after stenting [30]. Major complications occurred in four patients (19%), including one death within 30 days. In this high-risk group stenting appeared to be a relatively safe procedure to attempt to salvage a solitary kidney.

A recent Cochrane review analysed the effectiveness of balloon angioplasty on blood pressure control, renal function, frequency of renovascular complications and side effects in atherosclerotic renal artery stenosis [31]. It was concluded that there was insufficient data to confirm whether balloon angioplasty was superior to medical therapy in lowering blood pressure in patients in whom blood pressure could be controlled satisfactorily with medical therapy **(Ia/A)**. There was weak evidence that balloon angioplasty was more effective in lowering blood pressure in patients with refractory hypertension [31] **(Ia/A)**. There are currently two European trials that are well advanced and promise to provide the clinical evidence upon which to base decisions for choice of treatment for ARVD. The STAR trial, organised in the Netherlands, is relatively small and aims to randomise 140 patients, while the ASTRAL trial is randomising well and nearing its revised target of 700 patients.

Surgical revascularisation

In the context of improving techniques and results for endovascular intervention, the indications for surgery may be reducing. The problem with surgery is the peri-operative mortality rate which may reach 8%. The current indications for renal artery surgery are listed in Table 3. Each individual patient, however, needs to be considered according to the extent of the vascular disease and their risk factors.

Table 3. Indications for surgical renal artery revascularisation.
♦ Failed stent angioplasty
♦ Grossly atheromatous, hostile aorta thereby precluding percutaneous approach
♦ Occlusion of a renal artery origin with preservation of the kidney by collaterals
♦ Segmental renal arterial disease
♦ Solitary renal artery stenosis in patient fit for general anaesthetic
♦ Significant aortic aneurysm or aortic occlusive disease with concomitant symptomatic renal artery stenosis
♦ Patient fit for general anaesthesia

A number of surgical options are available: aortorenal bypass (Figure 2); renal endarterectomy (Figure 3); aortic resection and renal bypass (Figure 4); extra-anatomical bypasses - hepatorenal, splenorenal and supracoeliac (Figure 5). No randomised controlled comparisons of the various surgical procedures exist and the procedure should be tailored to individual circumstances.

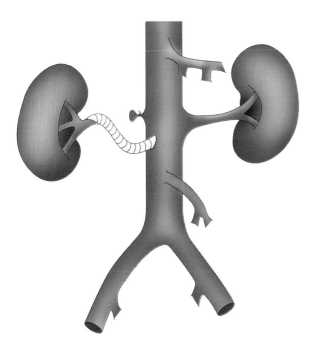

Figure 2. Aortorenal bypass is performed using either long saphenous vein, PTFE, Dacron or occasionally internal iliac artery.

The evidence for surgical treatment of ARVD

Since the advent of percutaneous techniques, surgery for renal artery stenosis has become less common. The only randomised trial comparing angioplasty and surgical reconstruction as initial therapy was conducted in 58 patients with unilateral atherosclerotic renal artery stenosis, and reported in 1993, thus predating the stent angioplasty era [32]. Technically successful angioplasty was achieved in 83%, whilst surgical success was recorded in 97% of patients. The primary patency rate after two years was 75% after angioplasty and 96% after surgery. There was no significant difference between the two groups with regard to hypertension, renal function or other secondary results. Nor was there any difference in the rates of major or minor complications. However, 17% of the angioplasty group required subsequent surgical reconstruction to achieve these results. The authors concluded that angioplasty could be recommended as the first choice revascularisation procedure for atherosclerotic renal artery stenosis, provided it was combined with intensive follow-up and aggressive re-intervention, as required **(Ib/A)**. There

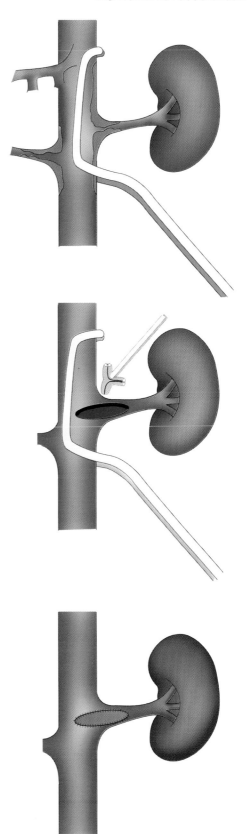

Figure 3. Renal endarterectomy with vein patch closure.

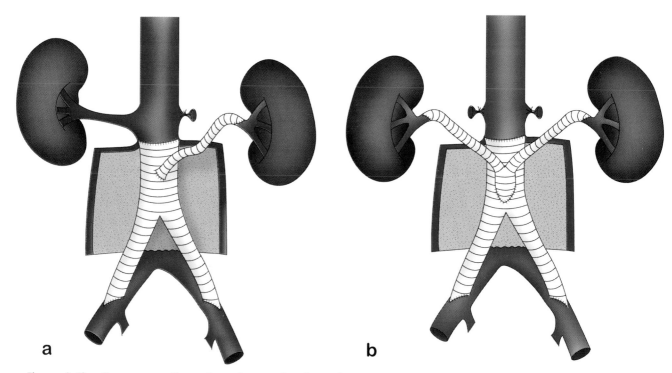

Figure 4. Simultaneous aortic and renal reconstruction. a) Renal bypass performed using 6-8mm PTFE or Dacron. The graft is sutured onto the aortic graft with an end-to-end renal anastomosis. b) In bilateral renal artery disease an inverted bifurcated graft is used.

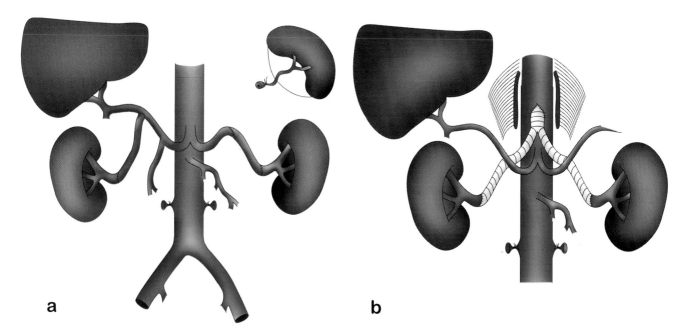

Figure 5 a) Extra-anatomic bypass grafts. The right kidney can be revascularised from the common hepatic artery. In approximately 40% of cases this can be via the gastroduodenal branch; alternatively an interposition saphenous vein graft is used. The left kidney can be revascularised using the splenic artery. The spleen remains *in situ* receiving blood from splenic collaterals and the short gastric arteries. b) Supracoeliac approach.

is still no reliable evidence comparing stent angioplasty and surgical revascularisation for ARVD.

The current arguments for surgical revascularisation for ARVD are based on several observational cohort studies **(IIa/B)**. Over the last five years even these have become less frequent as stent angioplasty has become dominant. Analysis of the available data suggests that surgery may be better in the fit patient, where it may be more cost-effective than angioplasty. This is especially so in light of the very low long-term restenosis rate of 3-4% after surgery, and better control of hypertension and renal failure [33-40] (Table 4).

Table 4. Summary of results after surgical revascularisation [33-40] (IIa/B).	
Treatment of hypertension (cure/improvement)	63-91%
Treatment of renal failure (cure/improvement)	33-91%
Primary patency rates	93-97%
Restenosis rate	3-4%
Morbidity	6-43%
Mortality	2-8%

The management of asymptomatic renal artery stenosis in patients requiring infrarenal aortic surgery remains controversial [41]. Some authors recommend simultaneous renal artery revascularisation, but others disagree [42]. At late follow-up (mean of 6.3 years), high-grade renal artery stenosis was associated with higher systolic blood pressure and the need for more antihypertensive medication. The outcome of arterial surgery is significantly worse in patients with pre-operative renal dysfunction [43]. Concomitant revascularisation with aortic surgery was more favourable as it was not associated with decreased survival, dialysis dependence or worsening serum creatinine levels [41], but it should probably only be performed where the renal artery stenosis is symptomatic, and in low-risk patients.

Failed endovascular renal revascularisation is an indication for surgical reconstruction. This surgical intervention is made more complex by the presence of the stent and the dense peri-arterial fibrosis around the juxtarenal aorta. Aortorenal bypass avoids the stented part of the proximal renal artery, and is technically possible in most cases, but with increased mortality (9.4 to 16%). More complex repairs are required in over 50% and the improvement in hypertension and renal function is less than after primary revascularisation [44]. This salvage scenario may become more of a problem to the vascular surgeon in the future if the use of stents in high-risk patients continues to escalate.

Nephrectomy

Nephrectomy is the oldest surgical procedure for the treatment of renovascular hypertension. It continues to be an appropriate option when there is a normal contralateral kidney, but the ipsilateral kidney is shrunken (<8cm) and driving the hypertension by excess rennin production. Contralateral nephrectomy may also be performed as part of revascularisation of a viable ipsilateral kidney. Such an operation is indicated when the renal vein renin ratio is greater than 1.5.

Conclusions

Unfortunately there is still a lack of good randomised trials available to determine which patients with renovascular disease benefit from best medical therapy alone, stent placement or surgery. The ASTRAL trial is nearing completion and preliminary results are expected in 2007. In it, the patients are randomised to either best medical therapy alone or best medical therapy with revascularisation by angioplasty and/or stent. The overwhelming majority randomised to intervention have undergone stent angioplasty and this large trial promises to define the role of intervention.

Surgery is now infrequently performed for ARVD, despite evidence of an improved functional outcome in survivors. A randomised comparison of endovascular and surgical revascularisation would be welcome, but it would be very difficult to establish because of the predominance of renal stent angioplasty and the gradual loss of surgical expertise in this area. Best medical therapy is the only treatment required for the majority of patients with ARVD; intervention should be reserved for specific indications **(Ia/A)**. At present, best care should continue to be delivered using a multidisciplinary team approach of nephrologist, endovascular and vascular surgeons, ideally in a centre involved in clinical trials.

Key points	Evidence level
◆ Renal artery stenosis, particularly when bilateral, is associated with a poor two-year survival.	IIa/B
◆ Renal artery stenosis >60% may be suitable for treatment if it is causing refractory hypertension, deteriorating or end-stage renal function.	IIa/B
◆ Angioplasty is the treatment of choice for renal artery fibromuscular hyperplasia.	Ib/A
◆ Renal artery stenting is the most common intervention, but there is limited evidence of its efficacy. The ASTRAL Trial is expected to clarify indications for treatment.	IIb/B
◆ Surgical renal artery revascularisation carries a higher mortality rate than stenting, but is indicated in selected patients. No randomised comparison with stenting exists.	III/B

References

1. Pascual A, Busch HS, Copley JB. Renal fibromuscular dysplasia in elderly persons. *Am J Kidney Dis* 2005; 45: E63-6.
2. Hansen KJ, Edwards MS, Craven TE, *et al*. Prevalence of renovascular disease in the elderly: a population-based study. *J Vasc Surg* 2002; 36: 443-51.
3. Farmer CKT, Reidy J, Kalra PA, *et al*. Individual kidney function before and after renal angioplasty. *Lancet* 1998; 352: 288-9.
4. Cheung CM, Hegarty J, Kalra PA. Dilemmas in the management of renal artery stenosis. *Br Med Bull* 2005; 73 & 74: 35-55.
5. Zierler RE, Berghelin RO, Davidson RC, *et al*. A prospective study of disease progression in patients with atherosclerotic renal artery stenosis. *Am J Hypertens* 1999; 12: 1-7.
6. Crowley JJ, Santos RN, Peter RH, *et al*. Progression of renal artery stenosis in patients undergoing cardiac catheterisation. *Am Heart J* 1998; 136: 913-18.
7. Connolly JO, Higgins RM, Mackie AD, *et al*. Presentation, clinical features and outcome in different patterns of atherosclerotic renovascular disease. *QJM* 1994; 87: 413-21.
8. Mailloux LU, Bellucci AG, Mossey RT, *et al*. Predictors of survival in patients undergoing dialysis. *Am J Med* 1988; 84: 855-62.
9. Harding MB, Smith LR, Himmelstein SI, *et al*. Renal artery stenosis: prevalence and associated risk factors in patients undergoing routine cardiac catheterisation. *J Am Soc Nephrol* 1992; 2: 1608-16.
10. Olin JW, Melia M, Young JR, *et al*. Prevalence of atherosclerotic renal artery stenosis in patients with atherosclerosis elsewhere. *Am J Med* 1990: 88; 46N-51N.
11. Herrara AH, Davidson RA. Renovascular disease in older adults. *Clin Geriatr Med* 1998; 14: 237-53.
12. Pickering TG, Herman L, Devereux RB, *et al*. Recurrent pulmonary oedema in hypertension due to bilateral renal artery stenosis: treatment by angioplasty or surgical revascularisation. *Lancet* 1998; ii: 551-2.
13. Wright JR, Shurrab A, Cooper A, *et al*. Left ventricular morphology and function in atherosclerotic renovascular disease. *J Am Soc Nephrol* 2005; 16: 2746-53.
14. Radermacher J, Chavan A, Bleck J, *et al*. Use of Doppler ultrasonography to predict the outcome of therapy for renal-artery stenosis. *N Engl J Med* 2001; 344: 410-7.
15. Patel ST, Mills JL, Tynan-Cuisinier G, *et al*. The limitations of magnetic resonance angiography in the diagnosis of renal artery stenosis: comparative analysis with conventional arteriography. *J Vasc Surg* 2005; 41: 462-8.
16. Fraioli F, Catalano C, Bertoletti L, *et al*. Multidetector-row CT angiography of renal artery stenosis in 50 consecutive patients: prospective interobserver comparison with DSA. *Radiol Med* (Torino) 2006; 111: 459-68.

17. Rashid ST, Salman M, Myint F, *et al.* Prevention of contrast-induced nephropathy in vascular patients undergoing angiography: a randomized controlled trial of intravenous N-acetylcysteine. *J Vasc Surg* 2005; 40: 1136-41.

18. Kalra PA, Gor H, Kausz AT, *et al.* Atherosclerotic renovascular disease in the US Medicare population: risk factors, revascularization and prognosis. *Kidney Int* 2005; 68: 293-301.

19. Tegtmeyer CJ, Kellum CD, Kron IL, *et al.* Percutaneous transluminal angioplasty in the region of the aortic bifurcation. The two-balloon technique with results and long-term follow-up study. *Radiology* 1985; 157: 661-5.

20. Martin LG, Price RB, Casarella WJ, *et al.* Percutaneous angioplasty in clinical management of renovascular hypertension: initial and long-term results. *Radiology* 1985; 155: 629-33.

21. Hamilton G. Early and late failure of endovascular renal artery repair. In: *Complications in vascular and endovascular surgery part 2.* Branchereau A, Jacobs M, Eds. Armonk, New York: Futura Publishing Company Inc., 2002: 195-206.

22. Kennedy DJ, Colyer WR, Brewster PS, *et al.* Renal insufficiency as a predictor of adverse events and mortality after renal artery stent placement. *Am J Kidney Dis* 2003; 42: 926-35.

23. Edwards MS, Craven BL, Stafford J, *et al.* Distal embolic protection during renal angioplasty and stenting. *J Vasc Surg* 2006; 44: 128-35.

24. Zeller T, Rastan A, Rothenpieler U, Muller C. Restenosis after stenting of atherosclerotic renal artery stenosis: is there a rationale for the use of drug-eluting stents? *Catheter Cardiovasc Interv* 2006; 68: 125-30.

25. White CJ. Catheter-based therapy for atherosclerotic renal artery stenosis. *Circulation* 2006; 113: 1464-73.

26. Webster J, Marshall F, Abdalla M, *et al.* Randomised comparison of percutaneous angioplasty vs. continued medical therapy for hypertensive patients with atheromatous renal artery stenosis. Scottish and Newcastle Renal Artery Stenosis Collaborative Group. *J Hum Hypertens* 1998; 12: 329-35.

27. Plouin PF, Chatellier G, Darne B, *et al.* Blood pressure outcome of angioplasty in atherosclerotic renal artery stenosis: a randomized trial. Essai Multicentrique Medicaments vs Angioplastie (EMMA) Study Group. *Hypertension* 1998; 31: 823-9.

28. van Jaarsveld BC, Krijnen P, Pieterman H, *et al.* The effects of balloon angioplasty on hypertension in atherosclerotic renal artery stenosis. *N Engl J Med* 2000; 341: 107-14.

29. van de ven PJG, Kaatee R, Beutler JJ, *et al.* Arterial stenting and balloon angioplasty in ostial atherosclerotic renovascular disease: a randomised trial. *Lancet* 1999; 353: 282-6.

30. Shannon HM, Gillespie IN, Moss JG. Salvage of the solitary kidney by insertion of a renal artery stent. *Am J Roentgenol* 1998; 171: 217-22.

31. Nordmann AJ, Logan AG. Balloon angioplasty versus medical therapy for hypertensive patients with renal artery obstruction. *Cochrane Database Syst Rev* 2003; 3: CD002944.

32. Weibull H, Bergqvist MD, Bergentz S-E, *et al.* Percutaneous transluminal renal angioplasty versus surgical reconstruction of atherosclerotic renal artery stenosis: a prospective randomized study. *J Vasc Surg* 1993; 18: 841-52.

33. Novick AC, Ziegelbaum M, Vidt DG, *et al.* Trends in surgical revascularization for renal artery disease. Ten years' experience. *JAMA* 1987; 257: 498-501.

34. Dean RH. Surgical reconstruction of atherosclerotic renal artery disease. In: *Long-term results of arterial interventions.* Branchereau A, Jacobs M, Eds. Armonk, New York: Futura Publishing Company, 1997: 205-16.

35. Benjamin ME, Hansen KJ, Craven TE, *et al.* Combined aortic and renal artery surgery. A contemporary experience. *Ann Surg* 1996; 223: 555-65.

36. Reilly JM, Rubin BG, Thompson RW, *et al.* Revascularization of the solitary kidney: a challenging problem in a high-risk population. *Surgery* 1996; 120: 732-6.

37. Steinbach F, Novick AC, Campbell S, *et al.* Long-term survival after surgical revascularization for atherosclerotic renal artery disease. *J Urol* 1997; 158: 38-41.

38. Cambria RP, Brewster DC, L'Italien G, *et al.* Renal artery reconstruction for the preservation of renal function. *J Vasc Surg* 1996; 24: 371-82.

39. Cherr GS, Hansen KJ, Craven TE, *et al.* Surgical management of atherosclerotic renovascular disease. *J Vasc Surg* 2002; 35: 236-45.

40. Marone LK, Clouse WD, Dorer DJ, *et al.* Preservation of renal function with surgical revascularization in patients with atherosclerotic renovascular disease. *J Vasc Surg* 2004; 39: 322-9.

41. Darling RC, III, Shah DM, Chang BB, *et al.* Does concomitant aortic bypass and renal artery revascularization using the retroperitoneal approach increase perioperative risk? *Cardiovasc Surg* 1995; 3: 421-3.

42. Williamson WK, Abou-Zamzam AM, Jr., Moneta GL, *et al.* Prophylactic repair of renal artery stenosis is not justified in patients who require infrarenal aortic reconstruction. *J Vasc Surg* 1998; 28: 14-22.

43. Black SA, Brooks MJ, Naidoo MN, *et al,* on behalf of the Joint Vascular Research Group. Assessing the impact of renal impairment on outcome after arterial intervention: a prospective review of 1559 patients. *Eur J Vasc Endovasc Surg* 2006; 32: 300-4.

44. Wong JM, Hansen KJ, Oskin TC, *et al.* Surgery after failed percutaneous renal artery angioplasty. *J Vasc Surg* 1999; 30: 468-82.

Chapter 26

The prevention and treatment of vascular graft infection

David A Ratliff MD FRCP FRCS (Eng & Ed), Consultant Vascular Surgeon
Northampton General Hospital, Northampton, UK

Introduction

Graft infection is a serious complication of arterial reconstructive surgery with high associated rates of amputation and mortality. Fortunately it is relatively uncommon, but problems in diagnosis and treatment create one of the most formidable of surgical challenges. The true incidence is uncertain but lies within the range 0.5-2.6% [1-4]. There are many differing approaches to management.

Recent initiatives in the prevention of graft infection have centred around the use of antibiotic-bonded grafts. There is also continuing interest in their use for treatment of this problem by graft excision and *in situ* replacement in selected cases, as an alternative to conventional surgical management. Another new approach to treatment is the replacement of infected aortic prostheses with autogenous deep lower extremity veins.

Pathogenesis

Graft infection may be divided into early (less than four months after surgery) and late infections [5]. Micro-organisms can infect the prosthesis through direct implantation at the time of surgery, through the wound if there is a complication of healing, or through haematogenous or lymphatic routes from remote sites of infection. It is thought that the majority of graft infections, both early and late, result from implantation at the time of initial surgery.

At operation a graft is placed in a closed system. An acute inflammatory reaction occurs, followed by a chronic inflammatory response and fibroblast infiltration of the perigraft space and graft interstices [6]. A concept termed 'the race for the surface' has been used to describe the events that arise at the surface-body interface after implantation of a prosthesis [7]. A contest between tissue cell integration and bacterial adhesion takes place. If human cells are the first to attach to the graft, it is likely that no prosthetic infection will occur. If bacteria adhere and form a nidus, however, a biofilm may develop which protects the bacteria from host defences and antibiotics. Some bacterial strains produce a slime layer in culture. *Staphylococcus aureus* and *epidermidis* produce a mucin that promotes their adherence to the prosthetic material, inhibits the action of phagocytes and antibodies, and reduces the penetration of antibiotics [8].

The pathological consequences of graft infection depend on the virulence of the organism, the host response and its site. Early graft infections are relatively uncommon and are usually associated with virulent pathogens such as *S. aureus* and the Gram-negative bacteria, *Streptococcus faecalis*, *Escherichia coli*, *Klebsiella*, *Pseudomonas aeruginosa* and *Proteus*. Multiple organisms may be present. They tend to be associated with serious complications such as systemic sepsis, infected false aneurysm, external drainage through wound infection and erosion into bowel (Figure 1). In contrast, late graft infections are commonly the result of less virulent bacteria, such as *S. epidermidis*, and are typically more difficult to diagnose. Clinical signs are usually absent but local signs develop as the infection progresses. These include tenderness and erythema of the skin overlying the graft, a perigraft mass or discharging sinus [9].

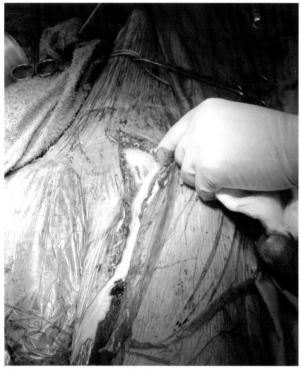

Figure 1. Infected aortobifemoral bypass graft with systemic sepsis and pus in the left groin. *Courtesy of Mr. Chris Gibbons, Swansea.*

The clinical manifestations of graft infection are the result of the balance between the pathogenicity of the organism and the host immunological defences. Bacteria such as *S. epidermidis* have been found frequently in prosthetic grafts removed for reasons other than sepsis [10], and it is possible that only a small proportion of grafts contaminated with this organism develop overt signs of infection [11].

The physiological status of bacterial cells living in biofilms is determined by the location of individual cells within them [12]. Cells located in the external layers are metabolically active and frequently reproducing, but highly susceptible to host defences and antibacterial agents. Cells in the deeper layers of the biofilm have scarce access to nutrients and oxygen, and are almost dormant. Their metabolism is differentiated towards the synthesis of glycocalyx (mucin) and they are extremely resistant to host defences and antibacterial agents. When the biofilm approaches its critical mass the cells in the outer layer may be released to cause acute episodes in the course of an otherwise almost silent infection. The degree of this cellular differentiation is proportional to the age of the biofilm and is an additional factor responsible for the complexity of the clinical syndrome of graft infection.

Identification of the infective organism

The causative organism may be difficult to identify. During acute episodes of systemic infection blood culture should be repeated at short intervals. Samples may also be obtained from wounds and perigraft fluid aspirated under ultrasound or CT control, or directly from the explanted graft. They must be transported to microbiology in a liquid medium and processed immediately. Sections of graft should then be extensively vortexed or sonicated by ultrasound to detach bacterial cells and disperse them in it [12]. The graft should be incubated with vigorous shaking for up to ten days, or until bacterial growth is observed. Therapeutic planning should be based on the bactericidal activity of antibiotics.

MRSA

There has been an epidemic of methicillin-resistant *Staphylococcus aureus* (MRSA) in many hospitals and

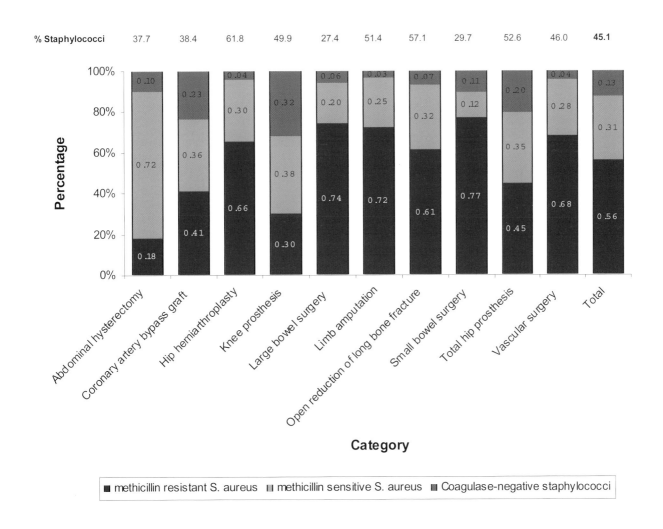

% Staphylococci   37.7   38.4   61.8   49.9   27.4   51.4   57.1   29.7   52.6   46.0   **45.1**

Legend: ■ methicillin resistant S. aureus   ▥ methicillin sensitive S. aureus   ■ Coagulase-negative staphylococci

Category

Figure 2. Surgical site infection caused by staphylococci by category of surgical procedure. For most categories of surgical procedure MRSA was the most common staphylococcus identified as causing surgical site infections [16]. *Reproduced with permission from the Health Protection Agency.*

countries since 1994, and a number of reviews have described its effect on vascular surgical practice [13-15]. MRSA is now the most common causative organism of surgical site infections in English hospitals, accounting for 25% of the total [16]. Vascular surgery and limb amputation are among the areas most affected, and this is accompanied by increased morbidity and mortality (Figure 2). MRSA aortic graft infection is almost uniformly fatal; patients with MRSA

infection of a prosthetic infra-inguinal bypass graft have a high incidence of amputation and MRSA can cause disruption of both native artery and vein grafts.

Prevention of MRSA infection is better than attempted cure. The most important elements of this approach are scrupulous hand washing, and effective communication and interaction with the hospital infection control team. Vascular surgical patients vary in risk, from those who are not colonised with MRSA having low-risk procedures, to those with known sepsis and possible but undocumented MRSA colonisation or infection (high risk), and others with established MRSA infection that need vascular surgery. The risks and problems are different in every hospital and co-operation with local microbiologists is essential in creating local protocols to deal with each category of patient, including antibiotic prophylaxis [15].

Predisposing factors

Graft infections are commonly associated with operative events leading to bacterial contamination of the graft, or with patient risk factors that predispose to infection due to impaired host defences (Table 1). The important association of graft infection with groin incisions has been well documented and the development of complications in a groin wound is frequently the precursor of an infected prosthesis [3]. The incidence of graft infection is increased with emergency surgery, early revision surgery, long operations and those associated with substantial blood loss. Simultaneous gastrointestinal, biliary and urological procedures also increase the risk.

Patients at increased risk of graft infection include those with malnutrition, diabetes mellitus, chronic renal failure, autoimmune disease, obesity and those who are immunocompromised due to malignancy or corticosteroid therapy. Infected or gangrenous lesions on the feet are associated with infection of groin wounds and grafts. The severity of the arterial ischaemia is an important risk factor; the risk of wound infection in patients undergoing lower limb vascular reconstruction is significantly increased in those with rest pain with or without skin necrosis [17].

The type of conduit is also important. Autogenous vein has inherent resistance to infection and graft infection is predominantly a feature of prosthetic grafts. Bacterial adherence to Dacron is 10-100 times greater than PTFE [18]. There is no clinical difference, however, in the incidence of graft infection between these two types of material [1, 3].

Table 1. Risk factors for infection.
Bacterial contamination of the graft
Faulty aseptic technique
Groin incision(s)
Emergency surgery
Early revision surgery
Long operations
Operations with substantial blood loss
Simultaneous gastrointestinal and other procedures
Prolonged pre-operative hospital stay
Severity of arterial ischaemia
Intercurrent remote infection
Postoperative superficial wound infection
Impaired host defences
Malnutrition
Diabetes mellitus
Chronic renal failure
Autoimmune disease
Obesity
Malignancy
Corticosteroid therapy

Prevention

Pre-operative measures

Antibiotic prophylaxis reduces both wound and early graft infection after vascular surgery and is mandatory [19] **(Ia/A)**. It is common practice to give the first dose of antibiotic on induction of anaesthesia, followed by two postoperative doses to provide cover for the first 24 hours. There is no evidence of significant benefit from more prolonged courses of antibiotics, which may be associated with the proliferation of resistant organisms [19]. There is also no hard data from clinical trials that antibiotic prophylaxis prevents late graft infection; this may be mainly due to the small incidence of infection and the large size of the study that would be necessary [20]. Therapeutic serum and tissue levels must be maintained throughout the operation to ensure adequate protection and intra-operative redosing is recommended if there is substantial blood loss, the procedure is prolonged or other circumstances occur which might increase the risk of infection (e.g. opening the bowel, synchronous procedures) [19]. There are no standard recommendations for prophylaxis in other situations where the risk is increased, such as active lower limb infection or tissue loss, emergency surgery or re-operations. It is reasonable to give a full course of antibiotics in this situation (five days), although this is not of proven benefit.

The choice of antibiotic will be determined by the sensitivities of the organisms most frequently encountered. Broad spectrum cover with augmentin (co-amoxiclav) or cefuroxime plus metronidazole is popular. Vancomycin or teicoplanin may be used in infections with MRSA. One of these agents and/or gentamicin may be used when the presence of resistant organisms is suspected, for example, after prolonged pre-operative hospital admission.

Antiseptic baths with chlorhexidine before surgery have not been shown to be beneficial [21]. Shaving of the skin should be carried out as close to the time of surgery as possible. Skin preparation with povidone-iodine or chlorhexidine is carried out immediately before surgery. There is no evidence to suggest that either solution is superior [5]. Sterile plastic adhesive drapes are widely used to separate the operative field from the pubic area and perineum. Their use has not been shown to reduce the incidence of wound infection, even in the groin [22], but they do prevent contact of the graft with the skin.

Intra-operative measures

General

Meticulous surgical and aseptic technique is of paramount importance in reducing the incidence of wound infection and the risk of graft infection [3, 23]. Tissues should be handled carefully with attention to haemostasis, to prevent haematoma formation. Groin incisions should be avoided whenever possible. When these are necessary, minimal dissection of the lymphatics should be carried out, divided channels should be ligated and the incisions closed in at least two layers with accurate approximation of the skin edges to eliminate the dead space, reduce seroma formation and promote primary healing. Avoidance of undercutting the skin edge is important in the

exposure of the femoral artery in the groin and the long saphenous vein in the thigh. This can result in skin flap necrosis and threaten the graft. Oblique groin incisions and pre-operative vein marking by duplex may help to reduce its incidence. Wound healing in the thigh is also improved by the use of three or four incisions with short intervening skin bridges, rather than one long continuous incision. Routine vacuum drainage of groin wounds does not prevent either lymphocoele or wound infection [24] **(Ib/A)**.

With regard to aortic grafts, simultaneous gastrointestinal procedures should be avoided if at all possible to prevent graft contamination with enteric organisms. If the bowel is inadvertently entered during division of adhesions or exposure of the aorta, the incision should be closed and the arterial reconstruction rescheduled for a second occasion a few days later, if feasible. If a bowel resection is necessary, the reconstruction may be delayed in cases of occlusive disease but, if the surgery is urgent, an extra-anatomic bypass may be considered as an option. Elective repair of aortic aneurysm is probably best delayed for a short interval until the patient has recovered from the bowel resection. An exception to this may occur in cases of large aneurysm when it may be preferable to carry out both procedures together. In this instance it is probably best to repair the aneurysm first and close the retroperitoneum before carrying out the bowel resection. Where symptomatic coincidental pathology of the 'clean contaminated' category is present, such as gallstones, a combined procedure may be appropriate. In this situation cholecystectomy should be performed only after the aortic graft has been implanted and the retroperitoneum closed. Most asymptomatic gallstones, however, can safely be left untreated at the initial operation.

After insertion of an aortic graft it is essential that the duodenum and remaining bowel are separated from the graft to prevent the development of a secondary aorto-enteric fistula (AEF). This requires complete closure of the retroperitoneum with interposition of greater omentum between the duodenum and the graft, if necessary.

Rifampicin-bonded and silver-coated grafts

The inclusion of antibiotic in graft material is one potential way to reduce graft infection in the immediate peri-operative period, when it is most at risk. Rifampicin binds to the surface of gelatin-coated Dacron and has good activity against both *S. epidermidis* and *aureus* [25, 26], although it is not effective against some Gram-negative and other virulent organisms such as MRSA and *E. coli* [27, 28]. Animal experiments have shown that rifampicin remains bound to grafts in an active concentration for at least 72 hours, and up to two weeks [27].

There have been three randomised trials of rifampicin bonding [29-31]. Six hundred patients having an aortofemoral graft were randomly allocated into two groups in an Italian study; the rifampicin-bonded group received a graft soaked for 15 minutes in a solution of rifampicin (1mg/ml saline) and the control group received the same untreated graft [29] (Figure 3). All patients received systemic antibiotic prophylaxis. The incidence of graft infection was 2% at two years, with no significant difference between the two groups.

A large European study with a similar design examined 2400 patients having aortofemoral or femorofemoral bypass [30]. A significant reduction in superficial and deep wound infections (Szilagyi grades I and II) was found in patients receiving rifampicin-bonded grafts (2.9% vs. 4.4% controls), but there was no significant difference in the rate of graft infection (0.3% vs. 0.6% controls). No late results have been reported.

In the JVRG study, 257 patients who had an extra-anatomic graft were randomised to rifampicin bonding or a control group [31]. The rate of early graft infection (within one month of surgery) was low (0.4%). Infective complications were similar in both groups, even in patients with one or more pre-operative risk factors for infection. The early and late results at two years showed no significant advantage from rifampicin bonding [32].

Despite these studies on over 3000 patients, there remains no scientific evidence therefore that rifampicin bonding reduces the incidence of vascular

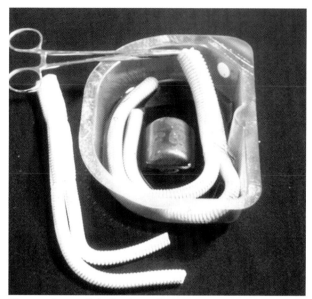

Figure 3. Antibiotic bonding of a gelatin coated bifurcation graft.

graft infection [19] **(Ia/A)**. This may be the result of an inadequate antibiotic delivery system (wrong drug or dose of drug) or the wrong concept, namely that the cause of graft infection is more complicated than originally thought [32]. New experimental evidence suggests that a higher concentration of 10-60mg/ml may be more effective [33]. It would take huge studies of any future graft with high costs, however, to prove any advantage.

Despite this lack of evidence many surgeons now use rifampicin-bonded grafts selectively in patients known to be at increased risk of infection, such as those with diabetes, distal skin necrosis or previous surgery [20]. This pragmatic approach seems reasonable as the technique is simple, rifampicin is relatively cheap and no disadvantages have been identified [34].

Silver-coated grafts have also recently been proposed as an alternative for prevention or treatment of prosthetic graft infections. Silver is a broad-spectrum bacteriostatic agent that shows antimicrobial activity *in vitro*, but several studies have shown that it is ineffective in animal models or *in vivo* [28, 35, 36]. Preliminary results in only one small series demonstrated a favourable outcome when *in situ* silver-coated grafts were used to treat aortic infections caused by organisms with low virulence [37].

Postoperative measures

Early recognition and aggressive treatment of postoperative wound infection is essential to avoid potential infection of the underlying graft. Graft coverage should be maintained at all times. Exposure of a graft section will inevitably lead to infection unless urgent action is taken to restore healthy overlying tissue. In the groin the simplest way to achieve this is by debridement and resuture, but sartorius myoplasty is an excellent alternative when this is not possible [38]. If there is any doubt clinically about the depth or extent of wound infection, simple palpation of the defect with a sterile glove will rapidly clarify the situation; not uncommonly a cavity may be detected with a pulsating graft in its base that was not initially evident.

Failure of prosthetic grafts to develop a protective endothelial lining renders them susceptible to late colonisation and infection through bacteraemia. After graft insertion patients should be informed of this potential risk. Interventional urological procedures, colonoscopy and dental treatment risk occult bacteraemia and antibiotic prophylaxis has been recommended in these circumstances [23, 39, 40]. The risk is very low, however, and other studies have shown no benefit from dental-style antibiotic prophylaxis [41].

Treatment

The management of graft infection (Figure 4) is controversial and depends on the site and extent of the infection, the virulence of the infecting organism, the need for distal revascularisation and involvement of anastomoses. There are many differing approaches to management, each of which may be appropriate in certain circumstances; each patient should be considered individually.

Total graft excision and extra-anatomic bypass

Traditional or standard treatment of aortic graft infection (AGI) has involved an aggressive surgical approach with total excision of the graft including

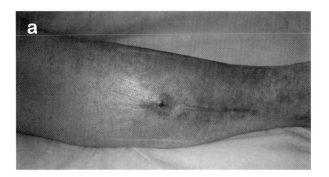

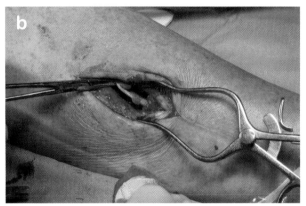

Figure 4. Infected occluded femorotibial PTFE graft. a) Sinus in the wound over the anterior compartment. b) On exploration the graft was infected, and was excised down to its anastomosis with the peroneal artery.

adjacent artery, and debridement of infected perigraft tissue, followed by extra-anatomic bypass to uninvolved arterial segments (the sequential technique). Culture-specific antibiotics are also administered. This has been associated historically with high mortality and amputation rates and a significant risk of secondary haemorrhage from the aortic stump, which is usually fatal [1]. In the staged technique revascularisation by extra-anatomic bypass is performed two to four days before graft excision. This approach is recommended whenever possible, providing the patient's condition is stable [42, 43]. The risk of recurrent graft infection is not increased. Not surprisingly, mortality in unstable patients requiring emergency repair is higher than those in whom urgent or elective repair is possible.

Considerable improvement in results with the traditional approach have been reported recently [43-46]. Reilly [43] and Kuestner [46] have reported extensive reviews of the current treatment of AGI and secondary AEF, the group with graft infection at highest risk. In 33 patients with AEF, peri-operative mortality, amputation and aortic stump disruption were 18%, 6% and 6%, respectively. Cumulative cure was 70% at three years, with 90% secondary patency of the extra-anatomic bypass at four years. The improved survival rate was attributed to the following factors: ongoing improvement in pre-operative preparation; intra-operative anaesthetic management and postoperative care; thorough debridement of the infected aorta, perigraft tissue and retroperitoneum; and the routine performance of the extra-anatomic revascularisation before the removal of the infected graft which avoids lower body ischaemia with all of its adverse metabolic consequences [46]. Complete excision of the graft with extra-anatomic bypass provides a satisfactory long-term outcome and remains the standard with which other approaches must be compared.

The endovascular approach seems a reasonable treatment option in unstable patients with bleeding secondary AEF, when aortic stent grafting can rapidly seal the aorto-enteric communication [47]. Secondary surgical repair is not always required and infection may be controlled by prolonged antibiotic therapy.

Total graft excision and in situ graft replacement

Previous dissatisfaction with the results of conventional surgical treatment and reports of success with various methods of conservative management led to the development of in situ graft replacement as an alternative option in selected cases [48]. Patients most suitable are those with negative cultures, no signs of systemic sepsis and minimal contamination at surgery, such as those with late graft infection due to S. epidermidis. In situ replacement is appealing because it is often less technically demanding than traditional graft excision and extra-anatomic bypass, particulary for AGI. Several techniques are available.

Dacron or PTFE

The first large series of in situ replacement was reported by Walker in patients with secondary AEF [49].

The proximal part of the graft was removed and replaced with a new section of Dacron, covered by an omentoplasty to separate it from the duodenum. Good results have been reported recently from Italy with in situ replacement with a standard PTFE graft in selected patients [50]. Before placement the surrounding necrotic tissues were debrided as thoroughly as possible, the field was washed repeatedly with a solution of 2% povidone iodine and an omental wrap was carried out.

Antibiotic-bonded graft

Recent attempts have focused on using rifampicin-bonded grafts (soaked with the higher concentration of 60mg/ml for 10-15 minutes [20]) for in situ reconstruction in AGI. In Leicester, initial optimism with this technique has been tempered by additional experience in 11 patients with longer follow-up, and concern particularly about its lack of efficacy in resisting MRSA infection [51]. Bandyk used rifampicin-bonded grafts selectively in 22 patients with low-grade graft infections due to Staphylococcus epidermidis or aureus (afebrile, sterile pre-operative perigraft culture, negative intra-operative Gram stain) [48]. Six (27%) died and 10% developed recurrent graft infections after a mean follow-up of 18 months, a much shorter time than the median of three years that AGIs may take to become apparent clinically. Reported series involve only small numbers of selected patients and many patients die before long-term follow-up, thus making the results difficult to interpret. No controlled trials exist. Although this technique has become a standard treatment option, its role therefore remains uncertain.

Autogenous vein

The use of autogenous superficial femoral and popliteal veins (SFPV) to create a neo-aortoiliac system in the treatment of AGI was first reported in 1993 by Clagett [52] and has been successfully adopted by others [53, 54]. This approach has the advantages that it avoids extra-anatomic revascularisation and uses autogenous vein with its ability to resist infection of all types. Clagett's group reported excellent results in 41 patients treated by this

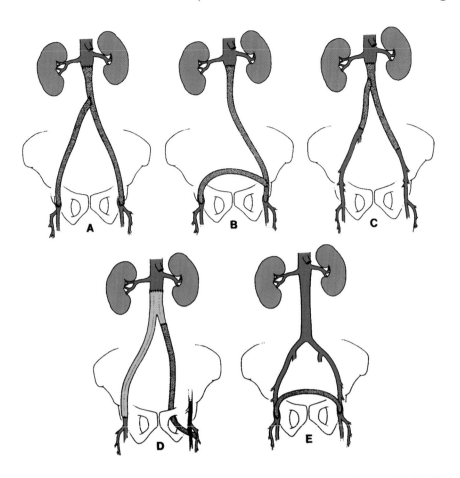

Figure 5. Aorto-iliac/femoral reconstructions using SFPV in 41 patients (31 with graft infection, 10 with regional infection, recurrent failure of standard vascular prostheses or young patients with small vessels). (A) 14 (34%) patients underwent SFPV aorto-unilateral bypass with a limb also fashioned from SFPV anastomosed end-to-side. (B) 13 (32%) patients underwent SFPV aortofemoral bypass with a SFPV femoral crossover bypass. (C) 3 (7%) patients underwent SFPV aorto-iliac reconstructions. (D) 6 (15%) underwent aortofemoral bypass single-limb replacement or iliofemoral bypass with SFPV grafts. (E) 5 (12%) patients had femoral crossover bypass alone performed with SFPV grafts. *Reproduced with permission from the Journal of Vascular Surgery. Clagett GP, Valentine RJ, Hagino RT. Autogenous aortoiliac-femoral reconstruction from superficial-femoral popliteal veins: feasibility and durability. J Vasc Surg 1997; 25: 255-70.*

technique (Figure 5) [55]. Peri-operative mortality was 7.3% and 5% required amputation. The problem of aortic stump disruption was removed and no patient developed haemorrhage or false aneurysm formation in relation to the proximal aortic anastomosis. At five years the cumulative secondary patency rate of the grafts was 100% and venous morbidity was surprisingly minimal. No reinfection or aneurysmal dilatation of the SFPV grafts occurred. The principal detraction was that the procedure was long and arduous, with a mean operative time of 7.9 hours. A two-team approach is therefore preferable. Poor

results were obtained in unstable patients with secondary AEF and total graft excision and extra-anatomic bypass were recommended in these circumstances, as well as in the sickest patients with severe medical comorbidities such as unstable angina. Otherwise, the procedure is an excellent alternative for the treatment of most other patients with AGI and is particularly useful in those where extra-anatomic reconstruction cannot be performed, due to extensive thigh sepsis. The operation is associated with gratifyingly low mortality and amputation rates that are far better than published rates associated with graft excision and extra-anatomic bypass [56].

Alternative autografting techniques include the use of long saphenous vein and endarterectomised superficial femoral artery. The long saphenous vein can be used when it is large (>8mm diameter), but it is usually not suitable for aorto-iliac replacement. Previous experience with such grafts has been disappointing with frequent failures due to focal and generalised neointimal hyperplasia; they are also prone to kinking. The proximal end of a SFPV graft is 1.0-1.5cm in diameter, however, which allows comfortable anastomosis to the aorta [55].

Arterial allografts

The treatment of AGI using fresh or cryopreserved aortic allografts has been available for approximately 40 years, with disappointing results overall. In addition, the natural history of the aortic homograft has been described as being one of progressive deterioration [44]. The peri-operative mortality and incidence of early and late complications are high [57, 58]. These include graft disruption and reinfection leading to persistent septic complications including aortic rupture, graft stenoses and thrombosis. Allograft replacement for AGI has therefore fallen into relative disfavour, although some authors consider it as a bridge to allow resolution of infection before *in situ* prosthetic graft replacement [58].

Additional techniques

Partial graft excision is effective for infection limited to one limb of an aortic graft, with revascularisation via an obturator foramen bypass [59]. There are other situations in which complete or partial graft preservation is reasonable in patients at very high risk [60].

Some surgeons have adopted a conservative approach, with antibiotic irrigation in selected cases [61, 62]. Despite successful results in a small number of patients, methods that involve leaving an infected aortic graft in place are unlikely to be widely adopted due to concern about the incidence of persistent infection

and death. Gentamicin beads and impregnated collagen mesh have been described in small series as alternative methods of treating localised graft infections, such as in the groin [63, 64].

Parenteral antibiotics are universally used in the management of graft infection but the optimal duration of treatment is unknown. Many surgeons continue oral antibiotics after a course of parenteral therapy for months, or even years.

Infection of endovascular stent grafts

The incidence of endovascular stent graft infection appears to be lower than following conventional surgery, although this will inevitably increase as the follow-up periods for endografts lengthen. The true incidence is not yet known. Fiorani reported an incidence of 0.4% in 24 centres with a short mean follow-up of 48 weeks, half of which were due to *S. aureus* [65]. Dattilo reported an incidence of two (0.6%) late infections in 362 patients that presented after an interval of 1.5 and 2.5 years, with an average follow-up of 1.5 years [66]. Both were thought to be due to bacteraemic seeding of the endoluminal device and were successfully treated by removal of the infected endograft, aortic ligation and extra-anatomic bypass. Three (2.2%) of 136 patients who underwent endovascular repair with an aorto-uni-iliac device in an earlier series from Nottingham, with a median follow-up period of seven months, developed infection in the associated femorofemoral crossover bypass [67]. One of these was due to MRSA and the patient died. Additional case reports of AEF following endoluminal repair have also been reported, occurring as a result of device failure following stent migration and fabric rupture [68-70].

When the diagnosis of stent graft infection is made, the principles of management are the same as for open AGI. Treatment is usually by graft excision and extra-anatomic bypass. Successful outcomes may be anticipated but the risks associated with removal of the stent graft can be expected to be higher; suprarenal fixation imposes additional risks of visceral and renal ischaemia. Management is challenging, particularly in patients at high risk.

Conclusions

The importance of prevention, and of meticulous surgical and aseptic technique in avoiding graft infection cannot be overemphasised. The use of antibiotic-bonded grafts to prevent contamination at the time of initial operation has become more widely adopted, particularly in patients at high risk of infection. When infection does occur each individual case requires careful consideration. There is unlikely ever to be a single best treatment option. Total graft excision with extra-anatomic bypass should be employed when there is gross contamination with obvious sepsis. A conservative approach such as *in situ* replacement with an antibiotic-bonded graft may be justified when there is minimal contamination. The results with autogenous vein are impressive, but experience with this technique to date is limited to a small number of centres and it has not yet gained widespread popularity.

Individual vascular surgeons have limited experience of graft infection. Improved results may be achieved by transfer of patients to large vascular centres whenever possible, where there may be greater experience of these complex problems and several surgeons may be available to operate simultaneously.

Key points	Evidence level
◆ Peri-operative parenteral antibiotic prophylaxis reduces wound and early graft infection.	Ia/A
◆ Overt sepsis, positive blood culture, extensive retroperitoneal infection and secondary aorto-enteric fistula are associated with a poor prognosis.	IIa/B
◆ Total graft excision and extra-anatomic bypass remains the standard treatment for aortic graft infection. Results have improved in the last decade.	IIa/B
◆ *In situ* graft replacement with an antibiotic-bonded graft is an alternative in selected patients with minimal contamination but late results are uncertain. *In situ* graft replacement with autogenous superficial femoral and popliteal veins may be more successful and durable, but is technically challenging.	IIa/B
◆ Antibiotic-bonded grafts have not been shown to reduce the incidence of graft infection.	Ia/A
◆ Prospective studies into the prevention of MRSA wound and graft infection are needed, including the role of specific antibiotic therapy and isolation techniques.	

References

1. Calligaro KD, Veith FJ. Diagnosis and management of infected prosthetic aortic grafts. *Surgery* 1991; 110: 805-13.
2. Yeager RA, Porter JM. Arterial and prosthetic graft infection. *Ann Vasc Surg* 1992; 6: 485-91.
3. Lorentzen JE, Nielsen OM, Arendrup H, *et al*. Vascular graft infection: an analysis of sixty-two graft infections in 2411 consecutively implanted synthetic vascular grafts. *Surgery* 1985; 98: 81-6.
4. O'Hara PJ, Hertzer NR, Beven EG, *et al*. Surgical management of infected abdominal aortic grafts: review of a 25-year experience. *J Vasc Surg* 1986; 3: 725-31.
5. Hicks RCJ, Greenhalgh RM. Pathogenesis of vascular graft infection. *Eur J Vasc Endovasc Surg* 1997; 14 (Suppl A): 5-9.
6. Olofsson P, Rabahie GN, Matsumoto K, *et al*. Histopathological characteristics of explanted human prosthetic arterial grafts: implications for the prevention and management of graft infection. *Eur J Vasc Endovasc Surg* 1995; 9: 143-51.

7. Gristina AG. Biomaterial-centred infection: microbial adhesion versus tissue integration. *Science* 1987; 237: 1588-95.

8. Levy MF, Schmitt DD, Edmiston CE, *et al.* Sequential analysis of staphylococcal colonisation of body surfaces of patients undergoing vascular surgery. *J Clin Microbiol* 1990; 28: 664-9.

9. Bandyk DF, Esses GE. Prosthetic graft infection. *Surg Clin North Am* 1994; 74: 571-90.

10. Vinard E, Eloy R, Descotes JR, *et al.* Human vascular graft failure and frequency of infection. *J Biomed Material Research* 1991; 25: 499-513.

11. Wooster DL, Louch RE, Kradjen S. Intraoperative bacterial contamination of vascular grafts: a prospective study. *Can J Surg* 1985; 28: 407-9.

12. Selan L, Passariello C. Microbiological diagnosis of aortofemoral graft infection. *Eur J Endovasc Surg* 1997; 14 (Suppl A): 10-2.

13. Nasim A, Thompson MM, Naylor AR, *et al.* The impact of MRSA on vascular surgery. *Eur J Vasc Endovasc Surg* 2001; 22: 211-4.

14. Naylor AR, Hayes PD, Darke S, on behalf of the Joint Vascular Research Group. A prospective audit of complex wound and graft infections in Great Britain and Ireland: the emergence of MRSA. *Eur J Vasc Endovasc Surg* 2001; 21: 289-94.

15. Earnshaw JJ. Methicillin-resistant *Stahylococcus aureus*: vascular surgeons should fight back. *Eur J Vasc Endovasc Surg* 2002; 24: 283-86.

16. Health Protection Agency. Surveillance of surgical site infection in England: October 1997-September 2005. London: Health Protection Agency, July 2006. Available online: www.hpa.org.uk/infections/topics_az/surgical_site_infection/SSIpubs.htm.

17. Earnshaw JJ, Slack RCB, Hopkinson BR, Makin GS. Risk factors in vascular surgical sepsis. *Ann R Coll Surg Engl* 1988; 70: 139-43.

18. Schmitt DD, Bandyk DF, Pequet AJ, Towne B. Bacterial adherence to vascular prostheses. *J Vasc Surg* 1986; 3: 732-40.

19. Stewart A, Eyers P, Earnshaw JJ. Prevention of infection in arterial reconstruction. *Cochrane Database Syst Rev* 2006; 3: CD 003073.

20. Strachan CJL. Antibacterial prophylaxis in peripheral vascular and orthopaedic prosthetic surgery. *J Antimicrob Chemother* 1993; 31 (Suppl B): 65-78.

21. Earnshaw JJ, Berridge DC, Slack RCB, *et al.* Do preoperative chlorhexidine baths reduce the risk of infection after vascular reconstruction? *Eur J Vasc Surg* 1989; 3: 323-6.

22. Cruse PJE, Foord R. The epidemiology of wound infection. A 10-year prospective study of 62,939 wounds. *Surg Clin North Am* 1980; 60: 27-40.

23. Bandyk DF, Bergamini TM. Infection in prosthetic vascular grafts. In: *Vascular Surgery*, 4th Ed. Rutherford RB, Ed. 1995: 588-604.

24. Dunlop MG, Fox JN, Stonebridge PA, *et al.* Vacuum drainage of groin wounds after vascular surgery: a controlled trial. *Br J Surg* 1990; 77: 562-3.

25. Strachan CJL, Newsom SWV, Ashton TR. The clinical use of an antibiotic-bonded graft. *Eur J Vasc Surg* 1991; 5: 627-32.

26. Zavasky D-M, Sande MA. Reconsideration of rifampicin. A unique drug for a unique infection. *JAMA* 1998; 279: 1575-7.

27. Koshiko S, Sasajima T, Muraki S, *et al.* Limitations in the use of rifampicin-gelatin grafts against virulent organisms. *J Vasc Surg* 2002; 35: 779-85.

28. Schmacht D, Armstrong P, Johnson B, *et al.* Graft infectivity of rifampicin and silver-bonded polyester grafts to MRSA contamination. *Vasc Endovasc Surg* 2005; 39: 411-20.

29. D'Addato M, Curti T, Freyrie A and Italian Investigators Group. Prophylaxis of graft infection with rifamcipin-bonded Gelseal graft: 2-year follow-up of a prospective clinical trial. *Cardiovasc Surg* 1996; 4: 200-4.

30. D'Addato M, Curti T and Freyrie A. The rifampicin-bonded Gelseal graft. *Eur J Vasc Endovasc Surg* 1997; 14 (Suppl A): 15-7.

31. Braithwaite BD, Davies B, Heather BP, Earnshaw JJ, on behalf of the Joint Vascular Research Group. Early results of a randomized trial of rifampicin-bonded Dacron grafts for extra-anatomic vascular reconstruction. *Br J Surg* 1998; 85: 1378-81.

32. Earnshaw JJ, Whitman B, Heather BP, on behalf of the Joint Vascular Research Group. Two-year results of a randomized controlled trial of rifampicin-bonded extra-anatomic Dacron grafts. *Br J Surg* 2000; 87: 758-9.

33. Vicaretti M, Hawthorne WJ, Ao PY, *et al.* An increased concentration of rifampicin bonded to gelatine-sealed Dacron reduces the incidence of subsequent graft infections following a staphylococcal challenge. *Cardiovasc Surg* 1998; 6: 268-73.

34. Earnshaw JJ. The current role of rifampicin-impregnated grafts: pragmatism versus science. *Eur J Vasc Endovasc Surg* 2000; 40: 409-12.

35. Hernandez-Richter T, Schardey HM, Wittman F, *et al.* Rifampicin and triclosan but not silver is effective in preventing bacterial infection of vascular Dacron graft material. *Eur J Vasc Endovasc Surg* 2003; 26: 550-7.

36. Goeau-Brissonniere OA, Fabre D, Leflon-Guibout V, *et al.* Comparison of the resistance to infection of rifampin-bonded gelatin-sealed and silver/collagen-coated polyester prostheses. *J Vasc Surg* 2002; 35: 1260-3.

37. Batt M, Magne J-L, Alric P, *et al. In situ* revascularisation with silver-coated polyester grafts to treat aortic infection: early and midterm results. *J Vasc Surg* 2003; 38: 983-9.

38. Maser B, Vedder N, Rodriguez D, Johansen K. Sartorius myoplasty for infected vascular grafts in the groin. Safe, durable and effective. *Arch Surg* 1997; 132: 522-6.

39. Stansby G, Byrne MTL, Hamilton G. Dental infection in vascular surgical patients. *Br J Surg* 1994; 81: 1119-20.

40. Wooster DL, Krajden S. Selection of antibiotic coverage in vascular patients undergoing cystoscopy. *J Cardiovasc Surg* 1990; 31: 469-73.

41. Jones L, Braithwaite BD, Heather BP, Earnshaw JJ. Mechanism of late prosthetic vascular graft infection. *Cardiovasc Surg* 1997; 5: 486-9.

42. Calligaro KD, DeLaurentis DA, Veith FJ. An overview of the treatment of infected prosthetic vascular grafts. *Advances in Surgery* 1996; 29: 3-16.

43. Reilly LM. Aortic graft infection: evolution in management. *Cardiovasc Surg* 2002; 10: 372-7.

44. Perera GB, Fujitani RM, Kubaska SM. Aortic graft infection: update on management and treatment options. *Vasc Endovasc Surg* 2006; 40: 1-10.

45. Armstrong PA, Back MR, Wilson JS, *et al*. Improved outcomes in the recent management of secondary aortoenteric fistula. *J Vasc Surg* 2005; 42: 660-6.

46. Kuestner LM, Reilly LM, Jicha DL, *et al*. Secondary aortoenteric fistula: contemporary outcome with use of extra-anatomic bypass and infected graft excision. *J Vasc Surg* 1995; 21: 184-96.

47. Kotsis T, Lioupis C, Tzanis A, *et al*. Endovascular repair of a bleeding secondary aortoenteric fistula with acute leg ischaemia: a case report and review of the literature. *J Vasc Interv Radiol* 2006; 17: 563-7.

48. Bandyk DF, Novotnel ML, Back MR, *et al*. Expanded application of *in situ* replacement for prosthetic graft infection. *J Vasc Surg* 2001; 34: 411-30.

49. Walker WE, Cooley DA, Duncan JM, *et al*. The management of aortoduodenal fistula by *in situ* replacement of the infected abdominal aortic graft. *Ann Surg* 1987; 205: 727-32.

50. Fiorani P, Speziale F, Rizzo L, *et al*. Long-term follow-up after *in situ* graft replacement in patients with aortofemoral graft infections. *Eur J Vasc Endovasc Surg* 1997; 14 (Suppl A): 111-4.

51. Hayes PD, Nasim A, London NJM, *et al*. *In situ* replacement of infected aortic grafts with rifampicin-bonded prostheses: The Leicester experience (1992 to1998). *J Vasc Surg* 1999; 30: 92-8.

52. Clagett GP, Bowers BL, Lopez-Viego MA, *et al*. Creation of a neo-aortoiliac system from lower extremity deep and superficial veins. *Ann Surg* 1993; 218: 239-49.

53. Daenens K, Fourneau I, Nevelsteen A. Ten-year experience in autogenous reconstruction with the femoral vein in the treatment of aortofemoral prosthetic infection. *Eur J Vasc Endovasc Surg* 2003; 25: 240-5.

54. Gibbons CP, Ferguson CJ, Fligelstone L, Edwards K. Experience with femoro-popliteal vein as a conduit for vascular reconstruction in infected fields. *Eur J Vasc Endovasc Surg* 2003; 25: 424-31.

55. Clagett GP, Valentine RJ, Hagino RT. Autogenous aortoiliac-femoral reconstruction from superficial-femoral popliteal veins: feasibility and durability. *J Vasc Surg* 1997; 25: 255-70.

56. Valentine RJ, Clagett GP. Aortic graft infections: replacement with autogenous vein. *Cardiovasc Surg* 2001; 9: 419-25.

57. Kieffer E, Gomes D, Chiche L, *et al*. Allograft replacement for infrarenal aortic graft infection: early and late results in 179 patients. *J Vasc Surg* 2004; 39: 1009-17.

58. Noel A, Gloviczki P, Cherry KJ, *et al*. Abdominal aortic reconstruction in infected fields: early results of the United States Cryopreserved Aortic Allograft Registry. *J Vasc Surg* 2002; 35: 847-52.

59. Miller JH. Partial replacement of an infected arterial graft by a new prosthetic polytetrafluoroethylene segment: a new therapeutic option. *J Vasc Surg* 1993; 17: 546-58.

60. Calligaro KD, Veith FJ, Yuan JG, *et al*. Intra-abdominal aortic graft infection: complete or partial graft preservation in patients at very high risk. *J Vasc Surg* 2003; 38: 1199-205.

61. Gordon A, Conlon C, Collin J, *et al*. An 8-year experience of conservative management for aortic graft sepsis. *Eur J Vasc Surg* 1994; 8: 611-16.

62. Morris GE, Friend PJ, Vassallo DJ, *et al*. Antibiotic irrigation and conservative surgery for major aortic graft infection. *J Vasc Surg* 1994; 20: 88-95.

63. Nielsen OM, Noer HH, Jorgensen LG, Lorentzen JE. Gentamicin beads in the treatment of localised vascular graft infection - long-term results in 17 cases. *Eur J Vasc Surg* 1991; 5: 283-5.

64. Jensen LP, Nielsen OM, Jorgensen L, Lorentzen JE. Conservative treatment of vascular graft infections in the groin. *Eur J Vasc Endovasc Surg* 1977; 14 (Suppl A): 43-6.

65. Fiorani P, Speziale F, Calisti A, *et al*. Endovascular graft infection: preliminary results of an international enquiry. *J Endovasc Ther* 2003; 10: 919-27.

66. Dattilo JB, Brewster DC, Fan C-M, *et al*. Clinical failures of endovascular abdominal aortic aneurysm repair: incidence, causes and management. *J Vasc Surg* 2002; 35: 1137-44.

67. Walker SR, Braithwaite B, Tennant WG, *et al*. Early complications of femorofemoral crossover bypass grafts after aorto uni-iliac endovascular repair of abdominal aortic aneurysms. *J Vasc Surg* 1998; 28: 647-50.

68. Ghosh J, Murray D, Khwaja N, *et al*. Late infection of an endovascular stent graft with septic embolisation, colonic perforation and aortoduodenal fistula. *Ann Vasc Surg* 2006; 20: 263-6.

69. Janne DB, Soula P, Otal P, *et al*. Aortoduodenal fistula after endovascular stent-graft of an abdominal aortic aneurysm. *J Vasc Surg* 2000; 31: 190-5.

70. Abou-Zamzam AM, Bianchi C, Mazraany W, *et al*. Aortoenteric fistula development following endovascular abdominal aortic aneurysm repair. *Ann Vasc Surg* 2003; 17: 119-22.

Chapter 27

Management of vascular trauma

Denis W Harkin MD FRCS EBSQ-VASC, Senior Lecturer & Consultant Vascular Surgeon

Regional Vascular Surgery Unit, Royal Victoria Hospital, Belfast, Northern Ireland

Epidemiology

Trauma is the leading cause of death in adults under 40 years in the developed world, and accounts for the greatest number of years of life lost. Information on the incidence and aetiology of vascular trauma is still scarce; epidemiological studies are largely based on the clinical experience accumulated with military campaigns and civilian trauma [1-3]. Overall, the civilian incidence of vascular injuries is relatively low, estimated at 0.9 to 2.3 per 100,000 of the population [4] **(III/B)**. Young adult males are more likely to suffer vascular trauma, elderly patients are most at risk of iatrogenic vascular injury, and although vascular injury is rare in children it is often iatrogenic [1-3, 5, 6] **(IIa/III/B)**.

Pathophysiology of vascular trauma

Historically there was a clear distinction between the mechanism of injury between military and civilian trauma; the former mainly arising from high velocity penetrating injury (bullets, missiles, shrapnel), the latter mainly high velocity blunt trauma (road traffic accidents) or low velocity penetrating injury (knife wounds). Much of our current management of vascular trauma owes origin to seminal studies arising from major conflict in World War II, the Korean and

Vietnam Wars, and the Bosnian War. The majority of these battlefield injuries were caused by high velocity penetrating injury from bullet, missile, or blast-associated shrapnel. High velocity weapons dissipate a large amount of energy as the projectile passes through the tissues; this cavitational effect can cause tissue destruction well beyond the path of the missile. Shockwave experiments have demonstrated significant damage to all layers of the vessel wall, beyond the immediate bullet trajectory; this 'percussion' effect may sufficiently displace and distort the vessel anatomy to produce thrombosis, embolism, and extravasation.

In civilian practice, vascular trauma is most commonly encountered following road traffic accidents, with vessel damage induced by blunt, deceleration-type, and penetrating injuries. There is a strong correlation between increasing severity of injury and the incidence of associated vascular injury [7] **(IIa/B)**. Major skeletal trauma is often associated with specific vascular injury patterns, for example: thoracic vascular injuries in the presence of first rib fractures [8, 9]; iliac arterial and venous injuries in the presence of major pelvic fractures or dislocations [10]; popliteal artery injury with knee dislocation [11]. These skeletal injuries in part reflect the degree of force transmitted, but also exemplify how bones can become secondary internal missiles in certain traumatic settings. In the urban environment low velocity penetrating injury from knives or other weapons remains common due to the proliferation of firearm crime and terrorism [4].

Currently, iatrogenic trauma is believed responsible for 5-75% of vascular injuries, an incidence that varies according to the type of vascular practice studied and the referral bias [4, 12] **(III/B)**. The trend for invasive monitoring, and percutaneous vascular intervention for diagnostic or therapeutic procedures has produced an inevitable increase in iatrogenic vascular injuries. Although the majority of catheter-based interventions are uncomplicated, dependent on the complexity of the procedure and on patient-specific factors, complications can include haemorrhage, pseudo-aneurysm, arteriovenous fistula, embolisation, and vessel dissection, occlusion, and rupture. Indwelling intravascular devices are another common source of iatrogenic vascular injury such as thrombosis, embolisation, or infection [12]. Surgical procedures carry an inherent risk of inadvertent trauma to adjacent vessels, in particular in the perihepatic, retroperitoneal and pelvic regions. Oncological surgery for advanced or recurrent tumours carries significant risk to the great arteries and veins of the abdomen [13]. Laparoscopic surgery has unique technical challenges, and although vessel injuries associated with blind insertion of laparoscopic insufflation devices are now essentially of historical interest with the adoption of open-insertion techniques [14], advanced laparoscopic procedures and even routine laparoscopic cholecystectomy are still associated with occasional vessel injuries [15] **(III/B)**.

Diagnosis of vascular trauma

Perhaps reassuringly for those treating trauma, clinical assessment by an experienced clinician with a high index of suspicion will identify the majority of clinically significant vascular injuries. In the acute phase clinical signs relate to haemorrhage, occlusion, or mass-effect. Clinical signs of vascular injury may be soft (history of bleeding, non-pulsatile haematoma) or hard (pulsatile haematoma, bruit, thrill, pulse deficit), (Table 1). With extremity injuries, signs may be overt from the outset, but deep in the cavities of the chest or abdomen, signs may be subtle and must be sought actively and excluded by investigation.

Table 1. The clinical manifestations of vascular injury.

Hard signs	Soft signs
Pulsatile bleeding	Haematoma (small)
Expanding haematoma	History of haemorrhage at scene
Absent distal pulses	Unexplained hypotension
Cold, pale limb	Peripheral nerve deficit
Palpable thrill	
Audible bruit	

At present, the available diagnostic modalities are clinical examination, ultrasound (US), computed tomography (CT), magnetic resonance (MR) imaging, and contrast angiography. The radiologist has a prime role in the management of trauma, and increasingly plays an active role in treatment, as interventional radiology affords therapeutic procedures alternative to surgery [16, 17] **(III/C)**. Ultrasonography can provide a rapid mode of bedside assessment in the unstable patient. Focused Assessment with Sonography for Trauma (FAST) has been widely adopted by many trauma units worldwide and can identify free fluid (suggestive of haemorrhage) by rapid assessment of key areas, namely the perihepatic and perisplenic spaces, the pelvis, and pericardium [18] **(Ib/A)**. In cervical or extremity trauma, ultrasound (duplex and Doppler) can also provide rapid confirmation of vessel integrity, blood flow, bleeding, and associated solid organ pathology. Transoesophageal echocardiography provides high-quality real-time images of the beating heart and mediastinal structures (thoracic aorta), which has a role in the critically ill patient with chest trauma, because of its portability, ease of insertion and ready accessibility [19] **(IIa/B)**. Contrast-enhanced computed tomography angiography (CTA) is becoming the examination of choice in major trauma, due to widespread availability, speed, ready interpretation, and three-dimensional capability. Helical contrast-enhanced CTA is a reliable method for screening patients with blunt chest trauma for vascular and visceral injuries [20] **(IIa/B)**. Even in patients who are haemodynamically unstable, but respond to initial resuscitation, CT evaluation is safe and can often indicate a non-operative or endovascular treatment option [20] **(IIa/B)**. MRI can provide superb images of vascular anatomy but is limited in the emergency setting by availability, acquisition speed, and by the confined space which makes it unsuitable for some patients with trauma. Contrast digital subtraction angiography (DSA) remains the gold standard for assessment of the vascular system [21], and modern endovascular theatres provide the optimal balance between endovascular imaging quality and access to full operative capability, although a portable fluoroscopy unit can provide adequate visualisation on-table in most instances.

Management principles for vascular trauma

Once the diagnosis of acute vascular trauma has been verified, the objectives of treatment are haemorrhage control, restoration of oxygenated blood flow, and prevention of recurrent stenosis or occlusion. Often the vascular injury is only one of several life- or limb-threatening injuries and the vascular clinician, as part of a multidisciplinary team, must address these injuries on the basis of clinical priority. In civilian trauma, all patients are evaluated by the general surgery/ trauma service upon arrival in the emergency department, and resuscitation is carried out in accordance with the Advanced Trauma Life Support (ATLS) guidelines [22] **(Ib/A)**. Resuscitation starts with temporary control of haemorrhage, which may be achieved by manual compression over the bleeding site with surface wounds, by pack or balloon catheter tamponade (Foley catheter) for deeper cavities, but with certain wounds is unachievable without immediate surgical exposure and pedicle or proximal control. Blind attempts at clamping artery or vein in deep cavities without adequate exposure inevitably fails. The underlying principles of vascular control dictate that proximal and distal control should be sought before exploration of the bleeding site or haematoma. Whilst it is a fact that bleeding always stops, it is vital that it stops on terms that the patient can tolerate; as such a graded response to haemorrhage control allows the surgeon to escalate his response from simple to complex until control is achieved. Excessive fluid resuscitation in the emergency department in an attempt to normalise blood pressure simply encourages clot dislodgement

and rebleeding [23] **(IIb/B)**. Common practice in most centres is to allow permissive hypotension, sufficient to maintain cerebral perfusion [24]. An experienced member of staff should stay with the patient to ensure adequate resuscitation, swift transport, adequate positioning, and patient preparation for intervention. A management strategy is considered using the available evidence from history, mechanism of injury, patient physiology, clinical symptoms and signs, and available diagnostic tests. At all stages the surgeon should consider non-operative management of a haemodynamically stable patient; observation must be carried out in a critical care environment and imaging undertaken to exclude serious associated injuries **(IV/C)**.

Surgical management principles for vascular trauma

The operative strategy is crucial to the successful management of vascular trauma, and should consider procedure sequencing and priority, to include any potential bail-out options. The full extent of the injury, including any possible missile tracts, as well as proximal vessel control access points must be prepared. Limbs should be draped transparently to allow assessment of distal perfusion. Often the other limbs are required for vein conduit harvest. In general, the approach follows standard exposure principles in the thorax, abdomen and extremities, and is dictated by the suspected site of injury. It is essential that the operating table should be compatible with the use of on-table angiography, for both diagnostic and therapeutic interventions.

Vascular injuries may be treated by simple repair (lateral repair and ligation), or complex repair (patch angioplasty, end-to-end anastomosis, interposition grafting, extra-anatomic bypass) (Figure 1). In general terms, a rapid simple repair is preferable to a lengthy complex repair, particularly in the unstable patient. Minor lacerations (less than 50% circumferential) may be treated rapidly by lateral suture, but in children with small elastic vessels, or for major lacerations (more than 50% circumferential) lateral repair will result in significant vessel narrowing, and patch angioplasty or interposition grafting is often advantageous. Complete lacerations or transection even without segmental

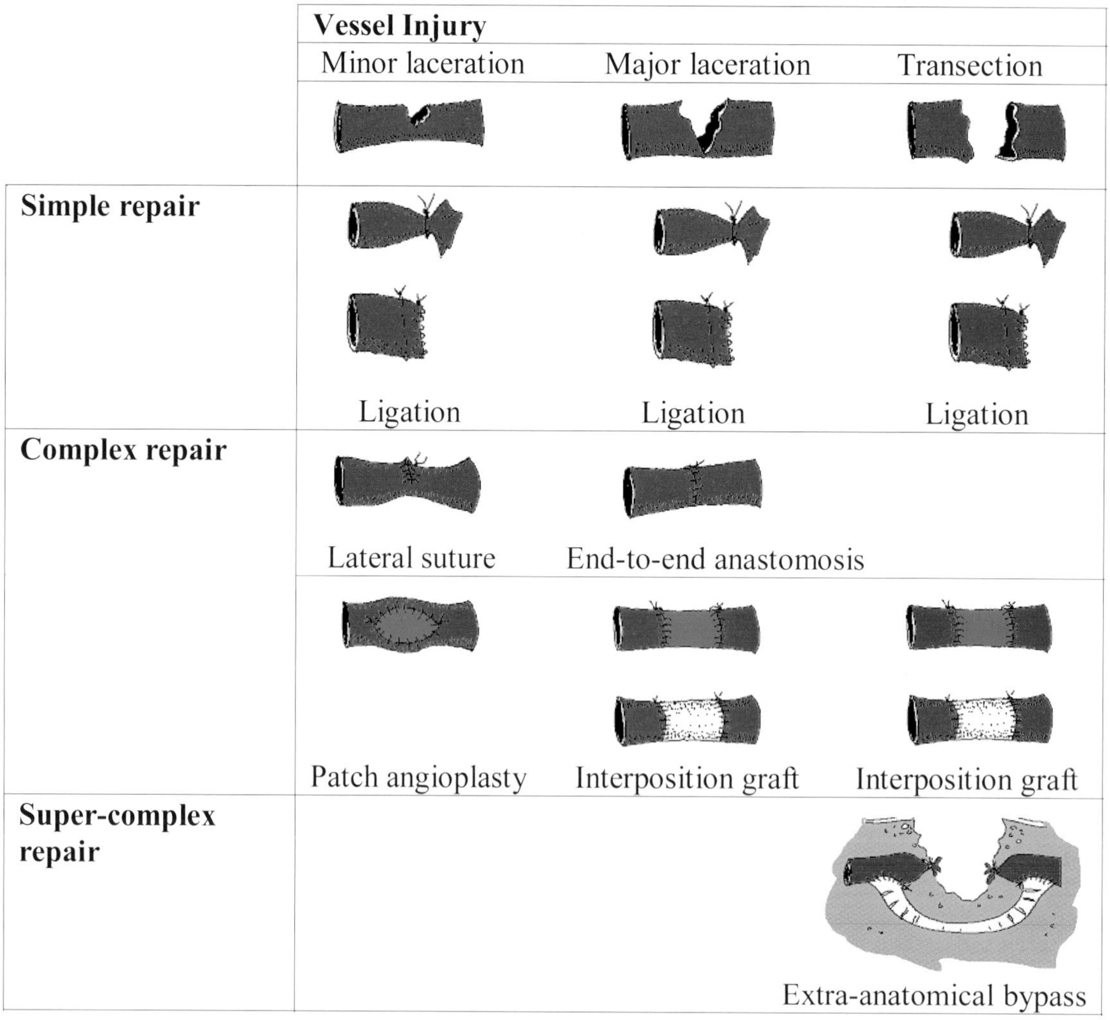

Vessel Injury		
Minor laceration	Major laceration	Transection

Figure 1. Vessel repair techniques for vascular trauma. The extent of vessel injury (minor laceration, major laceration, transection) influences the repair options (simple or complex).

loss, are best treated by interposition grafting, as vessel injury usually extends well beyond the laceration, such that mobilisation and debridement to healthy tissue rarely allows a tension-free primary repair. The choice of conduit includes autologous vein (usually long saphenous vein, rarely superficial femoral vein), synthetic graft (Dacron or PTFE), or rarely autologous artery (external carotid or internal iliac). Synthetic grafts are preferred for most large vessels, but perform poorly in the limbs, where vein grafts are superior. In grossly contaminated wounds, any anastomosis is at risk from sepsis with subsequent catastrophic failure. In these settings vessel ligation and extra-anatomic bypass is a good option if collateral circulation proves inadequate **(III/C)**. Complex reconstructions using composite vein grafts using a spiral or panelled graft technique, add substantially to operative time, and should only be considered in a stable patient with injuries to a single vascular territory **(IV/C)**.

Temporary intraluminal shunts have revolutionised the management of both arterial and venous trauma [25, 26] (Figure 2). This effect is most evident in the treatment of complex lower limb injuries as a result of blunt and penetrating trauma, where intraluminal shunting of the artery and vein decreases rates of fasciotomy, contractures, and amputation [27] **(IIa/B)**. A variety of

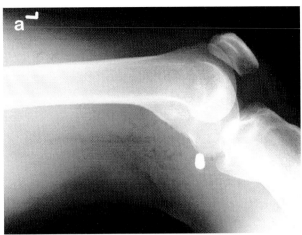
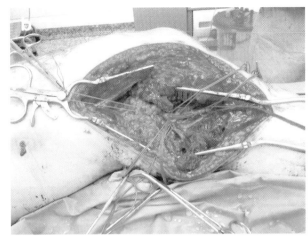

Figure 2. Intraluminal shunts in extremity vascular trauma. Multiple gunshot wounds to the left leg with acute ischaemia. a) The radiograph demonstrates one bullet lodged in the popliteal fossa. b) The entrance wound to the left medial thigh is seen; other entry wounds are incorporated in the exploratory medial leg incision. In the wound the transected popliteal artery is controlled with an intraluminal shunt; inferiorly, the popliteal vein has been repaired with a simple lateral suture.

commercial shunts are available, but even sterile heparinised polyethylene tubing or a chest tube will suffice for most vessel sizes encountered. Restoration of arterial inflow arrests tissue hypoxia and prevents further ischaemic damage, while restoration of venous outflow reduces capillary bed pressure and allows controlled release of cellular metabolites [28]. This allows time for a multidisciplinary approach to these complex multisystem injuries, adequate wound toilet, debridement, orthopaedic manipulation and fixation. Shunts are also used as part of damage control surgery; definitive repair can be delayed by 24 to 48 hours to allow transfer of a patient, and treatment of hypothermia, acidosis or coagulopathy.

In extremity trauma many surgeons elect to perform distal compartmental fasciotomy to prevent compartment syndrome, particularly if there are major associated injuries (bone, soft tissue), crush injuries, concurrent arterial and venous injury, or if presentation is delayed (greater than six hours) **(IV/C)**. In the lower limb a full four-compartment two-incision approach is recommended. Although there is some morbidity associated with these wounds, many can be closed incrementally on the ward using pre-placed sutures or skin grafts. Fasciotomy also has a role in protecting fragile arterial reconstructions or low-flow venous repairs, and is an essential adjunct if ligation of the main inflow vessel was done as part of damage limitation.

Endoluminal management of vascular trauma

The endovascular management of a haemodynamically stable patient with vascular trauma may avoid compounding physiological stress from injury with surgical stress. In particular, lesions that occur at anatomically inaccessible regions (base of the skull, infraclavicular or pelvic regions) often pose far less difficulty when managed by endoluminal techniques than by traditional surgical exposure. These procedures found an early role in proximal extremity vascular injury, where the ease of endoluminal access to the injury site contrasted with the difficulty of open surgery [29, 30]. Catheter-directed embolisation is an adaptable technique, whether with coils or procoagulants, and is particularly useful in the management of pelvic haemorrhage [31] **(IIb/B)**. One large single-centre experience has shown non-surgical management using transcatheter embolisation is safe for patients with blunt poly-trauma presenting with shock, provided they respond to initial resuscitation, with high success rates and low morbidity in the pelvic, splenic, hepatic and renal vascular territories [32]. One emerging area of interest is that of covered stents to treat major vascular trauma. Notable success has been achieved in the thoracic aorta, where it is now arguably the treatment of choice **(IIb/B)**. Endovascular techniques are an essential part of vascular trauma management, with endovascular specialists working in partnership with trauma teams [33] **(IV/C)**.

Extremity vascular trauma

The following summarises the principles of management of limb trauma:

- control of haemorrhage takes precedence over limb perfusion;
- in penetrating extremity injury, physical examination alone and a non-operative approach to clinically occult arterial injuries is associated with a low rate of early or late complications [34] **(IIa/B)**;
- in extremity trauma a positive duplex ultrasound scan or a reduced Doppler ankle-brachial pressure index (less than 0.9) is an absolute indication for an angiogram and possible intervention **(III/C)**;
- civilian extremity gunshot injuries are attended by a high amputation rate; prompt resuscitation and revascularisation is the key to successful outcomes [35] **(IIb/B)**;
- early shunting of artery and vein in complex limb vascular injuries has reduced morbidity and amputation rates [36] **(IIa/C)**;
- proximal vein ligation may be life-saving but is often followed by significant morbidity, and simple repair should be considered [37] **(III/C)**;
- in upper limb trauma, the brachial artery is most commonly injured; distal injuries result in more satisfactory outcomes, as proximal injuries are more commonly associated with severe neurological, soft tissue, and bony damage [38] **(III/C)**;
- selected proximal injuries may be treated by endovascular means [39] **(III/C)**;
- complete brachial plexus lesions result in uniformly poor outcomes;
- severely injured limbs for which attempted salvage would be futile can be identified using the Mangled Extremity Severity Score (MESS) [40], and require primary amputation.

Neck vascular trauma

The following summarises the principles of management of neck trauma:

- for the purposes of clinical assessment the neck is divided into three zones, based on anatomical landmarks:
  - base of the neck (zone 1);
  - mid-neck from clavicle to lower mandible (zone 2);
  - from the lower mandible to base of skull (zone 3) [41, 42];
- in an asymptomatic patient with penetrating trauma to zone 2, morbidity and mortality are low;
- zone 1 and 3 injuries require angiography (or contrast-enhanced CTA);
- the management of penetrating and blunt neck trauma has changed in recent years from mandatory exploration, which was frequently negative, to selective non-surgical management in a monitored environment after the reassurance of negative radiological investigation [43] **(IV/C)**;
- neurological status can be used to guide intervention; surgery does not affect outcome in a comatose patient [44] **(III/C)**;
- in selected cases of traumatic carotid artery dissections, endovascular stent-assisted angioplasty can immediately restore vessel integrity [45] **(IV/C)**;
- the majority of patients with a vertebral artery injury who are not exsanguinating can be managed non-operatively, or by angiographic embolisation [46].

Thoracic vascular trauma

The following summarises the principles of management of thoracic trauma:

- in the civilian setting, blunt thoracic aortic injuries are three-fold more common in men, particularly in their second and third decades of life [47, 48] **(III/C)**;
- in thoracic trauma, CT examination significantly affects the immediate clinical management and patient triage [20];

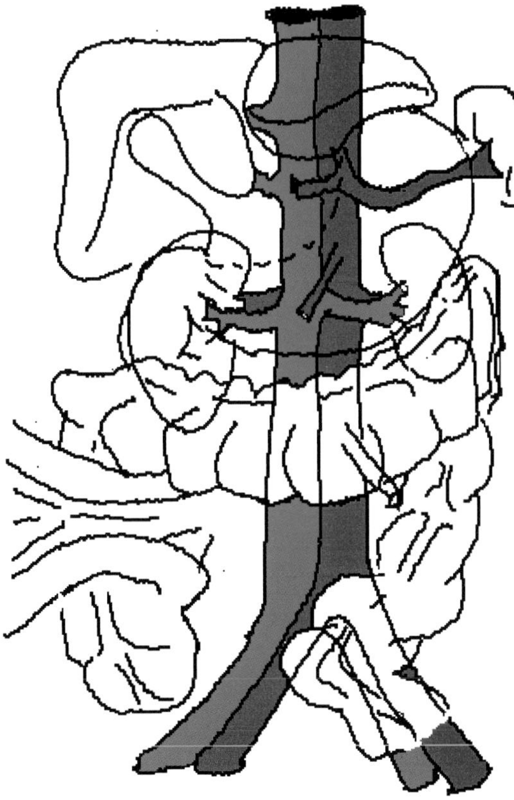

Right   Superior mesocolic compartment   Left

Suprarenal inferior vena cava or retrohepatic veins

Abdominal aorta, coeliac trunk, or proximal superior mesenteric artery

Right renal artery or vein

Left renal artery or vein

Infrarenal inferior vena cava or mesenteric vessels

Infrarenal abdominal aorta, distal superior mesenteric artery, and inferior mesenteric artery

Right iliac artery or vein

Left iliac artery or vein

Inferior mesocolic compartment

Figure 3. The great vessels in abdominal haemorrhage. The transverse mesocolon divides the abdomen into two compartments: supramesocolic and inframesocolic. When approaching intra-abdominal haemorrhage the site of the retroperitoneal haematoma in respect to these compartments allows the surgeon to consider the potential bleeding site and adopt the appropriate exposure.

- in stable rupture of the aorta, initial conservative treatment is safe and allows management of any major associated injuries and assessment of surgical and endovascular options [48] **(IIb/B)**;
- stable patients with aortic rupture distal to the left subclavian artery branch should be considered for endovascular thoracic stent grafting, if anatomically suitable, especially if high risk for conventional thoracotomy [49];
- the immediate outcome of patients treated with endovascular stent grafts appears to be better than with management by conventional surgical repair [50] **(IIb/B)**.

Abdominal vascular trauma

The following summarises the principles of management of abdominal trauma:

- abdominal vascular injuries are highly lethal; multiple arterial and venous injuries increase mortality, and mortality correlates with overall injury severity scores [51] **(III/C)**;
- CT is now a pre-requisite to modern management of abdominal trauma, in all but the most unstable patients. CT-based criteria help triage patients suitable for endovascular treatment, conservative management or surgical intervention and may also predict those at risk of post-traumatic complications [52] **(IIb/B)**;

Table 2. Clinical tips for vascular trauma.

Bleeding site	Approach	Technique
Extremity trauma ***The groin and femoral artery*** Perhaps most commonly injured iatrogenically from percutaneous catheter-based interventions.	The retroperitoneal approach allows proximal control of the external iliac artery. Incision 2cm above and parallel to the inguinal ligament is deepened through aponeurosis of external and internal oblique, transverses abdominis muscle and transversalis fascia to pre-peritoneal fat, cephalad reflection of which exposes the external iliac artery. In the extremis, proximal control can be gained by a midline laparotomy incision or by vertical groin incision extended through the inguinal ligament. Distal control is best achieved through the haematoma with blunt dissection, digital pressure, and by 'walking the clamps' into position. The profunda femoris artery may require insertion of a balloon catheter.	Damage control includes temporary shunting or ligation. If possible preserve the profunda femoral artery, as collateral flow from here will sustain the leg. Definitive repair may involve lateral suture, patch angioplasty, or interposition grafting. Repair of major veins is reasonable in a stable patient, but in the unstable almost all veins including the common femoral can be ligated, although resultant lower limb oedema may be severe. Essential soft tissue coverage may be achieved with a sartorius muscle flap (or quadriceps muscle flap) cover. Alternatively, interposition bypass are routed extra-anatomically through virgin tissue planes.
The knee and popliteal artery Injured with penetrating trauma (the classic 'knee-capping' gunshot wound) and blunt trauma such as fracture dislocations of the knee.	The medial approach to the popliteal vessels involves incision of the medial aspect of the lower thigh in the groove between vastus medialis and sartorius muscles, extended through deep fascia posterior to the femur bone to reveal popliteal vessels invested in fat. Distal extension of the primary incision or a separate medial incision 1cm posterior to the tibia extended through deep fascia to reveal the distal vessels immediately posterior to the tibia. The injury site may be exposed medially by connecting the incisions through the haematoma, dividing medial head of gastrocnemius, if necessary.	With total popliteal artery disruption collateral flow is inadequate to sustain the lower limb and rates of limb loss are high. Inflow and outflow vessel are cleared with proximal and distal passage of a balloon embolectomy catheter, followed by flushing with heparinised saline. Intraluminal shunts can be placed in both artery and vein, as required, revascularising the limb. With injuries below the knee, if all three vessels (anterior tibial, posterior tibial, and peroneal arteries) are disrupted, repair of one is usually sufficient and in view of its accessibility this is often the posterior tibial artery.
The upper limb, axillary and brachial artery The axillary artery is a thin, fragile, and unforgiving artery. Anatomically exposed, the brachial artery is the most frequently injured artery in the body.	The infraclavicular incision extending from the mid-clavicular region to the deltopectoral groove (arm in abduction), extended through pectoralis fascia and pectoralis minor, to pectoralis major, which invests the axillary incising clavipectoral fascia reveals axillary fat which invests the axillary vein with artery deep and superior. The brachial artery is exposed proximally through a medial upper arm incision in the groove between biceps and triceps muscle, extending proximal to the deltopectoral groove or distal across the antecubital fossa into the forearm. Deep extension, with anterior retraction of biceps muscle exposes the brachial sheath containing median nerve and brachial artery.	Damage control for the unstable patient can be achieved by ligation of the axillary artery, as collaterals are good around the shoulder, or by temporary intraluminal shunt insertion. However, definitive repair using interposition grafting (vein or synthetic) will avoid postoperative exertional arm claudication. If damage control is necessitated the brachial artery can be ligated, preferably distal to the take-off of the deep brachial artery, and this is often well tolerated but should be accompanied by upper limb fasciotomy. Definitive repair is best achieved by interposition vein graft repair using long saphenous vein harvested from the lower leg.
Neck trauma ***Carotid and vertebral arteries, and jugular veins*** Injuries to the larynx or trachea are common in penetrating injury, and prophylactic endotracheal intubation, may avoid subsequent need for emergency tracheostomy.	The preferred approach is an oblique skin incision anterior to the medial border of sternocleidomastoid (SCM) muscle (neck extended to the opposite side), extending deep to the medial border of the SCM, and internal jugular vein beneath (dividing facial vein anteriorly), exposes the carotid sheath (vagus nerve descending in the tracheo-oesophageal groove behind), opened longitudinally the artery can be dissected in the peri-adventitial plane. Extension inferiorly to the sternal notch and into a median sternotomy assists proximal control, and superiorly to the mastoid process (avoid the horizontally placed hypoglossal nerve), dividing digastric muscle, gains access to the internal carotid artery at base of skull.	Ligation for damage control carries a small risk of stroke but is generally safe with full collateral flow, and better tolerated in the common carotid as the external then gives retrograde flow to the internal carotid. Temporary shunts are useful after careful catheter thrombectomy, observing back bleeding from the distal stump. Definitive repair is best achieved with interposition reversed long saphenous vein graft. The vertebral artery is difficult to access surgically, and is often treatable by endovascular intervention. Lateral suture will suffice for most venous injuries, although ligation of any major neck vein is well tolerated. Careful inspection for associated injuries to the oesophagus, larynx, or nerves should follow vascular care.
Thorax trauma ***The heart and great vessels*** Deceleration injuries typically shear the proximal descending thoracic aorta with a contained or free rupture. Penetrating injuries may transect great vessels or cause cardiac disruption.	In the unstable patient the recommended approach is through a left anterolateral thoracotomy. In major penetrating injury exploration is best done in conjunction with a cardiothoracic surgeon, and access to extracorporeal cardiopulmonary bypass. Longitudinal incision of the pericardium (placed anterior to avoid the phrenic nerve) releases tamponade and allows delivery of the heart for inspection. Access to right-sided structures can be achieved by extension of the incision across the sternum to the other hemithorax, or by median sternotomy.	Temporary control is achieved with digital pressure, a balloon catheter, or if all else fails, very brief inflow control by manually compressing the right atrium or temporarily clamping the superior and inferior vena cava. A stopped heart may be restarted by warm fluid resuscitation, open cardiac compressions, adrenaline, and internal cardioversion. A simple wound in the heart may be repaired with interrupted deep partial thickness myocardial sutures, which may be supplemented with Teflon pledgets. Complex wounds involving the coronary arteries are often fatal if proximal, if distal they may be ligated accepting the consequence of myocardial infarction.

Table 2. Clinical tips for vascular trauma continued.

Bleeding site	Approach	Technique
Thoracic outlet and subclavian vessels With upper mediastinal haematoma, consider the great vessels of the aortic arch (right brachiocephalic, left common carotid, and subclavian artery).	Access is best achieved by median sternotomy incision, extended deep by ligating and dividing the thymus gland, revealing the left innominate vein, which can be ligated and divided, reconstructed later if necessary. This reveals the branches of the aortic arch; landmarks include the aortic root exposed by incising the superior pericardium, the right vagus nerve crosses the proximal right subclavian artery and the left vagus nerve crosses the arch between the left common carotid and subclavian arteries giving off its recurrent laryngeal branch.	Damage control may require ligation, with an attendant risk of stroke. Definitive repair is best achieved by bypass graft taken from the ascending aortic arch to the distal target vessel, with suture-ligation of the damaged portions. Extension into the neck by low division of the strap muscles exposes the carotid vessels. The subclavian vessels may be controlled by endovascular means through a brachial approach, but if surgery is necessary there are several approaches: third space anterolateral thoracotomy, median sternotomy, supraclavicular, and by clavicular resection.
Thoraco-abdominal injuries Penetrating midline injuries here associated with refractory hypotension suggest disruption of the main neurovascular complex, which is rarely survivable.	Entrance and exit wounds indicate the trajectory and likely injuries; in the emergency room radiological screening of chest and abdomen may identify any retained missile, pneumothorax, haemothorax. In the unstable patient this may be achieved through an upper midline or bilateral subcostal incision. FAST scan in the emergency room may suggest major intra-abdominal haemorrhage.	This junctional zone, separated by the diaphragm, extends from the costal margin to the nipple line anteriorly, the sixth intercostals space laterally, to the tip of scapula posterior. If after chest tube insertion bleeding is substantial or unabated, thoracotomy is required. If on the right the hemi-diaphragm is disrupted with bleeding from the underlying liver; do not explore this, but repair the defect with diaphragmatic sutures and reassess the situation.
Abdominal trauma **The supramesocolic compartment** Midline supramesocolic compartment haematomas often involve the suprarenal aorta, coeliac trunk or superior mesenteric vessels (SMA).	Enter the bleeding abdomen through a midline incision (from xiphoid sternum to pubis), removing clots and eviscerating the small bowel to the right. Rapidly place quadrant packs to right-upper quadrant and liver, left upper quadrant and spleen, both paracolic gutters and pelvis. Immediate haemorrhage control may be achieved by manual compression of the supracoeliac aorta. The left-medial visceral rotation will allow control of the lower thoracic aorta through the diaphragm and exposure of the aortic branches; extension to the left hemithorax may be required in extremis.	Temporary control may be achieved by manual compression, temporary packing (the liver sandwich technique), and inflow manoeuvres (Pringle manoeuvre: pinching or clamping the portal triad). Simple lacerations are best controlled with packs but deep liver sutures may be placed, if experienced. In damage control settings with injury to both portal vein and hepatic artery, one may be ligated, not both. The coeliac trunk may be ligated in most settings, but the SMA requires reconstruction by retrograde bypass, from distal aorta or right iliac artery to distal inframesocolic SMA.
The inframesocolic compartment Aortic injury is likely when haematoma is to the left of midline. A dark haematoma to the right behind the ascending colon suggests a caval injury.	If the haematoma is in the midline or to the left the infrarenal aortic injury may be approached and repaired by standard techniques used in aortic aneurysm rupture. It is prudent to obtain supracoeliac aortic control through the lesser omentum where the aorta may be clamped after division of the right crus of diaphragm. Alternatively, an endoluminal supracoeliac aortic balloon catheter may be placed by endovascular technique or guided through the aortic wall or injury site.	Damage control occasionally requires aortic ligation, in the presence of severe faecal contamination, with extra-anatomic revascularisation (axillo-femoral and femoro-femoral crossover graft). If exploration of the cava is required, after right medial rotation immediate control is achieved with proximal and distal manual compression, then placement of a single side-biting or standard clamp. Simple repair by lateral suture is often feasible, but if necessary the infrarenal cava may be ligated.
The pelvis Blunt pelvic trauma can result in significant blood loss from the fractured pelvis and associated extra-peritoneal pelvic veins. Orthopaedic stabilisation of the pelvis by external fixation will often control haemorrhage.	Pelvic angiography and embolisation should be considered. If laparotomy is indicated (other abdominal injuries) in blunt trauma, a contained pelvic haematoma in the presence of a pelvic fracture generally should not be explored, packs could be placed, and re-operation planned. In penetrating pelvic trauma injuries to the iliac vessels are common. With unilateral injuries access to the iliac vessels can be achieved, on the left by medial mobilisation and rotation of the sigmoid colon, and on the right by medial mobilisation and rotation of the caecum. In bilateral or proximal midline injuries both iliac systems can be exposed by a full Cattell-Braasch manoeuvre.	Temporary haemorrhage control may require manual compression, or clamping of the aorta or inferior vena cava. Proximal and distal control of iliac vessels will allow the clamps to be 'walked' to the injury site, with the internal iliac artery controlled by side-biting clamp or a balloon catheter. Approach to the confluence of the common iliac veins may require transection of overlying right iliac artery, with later repair. Damage control options include lateral suture, temporary shunting, or ligation. Ligation should be accompanied by ipsilateral lower limb fasciotomy, and if indicated extra-anatomic bypass by femoro-femoro crossover or axillofemoral bypass. This approach is also safer than anastomosis for iliac injury in the presence of gross intestinal contamination.

◆ intra-operative exsanguination is the primary cause of death in abdominal vascular trauma, and haemorrhage control should be the first priority;

◆ modern concepts include early exploration for suspected intra-abdominal bleeding and a conservative approach to liver injury [53] **(IV/C)**;

◆ injuries to the mesenteric vessels are daunting, with a high mortality often compounded by severe associated injuries [54];

◆ similarly, the outcome after iliac vessel injuries is also poor [55];

◆ the transverse mesocolon divides the abdomen into two compartments (supramesocolic and inframesocolic); considering the most likely vessel injury in each location can guide the surgical exposure (Figure 3).

Conclusions

The management of vascular trauma is challenging, where acute life- and limb-threatening scenarios require expedient, sometimes complex solutions. Management strategy should be based on correct interpretation of the pattern of injury, trauma burden and patient physiology, to create the optimal balance between damage control and definitive repair, within the constraints of the systems and resources available. Individualised management of the patient with multiple injuries requires a multidisciplinary approach and may include the co-ordinated activities of general, vascular, cardiothoracic, plastic and orthopaedic surgeons. Ideally, major vascular trauma should be dealt within a facility that combines appropriate expertise, access to diagnostic modalities, the full range of open and endovascular treatment options, and rehabilitation therapy. Some clinical tips for the management of vascular trauma are outlined in Table 2.

Key points	Evidence level
◆ Vascular trauma is grossly under-reported but more commonly accompanies penetrating trauma.	III/B
◆ Clinical examination alone by an experienced vascular surgeon has a high sensitivity and specificity for the detection of significant vascular trauma.	IIa/B
◆ In the unstable trauma patient contrast-enhanced CT provides important information on vascular and soft tissue architecture.	IIa/B
◆ Non-operative treatment of the stable patient with vascular trauma undoubtedly saves lives.	IIa/B
◆ Endoluminal treatments, such as embolisation and stenting, are effective treatments in thoracic and abdominal aortic trauma and proximal extremity vessels.	IIa/B
◆ In extremity vascular trauma the insertion of intraluminal vascular shunts to artery and vein reduces morbidity and amputation rates.	IIa/B
◆ Simple arterial repair, lateral suture or ligation, for haemorrhage control reduces mortality in unstable patients with multiple injuries.	IIa/B
◆ Complex repairs when indicated are best achieved with a synthetic tube graft in proximal vessels, and an autologous vein graft in distal extremities.	IIa/B
◆ In the extremity, vein ligation does not increase amputation rates.	IIa/B

References

1. Rich NM. Vascular trauma in Vietnam. *J Cardiovasc Surg (Torino)* 1970; 11: 368-77.

2. Mattox KL, Feliciano DV, Burch J, *et al*. Five thousand seven hundred sixty cardiovascular injuries in 4459 patients. Epidemiologic evolution 1958 to 1987. *Ann Surg* 1989; 209: 698-705.

3. Barros D'Sa AA. Twenty-five years of vascular trauma in Northern Ireland. *Br Med J* 1995; 310: 1-2.

4. Fingerhut A, Leppaniemi AK, Androulakis GA, *et al*. The European experience with vascular injuries. *Surg Clin North Am* 2002; 82: 175-88.

5. Thomson I, Muduioa G, Gray A. Vascular trauma in New Zealand: an 11-year review of NZVASC, the New Zealand Society of Vascular Surgeons' audit database. *NZ Med J* 2004; 117: U1048.

6. de Virgilio C, Mercado PD, Arnell T, *et al*. Noniatrogenic pediatric vascular trauma: a ten-year experience at a level I trauma center. *Am Surg* 1997; 63: 781-4.

7. Oller DW, Rutledge R, Clancy T, *et al*. Vascular injuries in a rural state: a review of 978 patients from a state trauma registry. *J Trauma* 1992; 32: 740-5.

8. Mattox KL. Contemporary issues in thoracic aortic trauma. *Semin Thorac Cardiovasc Surg* 1991; 3: 281-5.

9. Fisher RG, Oria RA, Mattox KL, *et al*. Conservative management of aortic lacerations due to blunt trauma. *J Trauma* 1990; 30: 1562-6.

10. Yelon JA, Scalea TM. Venous injuries of the lower extremities and pelvis: repair versus ligation. *J Trauma* 1992; 33: 532-6.

11. Bishara RA, Pasch AR, Lim LT, *et al*. Improved results in the treatment of civilian vascular injuries associated with fractures and dislocations. *J Vasc Surg* 1986; 3: 707-11.

12. Nehler MR, Taylor LM, Jr., Porter JM. Iatrogenic vascular trauma. *Semin Vasc Surg* 1998; 11: 283-93.

13. Oderich GS, Panneton JM, Hofer J, *et al*. Iatrogenic operative injuries of abdominal and pelvic veins: a potentially lethal complication. *J Vasc Surg* 2004; 39: 931-6.

14. Nordestgaard AG, Bodily KC, Osborne RW, *et al*. Major vascular injuries during laparoscopic procedures. *Am J Surg* 1995; 169: 543-5.

15. Fuller J, Ashar BS, Carey-Corrado J. Trocar-associated injuries and fatalities: an analysis of 1399 reports to the FDA. *J Minim Invasive Gynecol* 2005; 12: 302-7.

16. Poletti PA, Wintermark M, Schnyder P, *et al*. Traumatic injuries: role of imaging in the management of the polytrauma victim (conservative expectation). *Eur Radiol* 2002; 12: 969-78.

17. Wintermark M, Poletti PA, Becker CD, *et al*. Traumatic injuries: organization and ergonomics of imaging in the emergency environment. *Eur Radiol* 2002; 12: 959-68.

18. Yeo A, Wong CY, Soo KC. Focused abdominal sonography for trauma (FAST). *Ann Acad Med Singapore* 1999; 28: 805-9.

19. Tousignant C. Transesophageal echocardiographic assessment in trauma and critical care. *Can J Surg* 1999; 42: 171-5.

20. Gavant ML. Helical CT grading of traumatic aortic injuries. Impact on clinical guidelines for medical and surgical management. *Radiol Clin North Am* 1999; 37: 553-74.

21. Haage P, Krings T, Schmitz-Rode T. Nontraumatic vascular emergencies: imaging and intervention in acute venous occlusion. *Eur Radiol* 2002; 12: 2627-43.

22. Bell RM, Krantz BE, Weigelt JA. ATLS: a foundation for trauma training. *Ann Emerg Med* 1999; 34: 233-7.

23. Bickell WH, Wall MJ, Jr., Pepe PE, *et al*. Immediate versus delayed fluid resuscitation for hypotensive patients with penetrating torso injuries. *N Engl J Med* 1994; 331: 1105-9.

24. Martin RR, Bickell WH, Pepe PE, *et al*. Prospective evaluation of preoperative fluid resuscitation in hypotensive patients with penetrating truncal injury: a preliminary report. *J Trauma* 1992; 33: 354-61.

25. Barros D'Sa AA. The rationale for arterial and venous shunting in the management of limb vascular injuries. *Eur J Vasc Surg* 1989; 3(6): 471-4.

26. Barros D'Sa AA, Moorehead RJ. Combined arterial and venous intraluminal shunting in major trauma of the lower limb. *Eur J Vasc Surg* 1989; 3: 577-81.

27. Barros D'Sa AA, Harkin DW, Blair PH, *et al*. The Belfast approach to managing complex lower limb vascular injuries. *Eur J Vasc Endovasc Surg* 2006: in press.

28. Harkin DW, D'Sa AA, Yassin MM, *et al*. Reperfusion injury is greater with delayed restoration of venous outflow in concurrent arterial and venous limb injury. *Br J Surg* 2000; 87: 734-41.

29. McKinley AG, Carrim AT, Robbs JV. Management of proximal axillary and subclavian artery injuries. *Br J Surg* 2000; 87: 79-85.

30. Babatasi G, Massetti M, Bhoyroo S, *et al*. Non-penetrating subclavian artery trauma: management by selective transluminally placed stent device. *Thorac Cardiovasc Surg* 1999; 47: 190-3.

31. Maull KI, Sachatello CR. Current management of pelvic fractures: a combined surgical-angiographic approach to hemorrhage. *South Med J* 1976; 69: 1285-9.

32. Hagiwara A, Murata A, Matsuda T, *et al*. The usefulness of transcatheter arterial embolization for patients with blunt polytrauma showing transient response to fluid resuscitation. *J Trauma* 2004; 57: 271-6.

33. Nicholson AA. Vascular radiology in trauma. *Cardiovasc Intervent Radiol* 2004; 27: 105-20.

34. Dennis JW, Frykberg ER, Veldenz HC, *et al*. Validation of nonoperative management of occult vascular injuries and accuracy of physical examination alone in penetrating extremity trauma: 5- to 10-year follow-up. *J Trauma* 1998; 44: 243-52.

35. Nair R, Abdool-Carrim AT, Robbs JV. Gunshot injuries of the popliteal artery. *Br J Surg* 2000; 87: 602-7.

36. Barros D'Sa AA, Harkin DW, Blair PH, *et al*. The Belfast approach to managing complex lower limb vascular injuries. *Eur J Vasc Endovasc Surg* 2006: in press.

37. Parry NG, Feliciano DV, Burke RM, *et al*. Management and short-term patency of lower extremity venous injuries with various repairs. *Am J Surg* 2003; 186: 631-5.

38. Fitridge RA, Raptis S, Miller JH, *et al*. Upper extremity arterial injuries: experience at the Royal Adelaide Hospital, 1969 to 1991. *J Vasc Surg* 1994; 20: 941-6.

39. Danetz JS, Cassano AD, Stoner MC, et al. Feasibility of endovascular repair in penetrating axillosubclavian injuries: a retrospective review. J Vasc Surg 2005; 41: 246-54.

40. Johansen K, Daines M, Howey T, et al. Objective criteria accurately predict amputation following lower extremity trauma. J Trauma 1990; 30: 568-72.

41. Pearce WH, Whitehill TA. Carotid and vertebral arterial injuries. Surg Clin North Am 1988; 68: 705-23.

42. Monson DO, Saletta JD, Freeark RJ. Carotid vertebral trauma. J Trauma 1969; 9: 987-99.

43. Beitsch P, Weigelt JA, Flynn E, et al. Physical examination and arteriography in patients with penetrating zone II neck wounds. Arch Surg 1994; 129: 577-81.

44. Teehan EP, Padberg FT, Jr., Thompson PN, et al. Carotid arterial trauma: assessment with the Glasgow Coma Scale (GCS) as a guide to surgical management. Cardiovasc Surg 1997; 5: 196-200.

45. Cohen JE, Ben Hur T, Rajz G, et al. Endovascular stent-assisted angioplasty in the management of traumatic internal carotid artery dissections. Stroke 2005; 36: e45-7.

46. Roberts LH, Demetriades D. Vertebral artery injuries. Surg Clin North Am 2001; 81: 1345-56.

47. Symbas PN, Sherman AJ, Silver JM, et al. Traumatic rupture of the aorta: immediate or delayed repair? Ann Surg 2002; 235: 796-02.

48. Kodali S, Jamieson WR, Leia-Stephens M, et al. Traumatic rupture of the thoracic aorta. A 20-year review: 1969-1989. Circulation 1991; 84 (Suppl): 40-6.

49. Ott MC, Stewart TC, Lawlor DK, et al. Management of blunt thoracic aortic injuries: endovascular stents versus open repair. J Trauma 2004; 56: 565-70.

50. Amabile P, Collart F, Gariboldi V, et al. Surgical versus endovascular treatment of traumatic thoracic aortic rupture. J Vasc Surg 2004; 40: 873-9.

51. Asensio JA, Chahwan S, Hanpeter D, et al. Operative management and outcome of 302 abdominal vascular injuries. Am J Surg 2000; 180: 528-33.

52. Poletti PA, Mirvis SE, Shanmuganathan K, et al. CT criteria for management of blunt liver trauma: correlation with angiographic and surgical findings. Radiology 2000; 216: 418-27.

53. Defore WW, Jr., Mattox KL, Jordan GL, Jr., et al. Management of 1,590 consecutive cases of liver trauma. Arch Surg 1976; 111: 493-7.

54. Asensio JA, Britt LD, Borzotta A, et al. Multi-institutional experience with the management of superior mesenteric artery injuries. J Am Coll Surg 2001; 193: 354-65.

55. Haan J, Rodriguez A, Chiu W, et al. Operative management and outcome of iliac vessel injury: a ten-year experience. Am Surg 2003; 69: 581-6.

Chapter 28

Non-surgical factors that affect surgical outcome

Tom Carrell MA MChir FRCS, Consultant Vascular Surgeon

Peter R Taylor MA MChir FRCS, Consultant Vascular Surgeon

Department of General and Vascular Surgery, Guy's and St. Thomas' Hospitals NHS Foundation Trust, London, UK

Introduction

There has been considerable focus on the published outcomes of cardiac surgery following well-publicised failings and it seems certain that similar open accountability will be demanded of other surgical specialties. In vascular surgery, the outcomes of death, stroke and amputation are particularly easy to record. In trying to optimise results, it is tempting to concentrate on individual technical aspects of the common procedures, for example the relative merits of patching or of local anaesthesia in carotid surgery, but optimising non-surgical factors can have a more powerful overall influence on final outcome.

The effect of volume on outcome

Historically, many patients undergoing major vascular surgery have been managed in non-specialised general surgical wards. In this setting, there may be poor recognition by medical and nursing staff that patients with arterial disease are at greater risk than general surgical patients because of their frequent, and often occult, medical comorbidity. There may also be delay in recognising complications specific to vascular surgery. The development of vascular surgery as a specialty and the growth of dedicated vascular units has addressed these problems but at the cost of extra demand on local resources, such as intensive care, cardiology, renal medicine, physiotherapy and rehabilitation services. There is increasing centralisation of vascular surgery in the UK, driven by a number of factors, and there is some evidence to support the assumption that outcomes are improved in centres with a large throughput of patients (high-volume centres).

The evidence that volume influences outcome comes from retrospective cohort studies. The Finnvasc national registry examined 17,465 vascular interventions over a four-year interval, with 97% of operations performed in teaching or central hospitals and 3% in district hospitals. The workload and the number of elective aortic aneurysm repairs performed by an individual surgeon were highly significant indicators of reduced mortality ($p<0.01$) [1]. A study of 9847 elective abdominal aortic aneurysm repairs in New York State showed a significant positive relationship between hospital volume and in-hospital mortality [2]. A large series from the state of Florida examined over 90,000 patients undergoing abdominal aortic aneurysm surgery, carotid endarterectomy and lower limb bypass procedures. It found that high hospital volume was strongly associated with better outcomes for aortic aneurysm surgery and carotid endarterectomy, but not for lower limb arterial bypass operations. Certified vascular surgeons had consistently lower mortality and morbidity rates than surgeons with low volumes of vascular activity; a 15% lower risk of death or complications after carotid surgery (p=0.002) and a 24% lower risk of death or complications after aneurysm surgery (p=0.009) [3]. A systematic review of vascular surgical practice has supported the finding of improved outcome in high-volume centres for elective aortic surgery, and for high-volume surgeons for carotid endarterectomy [4].

It is reasonable to conclude from these studies that outcome, particularly for elective aortic aneurysm surgery, is improved in high-volume centres **(III/B)**. This is probably due to focused patient care by non-surgical staff, as well as being related to the number of operations performed by any individual surgeon. It is interesting that similar effects have been observed in other fields of medicine, notably with the establishment of specialised stroke units, where patient outcome improves independently of any specific therapeutic intervention [5].

Patient physiology

Most major arterial operations are performed for prognostic benefit to prevent aortic rupture, stroke, or limb loss in patients with severe atherosclerosis. Atherosclerosis is a systemic disease and the commonest cause of postoperative death after vascular surgery is myocardial infarction [6]. In addition, a major cause of arterial disease is smoking, so it is hardly surprising that other smoking-related illnesses, notably chronic obstructive pulmonary disease, are prevalent in patients undergoing vascular intervention.

Assessment of risk

There is much controversy and little consensus about how to assess risk before arterial surgery. A good example is the EVAR-2 trial, which studied patients considered 'unfit' for aortic surgery, but left the assessment and decision on fitness to the individual surgeon. It is clear that the criteria determining 'unfitness' varied widely between centres, which has made it difficult to apply the EVAR-2 results in clinical practice [7].

Appropriate pre-operative assessment is further complicated by the fact that nearly half of all vascular operations are urgent or emergency procedures. Only in elective cases is there sufficient opportunity for full assessment and medical optimisation. Pre-operative assessment has concentrated on open surgery for abdominal aortic aneurysm because it is one of the commonest vascular surgical procedures and places considerable stress on the heart due to the increased afterload of aortic cross-clamping, blood loss and ischaemic reperfusion. The prevalence of severe coronary artery disease in those undergoing open aortic surgery may be as high as 30% [8], but there is little evidence to support a policy of routine pre-operative invasive cardiological investigation of all patients. A history of ischaemic heart disease or significant electrocardiogram abnormality warrants further pre-operative investigation, and non-invasive screening with stress echocardiography or scintigraphy may be justified, with progression to coronary angiography and intervention if appropriate [9] **(III/C)**.

Cardiopulmonary exercise testing

An alternative approach to a purely cardiological assessment for stratifying risk employs a more holistic test of the reserve capacity of the cardiopulmonary system in exercise. Historically, many surgeons have used the question 'can you walk up two flights of stairs?' as a screening test for fitness for aortic surgery. A recent study has validated this approach by showing an 82% positive predictive value for inability to walk up two flights of stairs to predict postoperative cardiopulmonary complications in thoracic and upper abdominal surgery [10]. Cardiopulmonary exercise testing (Figure 1) quantifies fitness more objectively by measuring the maximum capacity of oxygen delivery during exercise, as defined by the anaerobic threshold. This is expressed as oxygen (ml) / body weight (kg) / time (min). Initially developed for use in general surgery, cardiopulmonary exercise testing can stratify risk and so help identify those patients who may benefit from further pre-operative assessment and optimisation [11] **(III/C)**. While the applicability of the technique may seem limited in those with impaired mobility (e.g. severe claudicants), arm exercise is as valid as the more conventional leg exercise on a stationary exercise cycle.

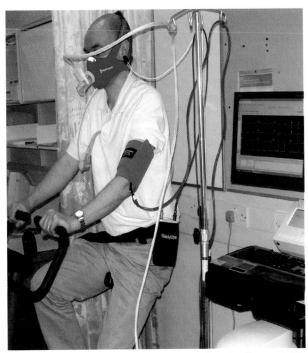

Figure 1. Cardiopulmonary exercise testing at St. Thomas' Hospital in London. Oxygen uptake during exercise, combined with synchronous ECG measurement, allows assessment of a subject's anaerobic threshold and provides an estimate of operative risk. *Consent obtained.*

Scoring systems in major abdominal and vascular surgery have been used to aid patient selection. A good scoring system should allow accurate stratification of the risk of peri-operative complications and death for an individual patient, as well as providing a suitable audit instrument for risk-adjustment, as is necessary to compensate for adverse case mix in any 'league-table' results. The Physiological and Operative Severity Score for the enUmeration of Morbidity and mortality (POSSUM) was invented for general surgical patients and tended to overestimate the risk of death when applied to vascular patients. This system has been refined as the Portsmouth (P-POSSUM) [12] and vascular modification (V-POSSUM) [13, 14].

The scoring systems were derived using Bayesian analysis of one half of a dataset and then validating the mathematical model by testing it against the other half. The relative weights of the different risk factors are summarised in Table 1. Increasing age, female gender, insulin-dependent diabetes, emergency admission and aortic surgery are adverse factors; smoking seems to have little effect. Of all the risk factors, the most powerful weighting was that for emergency admission. This corresponds well with a prospective study of a single surgeon's arterial workload in the authors' own hospital that showed a mortality of 4.3% for 1149 elective operations, 10.6% for 376 urgent operations and 23.9% for 188 emergency operations [15]. Despite reasonable accuracy across a cohort, the POSSUM-derived scoring systems have proved too complex and not specific enough for widespread use in individual prospective risk assessment. Such systems will, however, be of great value in individual and institutional audit.

Medical management of atherosclerosis

The term best medical therapy has often been loosely applied or ignored in vascular surgical practice. It is clear from several studies that a large proportion of patients with arterial disease do not receive appropriate antiplatelet, statin and antihypertensive therapies [16]. In the EVAR-2 trial, there was no stipulation as to best medical treatment in the conservative arm [7]. In the EVAR-1 trial of open versus endovascular aneurysm repair, there was a significant increase in non-aneurysm-related death one year after endovascular repair, suggesting that some of the benefit in early mortality seen in the endovascular arm was being lost by late cardiovascular death [17]. A likely explanation is that there were proportionately more early deaths in patients with occult high cardiovascular risk in the open arm, with the analagous survivors in the endovascular arm dying later of their cardiac disease. It is the responsibility of vascular surgeons to ensure that the risks of late, as well as peri-operative, death are minimised. Many trials have clearly demonstrated the large relative risk reductions that can be achieved through good medical management of atherosclerosis; aggressive medical treatment is an absolute requirement for all patients undergoing vascular surgery for atherosclerosis (see Chapter 5).

Table 1. Bayes Probability Table. Weight refers to the importance of the factor. Negative marks are associated with poor outcome, positive with good outcome. *Data taken from the first Vascular Society National Vascular Database report.*

Risk Factor		Number	Odds ratio	Weight
Age	0-60	262	2.9	10.7
	61-70	388	1.38	3.2
	71-75	284	0.94	-0.6
	76-80	199	0.56	-5.8
	81-85	90	0.61	-4.9
	86-90	44	0.46	-7.7
	>90	12	0.21	-15.8
Sex	male	892	1.11	1.0
	female	409	0.81	-2.1
Smoking				
	current	459	0.97	-0.3
	ex	607	1.18	1.6
	never	204	0.9	-1.1
Diabetes				
	none	1073	1	0.0
	diet	42	0.76	-2.7
	tablet	98	1.92	6.5
	insulin	66	0.65	-4.3
Admission				
	elective	1051	2.07	7.3
	urgent	149	0.45	-8.1
	emergency	95	0.14	-19.5
Aortic aneurysm				
	yes	320	0.57	-5.6
	no	984	1.29	2.5
Carotid surgery				
	yes	226	4.56	15.2
	no	1078	0.85	-1.7

Antiplatelet agents

A meta-analysis by the Antiplatelet Trialists' Collaboration of 145 randomised trials containing over 70,000 patients with vascular disease showed a reduction of about one third in non-fatal myocardial infarction and vascular death in those on low-to-medium-dose aspirin therapy (75-325mg daily) [18]. All patients with clinical evidence of arterial disease should have antiplatelet therapy **(Ia/A)**. The CAPRIE trial showed a marginal advantage for clopidogrel over aspirin in reducing a composite outcome of stroke, myocardial infarction and vascular death [19], but the higher cost of clopidogrel has precluded its widespread use. The recent MATCH trial has shown no significant advantage for a combination of aspirin and clopidogrel therapy over clopidogrel alone in preventing vascular events in patients with recent transient ischaemic attack or stroke [20]. The European Stroke Prevention Study-2 showed that a combination of dipyridamole and aspirin was superior to aspirin alone in reducing subsequent stroke in patients who have had a recent cerebral ischaemic event [21, 22].

The National Institute for Clinical Excellence (NICE) issued guidelines in 2005 recommending that all patients who have had an occlusive vascular event or have symptomatic peripheral arterial disease should receive antiplatelet therapy, usually low-dose aspirin. A combination of modified-release dipyridamole and aspirin is recommended for those who have had an ischaemic stroke or a transient ischaemic attack and this treatment should continue for a period of two years from the most recent event **(Ib/A)**; thereafter, or if dipyridamole is not tolerated, preventative therapy should revert to standard care. Clopidogrel alone is recommended for patients who are intolerant of low-dose aspirin and have experienced an occlusive vascular event or have symptomatic peripheral arterial disease.

Statins

Statins confer benefit through both a lipid-lowering effect and a plaque-stabilising effect. The Scandinavian Simvastatin Survival Study (4S) was the first to demonstrate that lipid-lowering treatment with simvastatin was safe and significantly improved survival in patients with coronary heart disease [23]. Since then, many large prospective randomised controlled trials have confirmed the significant benefit that can be obtained with statin therapy in patients with symptomatic cardiovascular disease. This benefit occurs irrespective of the baseline cholesterol level, in both the elderly and younger patients, and is reflected in a reduction in all-cause mortality, coronary events and peripheral arterial complications. The Anglo-Scandinavian Cardiac Outcomes Trial - Lipid Lowering Arm (ASCOT-LLA) was stopped early in 2002 by its data monitoring committee because the advantage of statin therapy was so significant [24]. The Medical Research Council / British Heart Foundation

Heart Protection Study (HPS) showed a reduction in all-cause mortality of 13% and a reduction in coronary events of 25% in patients treated with simvastatin 40mg daily [25]. The MIRACL [26] and PROSPER [27] trials showed similar beneficial effects, respectively, with atorvastatin 80mg daily and pravastatin 40mg daily. The benefits of statin therapy in reducing cardiovascular and all-cause mortality have been confirmed in patients undergoing major vascular surgery [28, 29]. In 2006, NICE published guidelines on the prescription of statins. The term 'cardiovascular disease' includes coronary, carotid and peripheral arterial disease and aortic aneurysm. NICE TA96 Guidance 1.1 is 'Statin therapy is recommended for patients with clinical evidence of cardiovascular disease' [30] **(Ia/A)**.

Antihypertensive agents

Hypertensive patients with a systolic blood pressure greater than 140mmHg or diastolic greater than 90mmHg should be treated with appropriate blood pressure-lowering medication.

Beta-blockers

There is some evidence that patients receiving ß-blockade who undergo major non-cardiac surgery have a lower incidence of peri-operative myocardial infarction and death [31]. A recent study examined over 780,000 patients undergoing surgery in the USA and found a significant risk reduction in high-risk patients who were receiving a ß-blocker [32]. However, two recent trials, DIPOM [33] and POBBLE [34], failed to show any benefit from short-acting ß-blockade with metoprolol. A recent meta-analysis of 22 trials suggested some benefit, but recommended further studies [35]. Guidelines from the American College of Cardiologists and the American Heart Association are that a ß-blocker should be given before operation to all patients thought to be at high risk, unless there are contraindications. If indicated, ß-blockade should probably be started a week or more before surgery, the dose titrated to a pre-operative heart rate of 50 to 60 beats per minute and continued for at least two weeks after surgery [36] **(IV/C)**.

Calcium-channel blockers and angiotensin-converting enzyme inhibitors

Management of hypertension is a major part of any strategy to modify atherosclerotic risk factors and reduce cardiovascular morbidity. The recently published Anglo-Scandinavian Cardiac Outcomes Trial - Blood Pressure Lowering Arm (ASCOT-BPLA), compared two antihypertensive regimens in patients with hypertension and at least three other cardiovascular risk factors [37]. The study found a reduced incidence of major cardiovascular events, including fatal and non-fatal stroke, and all-cause mortality in those receiving the regimen consisting of a calcium-channel blocker (amlodipine) plus an angiotensin-converting enzyme (ACE) inhibitor (perindopril) as required; the regimen for comparison was a thiazide diuretic plus ß-blocker **(Ib/A)**. Interestingly, the advantages of the former regimen occurred despite the control of blood pressure being similar in both groups. ACE inhibitors should, however, be given with caution to those with aortic disease as they have a 30-50% chance of having underlying renal artery stenosis and so may be at risk of renal failure [38].

Smoking cessation

Smoking is particularly closely associated with peripheral arterial disease [39] and up to 78% of intermittent claudication can be attributed to smoking [40]. The outcomes of arterial intervention are worse in smokers [41]. Patients should be offered access to a smoking cessation clinic and nicotine replacement therapy [42] **(IV/C)**.

Peri-operative care

Pre-operative fluid optimisation

Pre-operative saline loading has been shown in a non-randomised study to reduce pulmonary complications in patients having aortic reconstructive procedures [43]. However, in a prospective randomised trial of pulmonary artery catheterisation with optimisation of haemodynamics in patients having elective vascular surgery, there was no significant difference in morbidity or mortality. It was noted, however, that patients with a pulmonary catheter received more fluid volume [44].

Type of anaesthesia

The stress of surgery can be minimised by reducing the cardiovascular stress of the operation and providing good postoperative analgesia. Regional anaesthetic techniques, such as spinal and epidural anaesthesia, allow many leg operations to be performed under sedation without general anaesthesia. Epidural analgesia can provide effective relief from the pain of an abdominal incision after aortic surgery and may allow patients to be extubated earlier, reducing postoperative stress; on this latter point, however, there is no robust evidence available from trials **(IV/C)**. Endovascular aneurysm repair can be performed under epidural anaesthesia or local anaesthesia and it is possible that the advantages of these techniques over general anaesthesia may contribute to the three-fold reduction in early mortality noted in the EVAR-1 trial (1.7% vs 4.7%) [17].

Carotid surgery can be performed under local anaesthesia, although there is not yet any published evidence from the prospective randomised controlled GALA trial to confirm any theoretical advantage over general anaesthesia. As the trial is continuing to recruit, it seems reasonable to conclude that no major demonstrable difference in outcome between general and local anaesthesia has yet been substantiated.

Normothermia

Two studies have shown a protective effect of normothermia during vascular procedures. The first was a randomised trial of 300 patients, with coronary artery disease or otherwise at high risk of a cardiac event, undergoing abdominal, thoracic or vascular surgical procedures. The patients had either routine warming care or additional warming care to maintain normothermia; cardiac events and ventricular tachycardia were reduced in the latter group [45]. The second study was a randomised trial of a circulating water mattress compared with a forced air blanket in 100 patients having infrarenal aortic aneurysm repair [46]. The forced air blanket was much more effective in keeping the core temperature normal, both during and after surgery, and patients so treated had significantly less metabolic acidosis. There was, however, no difference in mortality, cardiac complications or length of stay between the groups. Patients who became hypothermic had a lower cardiac output, thrombocytopenia, an elevated prothrombin time and inferior APACHE II scores compared with normothermic patients, confirming benefit for maintaining normothermia **(Ib/A)**.

Autotransfusion

Autotransfusion has several theoretical benefits during aortic surgery, including reductions in net blood loss, transmission of infection, transfusion reactions and demand on the blood transfusion service (and, possibly, cost). However, in one randomised prospective trial of autotransfusion for aortic surgery no significant difference was noted between groups in the number of units of banked blood transfused, the proportion of patients that did not need banked blood, postoperative haemoglobin and haematocrit, and complications [47].

Postoperative care

Although many patients having arterial operations can be adequately nursed in high dependency units, there is still a role for intensive care, particularly after thoraco-abdominal aneurysm repair and emergency open infrarenal aortic surgery. Intensive care unit protocols may affect the outcome in such patients. In a unique study, a consecutive series of patients having non-elective aortic aneurysm surgery were admitted to one of two different hospitals under the care of a single consultant surgeon. The intensive care units had different protocols. Pulmonary artery catheters were inserted in 96% of patients in one hospital and in 18% in the other; the former group received much larger volumes of fluid and more inotropes, presumably to achieve set targets. In spite of this, a greater proportion of patients experienced acute renal failure in the former hospital, which also had a higher mortality rate [48]. This confirms the findings of other studies on pre-operative loading; it is now well established that pulmonary artery catheter insertion is associated with an increase in the amount of fluid that patients are given [44]. If they are used incorrectly in order to achieve goals that are more suited to younger trauma victims, their use may be harmful [49].

Conclusions

Factors other than the operative skill of the surgeon can have a large influence on the outcome of vascular surgery. It is essential that patients with significant arterial disease are recognised as being at high risk from cardiovascular and respiratory complications. Attempts should be made to identify those patients at highest risk, thereby allowing appropriate counselling on the risks of operation and providing an opportunity for pre-operative optimisation.

The publication of many large randomised controlled trials including patients with peripheral arterial disease has highlighted the benefits of aggressive medical management of atherosclerosis. The vascular surgeon should act to ensure that these patients are identified and treated with appropriate antiplatelet, statin and antihypertensive therapy.

Less invasive operative techniques and refinements in anaesthetic techniques promise to reduce the stress of major vascular surgery. However, close co-operation and good communication between surgeon, anaesthetist, intensivist, ward staff and primary care practitioner is more important than ever.

Key points	Evidence level

- All patients with clinical evidence of atherosclerosis should be treated with a statin. — Ia/A
- All patients with clinical evidence of atherosclerosis should be treated with an antiplatelet agent. — Ia/A
- Hypertension should be treated. Calcium-channel blockers and angiotensin-converting enzyme inhibitors may improve survival. — Ib/A
- High-volume centres have better results than low-volume centres. — III/B
- Patients with a pre-operative history suggesting cardiac disease or with electrocardiogram abnormalities should be assessed further before elective major vascular surgery. — III/B
- Cardiopulmonary exercise testing can identify patients at high risk. — III/B

References

1. Kantonen I, Lepantalo M, Salenius JP, et al. Mortality in abdominal aortic aneurysm surgery: the effect of hospital volume, patient mix and surgeon's case load. Eur J Vasc Endovasc Surg 1997: 14: 375-9.
2. Sollano JA, Gelijns AC, Moskowitz AJ, et al. Volume-outcome relationships in cardiovascular operations: New York State, 1990-1995. J Thor Cardiovasc Surg 1999; 117: 419-28.
3. Pearce WH, Parker MA, Feinglass J, et al. The importance of surgeon volume and training in outcomes for vascular surgical procedures. J Vasc Surg 1999; 29: 768-78.
4. Shackley P, Slack R, Booth A, Michaels J. Is there a positive volume-outcome relationship in peripheral vascular surgery? Results of a systematic review. Eur J Vasc Endovasc Surg 2000; 20: 326-35.
5. Kwan J, Sandercock P. In-hospital care pathways for stroke. Cochrane Database Syst Rev 2002; 2: CD002924.
6. Johnston K. Non-ruptured abdominal aortic aneurysm: six-year follow-up results from the multicentre prospective Canadian aneurysm study. J Vasc Surg 1994; 20: 163-70.
7. EVAR trial participants. Endovascular aneurysm repair and outcome in patients unfit for open repair of abdominal aortic aneurysm (EVAR trial 2): randomised controlled trial. Lancet 2005; 365: 2187-92.
8. Young JR, Hertzer NR, Beven EG, et al. Coronary artery disease in patients with aortic aneurysm: a classification of 302 coronary angiograms and results of surgical management. Ann Vasc Surg 1986; 1: 36-42.
9. Cambria RP, Brewster DC, Abbott WM, et al. The impact of selective use of dipyridamole-thallium scans and surgical factors on the current morbidity of aortic surgery. J Vasc Surg 1992; 15: 43-51.
10. Girish M, Trayner E Jr, Dammann O, et al. Symptom-limited stair climbing as a predictor of postoperative cardiopulmonary complications after high-risk surgery. Chest 2001; 120: 1147-51.
11. Older P, Hall A, Hader R. Cardiopulmonary exercise testing as a screening test for perioperative management of major surgery in the elderly. Chest 1999; 116: 355-62.
12. Midwinter MJ, Tytherleigh M, Ashley S. Estimation of mortality and morbidity risk in vascular surgery using POSSUM and the Portsmouth predictor equation. Br J Surg 1999; 86: 471-4.
13. Bown MJ, Cooper NJ, Sutton AJ, et al. The postoperative mortality of ruptured abdominal aortic aneurysm repair. Eur J Vasc Endovasc Surg 2004; 27: 65-74.
14. Harris JR, Forbes TL, Steiner SH, et al. Risk-adjusted analysis of early mortality after ruptured abdominal aortic aneurysm repair. J Vasc Surg 2005; 42: 387-91.
15. Lagattolla NRF, McGuinness CL, Taylor PR. Influence of case mix and priority on outcome following arterial surgery. Br J Surg 1999; 86 Suppl 1: 110-1.
16. Lloyd GM, Newton JD, Norwood MG, et al. Patients with abdominal aortic aneurysm: are we missing the opportunity for cardiovascular risk reduction? J Vasc Surg 2004; 40: 691-7.
17. EVAR trial participants. Endovascular aneurysm repair versus open repair in patients with abdominal aortic aneurysm (EVAR trial 1): randomised controlled trial. Lancet 2005; 365: 2179-86.
18. Collaborative overview of randomised trials of antiplatelet therapy - I: Prevention of death, myocardial infarction, and stroke by prolonged antiplatelet therapy in various categories of patients. Antiplatelet Trialists' Collaboration. Br Med J 1994; 308: 81-106.
19. A randomised, blinded, trial of clopidogrel versus aspirin in patients at risk of ischaemic events (CAPRIE). CAPRIE Steering Committee. Lancet 1996; 348: 1329-39.
20. Diener HC, Bogousslavsky J, Brass LM, et al; MATCH investigators. Aspirin and clopidogrel compared with

clopidogrel alone after recent ischaemic stroke or transient ischaemic attack in high-risk patients (MATCH): randomised, double-blind, placebo-controlled trial. *Lancet* 2004; 364: 331-7.

21. Diener HC, Cunha L, Forbes C, *et al.* European Stroke Prevention Study. 2. Dipyridamole and acetylsalicylic acid in the secondary prevention of stroke. *J Neurol Sci* 1996; 143: 1-13.

22. Sivenius J, Cunha L, Diener HC, *et al.* Second European Stroke Prevention Study: antiplatelet therapy is effective regardless of age. *Acta Neurol Scand* 1999; 99: 54-60.

23. Randomised trial of cholesterol lowering in 4444 patients with coronary heart disease: the Scandinavian Simvastatin Survival Study (4S). *Lancet* 1994; 344: 1383-9.

24. Sever PS, Dahlof B, Poulter NR, *et al*; ASCOT investigators. Prevention of coronary and stroke events with atorvastatin in hypertensive patients who have average or lower-than-average cholesterol concentrations, in the Anglo-Scandinavian Cardiac Outcomes Trial - Lipid Lowering Arm (ASCOT-LLA): a multicentre randomised controlled trial. *Lancet* 2003; 361: 1149-58.

25. Heart Protection Study Collaborative Group. MRC/BHF Heart Protection Study of cholesterol lowering with simvastatin in 20,536 high-risk individuals: a randomised placebo-controlled trial. *Lancet* 2002; 360: 7-22.

26. Schwartz GG, Olsson AG, Ezekowitz MD, *et al.* Effects of atorvastatin on early recurrent ischemic events in acute coronary syndromes: the MIRACL study: a randomized controlled trial. *JAMA* 2001; 285: 1711-8.

27. Shepherd J, Blauw GJ, Murphy MB, *et al.* Pravastatin in elderly individuals at risk of vascular disease (PROSPER): a randomised controlled trial. *Lancet* 2002; 360: 1623-30.

28. Poldermans D, Bax JJ, Kertai MD, *et al.* Statins are associated with a reduced incidence of perioperative mortality in patients undergoing major noncardiac vascular surgery. *Circulation* 2003; 107: 1848-51.

29. Kertai MD, Boersma E, Westerhout CM, *et al.* Association between long-term statin use and mortality after successful abdominal aortic aneurysm surgery. *Am J Med* 2004; 116: 96-103.

30. National Institute for Clinical Excellence. Statins for the prevention of cardiovascular events. Technology Appraisal Guidance 96: 2006.

31. Abir F, Kakisis I, Sumpio B. Do vascular surgery patients need a cardiology work-up? A review of pre-operative cardiac clearance guidelines in vascular surgery. *Eur J Vasc Endovasc Surg* 2003; 25: 110-7.

32. Lindenauer PK, Pekow P, Wang K, *et al.* Perioperative beta-blocker therapy and mortality after major noncardiac surgery. *N Engl J Med* 2005; 353: 349-61.

33. Juul AB, Wetterslev J, Gluud C, *et al.* Effect of perioperative beta blockade in patients with diabetes undergoing major non-cardiac surgery: randomised placebo controlled, blinded multicentre trial. *Br Med J* 2006; 332: 1482.

34. Brady AR, Gibbs JS, Greenhalgh RM, *et al*; POBBLE trial investigators. Perioperative beta-blockade (POBBLE) for patients undergoing infrarenal vascular surgery: results of a randomized double-blind controlled trial. *J Vasc Surg* 2005; 41: 602-9.

35. Devereaux PJ, Beattie WS, Choi PT, *et al.* How strong is the evidence for the use of perioperative beta blockers in non-cardiac surgery? Systematic review and meta-analysis of randomised controlled trials. *Br Med J* 2005; 331: 313-21.

36. Eagle KA, Berger PB, Calkins H, *et al.* American College of Cardiology/American Heart Association Task Force on Practice Guidelines (Committee to Update the 1996 Guidelines on Perioperative Cardiovascular Evaluation for Noncardiac Surgery). *Circulation* 2002; 105: 1257-67.

37. Dahlof B, Sever PS, Poulter NR, *et al*; ASCOT Investigators. Prevention of cardiovascular events with an antihypertensive regimen of amlodipine adding perindopril as required versus atenolol adding bendroflumethiazide as required, in the Anglo-Scandinavian Cardiac Outcomes Trial - Blood Pressure Lowering Arm (ASCOT-BPLA): a multicentre randomised controlled trial. *Lancet* 2005; 366: 895-906.

38. Choudhri AH, Cleland JG, Rowlands PC, *et al.* Unsuspected renal artery stenosis in peripheral vascular disease. *Br Med J* 1990; 301: 1197-8.

39. Doll R, Peto R, Wheatley K, *et al.* Mortality in relation to smoking: 40 years' observations on male British doctors. *Br Med J* 1994; 309: 901-11.

40. Leng GC, Lee AJ, Fowkes FGR, *et al.* The relationship between cigarette smoking and cardiovascular risk factors in peripheral arterial disease compared with ischaemic heart disease. The Edinburgh Artery study. *Eur Heart J* 1995; 16: 1542-8.

41. Cavender JB, Rogers WJ, Fisher LD, *et al.* Effects of smoking on survival and morbidity in patients randomized to medical or surgical therapy in the Coronary Artery Surgery Study (CASS): 10-year follow-up. *J Am Coll Cardiol* 1992; 20: 287-94.

42. Joseph AM, Norman SM, Ferry LH, *et al.* The safety of transdermal nicotine as an aid to smoking cessation in patients with cardiac disease. *N Engl J Med* 1996; 335: 1792-8.

43. Garrison RN, Wilson MA, Matheson PJ, Spain DA. Preoperative saline loading improves outcome after elective, noncardiac surgical procedures. *American Surgeon* 1996; 62: 223-31.

44. Bender JS, Smith-Meek MA, Jones CE. Routine pulmonary artery catheterization does not reduce morbidity and mortality after elective vascular surgery: results of a prospective, randomised trial. *Ann Surg* 1997; 226: 229-36.

45. Frank SM, Fleisher LA, Breslow MJ, *et al.* Perioperative maintenance of normothermia reduces the incidence of morbid cardiac events. A randomised clinical trial. *JAMA* 1997; 277: 1127-34.

46. Elmore JR, Franklin DP, Youkey JR, *et al.* Normothermia is protective during infrarenal aortic surgery. *J Vasc Surg* 1998; 28: 984-92.

47. Claggert GP, Valentine RJ, Jackson MR, *et al.* A randomized trial of intraoperative autotransfusion during aortic surgery. *J Vasc Surg* 1999; 29: 22-31.

48. Sandison AJP, Wyncoll DLA, Edmondson RC, *et al.* ICU protocol may affect the outcome of non-elective abdominal aortic aneurysm repair. *Eur J Vasc Endovasc Surg* 1998; 16: 356-61.

49. Hayes MA, Timmins AC, Yau EHS, *et al.* Elevation of systemic oxygen delivery in the treatment of critically ill patients. *N Engl J Med* 1994; 33: 1717-22.

Chapter 29

Vascular research in progress - the horizon scanned

Matt Thompson MD FRCS, Professor of Vascular Surgery

Ian Loftus MD FRCS, Consultant Vascular Surgeon

Gillian Cockerill PhD, Senior Lecturer in Vascular Biology

St. George's Vascular Institute, London, UK

Introduction

The philosophy behind current research into vascular disease was encapsulated by George Hunter who stated in the introduction to *Principles of Surgery* (1806):

"This last part of surgery, namely operations, is a reflection on the healing art; it is a tacit acknowledgement of the insufficiency of surgery is like an armed savage who attempts to get that by force which a civilized man would get by strategem."

The sentiment behind this statement may be reflected in a pyramidal approach to the treatment of traditional surgical disease (Figure 1). Open surgical procedures are gradually being superseded by minimally invasive alternatives (e.g. laparoscopic cholecystectomy). In some cases, surgical operations (vagotomy), have been replaced by pharmacotherapy, and it is likely that cell and gene-based therapy will become commonplace in the next ten years.

Progress in vascular surgery mirrors other surgical disciplines. The traditional open operations of aneurysm repair, carotid endarterectomy and lower limb bypass are being replaced gradually with endovascular aneurysm repair, carotid stenting and limb angioplasty. The importance of pharmacotherapy for vascular disease has belatedly been recognised, with more attention being directed towards medical management.

In the next decade, progress in the treatment of vascular disease is likely to accelerate. The minimally invasive approach to endoluminal treatment will receive more and more attention and progress in this area is expected. There will be increasing technological advancement in the design of endovascular prostheses and stents that will address some of the durability issues that currently affect these

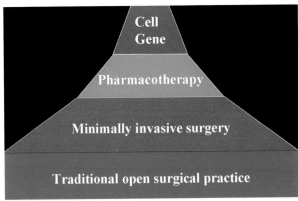

Figure 1. Pyramidal approach to the future of vascular surgery.

procedures. The place of endovascular surgery will be better defined by registry data, and some well-directed randomised trials. This process is inevitable, and research in this field will be directed towards defining specific indications for endovascular surgery, rather than comparing practice to traditional surgery.

Despite the endovascular revolution, significant progress in vascular therapy is likely to come from basic scientific research into the molecular mechanisms underlying vascular disease. The investigative tools available to study vascular pathology have become increasingly sophisticated and sensitive in the last few years. Stimulated by the human genome project, the fields of genomics, proteomics and metabolomics [1] have now been applied to many disease processes and have defined the molecular events that characterise atherosclerotic and aneurysmal tissue. Once the disease state is understood, cell, gene or drug-based therapy becomes a possibility. The rest of this chapter will concentrate on four areas of basic vascular research where progress appears probable within the next decade.

Cell therapy for cardiovascular disease

Experimental and human studies have demonstrated that progenitor cells have the ability to regenerate tissue. The therapeutic promise of these cells is based on the cell plasticity hypothesis: namely, that progenitor cells can transdifferentiate across traditional lineage barriers. It is therefore possible that progenitor cells may offer therapeutic potential to generate new blood vessels in ischaemia, and to allow remodelling in arteries degraded by atherosclerosis or during aneurysm genesis [2].

Potential sources of progenitor cells for cardiovascular therapy exist within the human body; these include stem cells derived from the bone marrow, circulating progenitor cells and resident cells in adipose tissue (Figure 2). The most promising cell types appear to be bone marrow-derived stem cells which have the potential to differentiate into haemopoietic, vasculogeneic or contractile

phenotypes. In addition, endothelial progenitor cells can be isolated from the circulation and may offer potential for neovascularisation in ischaemic tissues [3].

The concept of cell-based therapy for cardiovascular disease originated with the theory that stem cell injection might offer some reparative potential to damaged myocardium during coronary bypass surgery. After that initial concept, experimental results have suggested that stem cells might be useful in much broader situations where vascular disease is being propagated by tissue degradation. Many of the key cellular events that characterise both atherosclerosis and aneurysm formation involve cellular apoptosis and remodelling of the extracellular matrix. In theory, stem cells have the potential to reverse these processes by differentiation into mature cell types and engrafting the damaged tissue with fully functioning resident cells. The key steps in such a therapeutic process would include harvesting the progenitor cells, delivering them to the target tissue, ensuring appropriate differentiation and monitoring disease progression or reversal. The last point is particularly crucial as transplanted stem cells that functioned abnormally might accelerate the disease process rather than provide amelioration [4].

At the present time, clinical studies on the use of stem cell therapy in vascular disease are unconvincing

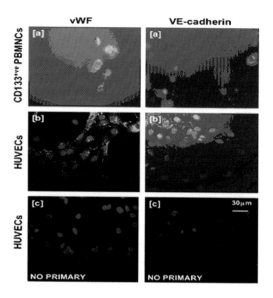

Figure 2. CD34+ve/CD133+ve mononuclear cells express endothelial cell markers following five days in culture.

and sparse. However, clinical data have suggested that progenitor cells play an important role in vascular homeostasis and that the normal stem cell population is affected by disease states. In healthy men, circulating progenitor cell concentration correlated with vascular function and inversely with cumulative cardiovascular risk [5]. Most chronic disease states associated with vascular pathology will deplete the concentration and function of progenitor cells (e.g. age, diabetes, renal failure), whilst statins mobilise progenitor cell number [6].

There are a significant number of challenges to be overcome before stem cell therapy may be used to modify the atherosclerotic or aneurysmal process. At the present time, there is considerable research effort investigating the role of progenitor cells in vascular pathology, and several Phase I trials have reported success with angiogenesis [7]. Stem cell therapy is probably ten years away from clinical application but offers considerable promise.

Gene therapy for cardiovascular disease

Gene therapy for vascular disease was thought to be the next big thing some ten years ago. Unfortunately, problems with *in vivo* gene transfer hampered the technology, and research slowed. Recent advances in DNA technology have stimulated further interest in this subject. Current approaches to gene therapy may be divided into two broad categories: strategies aimed at increasing angiogenesis in ischaemic tissue and strategies aimed at targeting specific areas within vascular disease processes.

In past years the processes involved in new vessel formation and maturation have been unravelled and the growth factors involved in these processes have been identified. Based on this work, investigators suggested that gene therapy could be used to initiate therapeutic angiogenesis and arteriogenesis in patients with critical leg ischaemia, who were not suitable for vascular reconstruction. The initial trials concentrated on using Vascular Endothelial Growth Factor (VEGF) to initiate angiogenesis in ischaemic

limbs [8]. In these studies an appropriate growth factor was usually delivered directly into the ischaemic leg using intramuscular injections of plasmid DNA, adenoviral vectors, or lysosomes. In addition, local catheter-mediated gene delivery of VEGF 165 was achieved following balloon angioplasty [9]. The initial trials had mixed results with some improvement of haemodynamic indices and some clinical improvement [10].

More recent theories have suggested that angiogenesis has a limited ability to compensate for loss of conductance vessels and that arteriogenesis should be the aim of gene therapy in ischaemic legs, as this has the greater potential to deliver high volume blood flow. Angiogenesis may still be appropriate for conditions of microvascular loss (e.g. Buerger's disease). Less is known about the mediators of arteriogenesis than angiogenesis, and research in this field is clearly crucial. Transforming growth factor-beta (TGF-β) is increased in collateral vessel formation, and may provide an appropriate therapeutic spectrum of activity. Gene therapy to initiate arteriogenesis is still at an early stage and has probably been set back by the early rush to trial of many angiogenic factors. A significant amount of research is still required in identification of appropriate gene products and delivery systems before widespread clinical application. The ultimate goal must be to develop mature microvessel networks with appropriate safety margins. This remains a realistic goal within the next decade.

An alternative approach to gene therapy involves the targeting of specific molecular events within pathological arterial disease. Powerful molecular tools are now available to determine key molecular processes that drive common arterial pathologies. Once identified, these processes can be targeted by delivering gene products to the molecular processes causing disease. Key proteins within the pathological process may be inhibited either by delivering genetic products coded for inhibitors of the protein [11] or by directly inhibiting production of the protein at a genetic level using specific antisense oligonucleotides or small interfering RNA (siRNA) [12]. Clinical trials for any such agents are still a long way off. The principal hurdles to be overcome include effective delivery of gene products and overcoming the redundancy of complex biological pathways.

Modern pharmacotherapy - towards regression?

Most basic research into atherosclerosis and aneurysms aims to delineate crucial cellular and molecular events in the disease process that can be targeted by effective pharmacotherapy. The importance of effective medical therapy for patients with vascular disease has been highlighted in many recent trials [13]. The main goal of medical therapy has been to stabilise existing disease, modify risk factors and therefore reduce the incidence of major vascular events including myocardial infarction and stroke. The strategy of current pharmacotherapy is to contain the disease burden and halt disease progression. In atherosclerosis this is manifest by the current treatment goals of stabilising vulnerable atherosclerotic plaques, preventing plaque rupture and thus reducing complications. In aneurysm research the current goal is to define a pharmacotherapeutic strategy to reduce aneurysm expansion rates and so defer surgical repair [14].

In the next few years, there is likely to be a reappraisal of these aims, with the overall strategy becoming one of inducing regression of arterial lesions. The ultimate aim of pharmacotherapy within the vascular tree will be to attempt to reverse the atherosclerotic and aneurysmal processes. These goals are perhaps closer with pharmacotherapy than with either cell or gene-based treatments. Until recently, most trials of treatments for atherosclerosis demonstrated disease stabilisation, but no regression. The ASTEROID trial was designed to test the hypothesis that intensive rosuvastatin therapy would result in atheroma regression, as assessed by intravascular ultrasound. The trial reported the outcome of 349 patients, and revealed that significant reductions were observed in atheroma volume [15]. This is the first trial reporting atheroma regression and sets the benchmark for future agents developed for this purpose. The next few years are likely to see a large number of trials testing existing and new agents aimed at atheroma regression therapy.

A similar landmark study has recently been applied to aneurysm research. Abdominal aneurysms are characterised by proteinase-mediated degradation of the extracellular matrix, apoptosis and widespread inflammation [16]. These cellular events have been targeted by agents aiming to reduce aneurysm expansion rates. Many agents have been applied successfully in experimental models and there is now reasonable clinical evidence that statins and doxycycline may reduce aneurysm growth rates in the clinical setting, principally by inhibiting matrix metalloproteinase-9 (MMP-9) and other pro-inflammatory mediators.

In the aneurysm wall, inflammatory stimuli activate protease activity through activating protein-1, a downstream target of c-Jun N-terminal kinase (JNK). In a recent study, it was demonstrated that human aneurysms expressed high levels of JNK and that activated JNK localised to the site of protease activity. Experimental models then revealed that established aneurysms regressed when treated with a synthetic JKN inhibitor [17]. These findings are potentially revolutionary as they indicate for the first time that aneurysm regression may be a valid clinical goal, and that manipulation of the extracellular matrix may be one way to achieve this. Unfortunately, inhibition of JNK is not a reasonable clinical strategy, but selecting targets from the JNK pathway may offer a prospect of regressing small aneurysms.

Genetic influences in vascular disease

Family history is an important risk factor for both peripheral vascular disease and aneurysm formation. The advances in genomics that accompanied the human genome project have been enthusiastically applied to complex diseases, such as coronary artery disease [18]. These studies are now yielding important results and are likely to continue for a number of years. The uptake of these techniques in the vascular community has been slow. This is perhaps surprising as abdominal aneurysms have a much stronger inheritance than ischaemic heart disease.

First degree relatives of individuals with an aneurysm have an eight-fold increased risk of the disease and pedigree studies have suggested a multifactorial genetic mode of inheritance for AAA. Research into the genetics of AAA has concentrated on a candidate gene approach. This relies on existing research to generate a hypothesis that a particular gene may be associated with aneurysm formation or expansion. Common polymorphisms of the candidate gene are then examined, and associations defined. The candidate gene approach has not been particularly successful. Several associations with presence and expansion rates of AAA have been found and many have some biological plausibility. However, many studies have given negative results and often the positive associations are weak.

With recent advances in technology, it is now possible to perform a genome-wide association study for AAA to look throughout the genome and identify any associated single nucleotide polymorphisms with either aneurysm pathogenesis or expansion. This type of study can give a unique insight into the mechanisms causing aneurysm disease and help to formulate a therapeutic strategy.

Conclusions

The rapid advances in understanding of vascular biology are likely to lead to new and innovative treatments within the next decade. Trials of gene and cell-based therapy have started at a low level and these are likely to increase. The aim of pharmacotherapy that currently acts to stabilise disease may change to regression therapy. The main focus of these treatments is likely to be aneurysm regression, plaque regression and angiogenesis.

Key points	Evidence level
◆ Rapid improvements in the techniques of molecular biology, genomics, proteomics and metabolomics have led to a better understanding of vascular pathology.	IV/C
◆ These advances are now being used to design therapeutic strategies that should change the treatment algorithm for vascular disease.	IV/C
◆ In the next decade, the aim should be to treat vascular disease by early identification and implementation of a therapeutic strategy to cause disease regression.	IV/C
◆ Open surgical and endovascular techniques may then only be applicable to highly advanced pathology.	IV/C

References

1. Mayr M, Mayr U, Chung YL, *et al*. Vascular proteomics: linking proteomic and metabolomic changes. *Proteomics* 2004; 4: 3751-61.
2. Caplice NM, Gersh BJ, Alegria JR. Cell therapy for cardiovascular disease: what cells, what diseases and for whom? *Nat Clin Pract Cardiovasc Med* 2005; 2: 37-43.
3. Xu Q. The impact of progenitor cells in atherosclerosis. *Nat Clin Pract Cardiovasc Med* 2006; 3: 94-101.
4. Caplice NM, Doyle B. Vascular progenitor cells: origin and mechanisms of mobilization, differentiation, integration, and vasculogenesis. *Stem Cells Dev* 2005; 14: 122-39.
5. Hill JM, Zalos G, Halcox JP, *et al*. Circulating endothelial progenitor cells, vascular function, and cardiovascular risk. *N Engl J Med* 2003; 348: 593-600.
6. Walter DH, Dimmeler S, Zeiher AM. Effects of statins on endothelium and endothelial progenitor cell recruitment. *Semin Vasc Med* 2004; 4: 385-93.
7. Tateishi-Yuyama E, Matsubara H, Murohara T, *et al*. Therapeutic angiogenesis for patients with limb ischaemia by

autologous transplantation of bone-marrow cells: a pilot study and a randomised controlled trial. *Lancet* 2002; 360: 427-35.

8.   Isner JM, Pieczek A, Schainfeld R, *et al*. Clinical evidence of angiogenesis after arterial gene transfer of phVEGF165 in patient with ischaemic limb. *Lancet* 1996; 348: 370-4.

9.   Comerota AJ, Throm RC, Miller KA, *et al*. Naked plasmid DNA encoding fibroblast growth factor type 1 for the treatment of end-stage unreconstructable lower extremity ischemia: preliminary results of a phase I trial. *J Vasc Surg* 2002; 35: 930-6.

10. Morishita R, Aoki M, Ogihara T. Does gene therapy become pharmacotherapy? *Exp Physiol* 2005; 90: 307-13.

11. Allaire E, Forough R, Clowes M, *et al*. Local overexpression of TIMP-1 prevents aortic aneurysm degeneration and rupture in a rat model. *J Clin Invest* 1998; 102: 1413-20.

12. Herweijer H, Wolff JA. Progress and prospects: naked DNA gene transfer and therapy. *Gene Ther* 2003; 10: 453-8.

13. Hankey GJ, Norman PE, Eikelboom JW. Medical treatment of peripheral arterial disease. *JAMA* 2006; 295: 547-53.

14. Dawson J, Choke E, Sayed S, *et al*. Pharmacotherapy of abdominal aortic aneurysms. *Curr Vasc Pharmacol* 2006; 4: 129-49.

15. Nissen SE, Nicholls SJ, Sipahi I, *et al*. Effect of very high-intensity statin therapy on regression of coronary atherosclerosis: the ASTEROID trial. *JAMA* 2006; 295: 1556-65.

16. Choke E, Cockerill G, Wilson WR, *et al*. A review of biological factors implicated in abdominal aortic aneurysm rupture. *Eur J Vasc Endovasc Surg* 2005; 30: 227-44.

17. Yoshimura K, Aoki H, Ikeda Y, *et al*. Regression of abdominal aortic aneurysm by inhibition of c-Jun N-terminal kinase. *Nat Med* 2005; 11: 1330-8.

18. Watkins H, Farrall M. Genetic susceptibility to coronary artery disease: from promise to progress. *Nat Rev Genet* 2006; 7: 163-73.

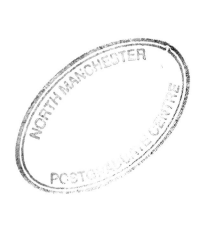
NORTH MANCHESTER

POSTGRADUATE CENTRE